FOREWORD

Surgical skills are commonly thought of as those
enable the surgeon to safely and effectively perform ~~~~~
however, a very narrow definition. The fundamental surgical skills are not only
basic instrument, tissue handling and suturing techniques, but a wide range of
non-technical skills as well.

In this text, authored by the ASSET committee of the Board of Basic
Surgical Training of the Royal Australasian College of Surgeons, the full range
of fundamental surgical skills is explored. Chapters on surgical conduct, surgical
decision making and surgical safety clearly outline some of the skills that the
trainee surgeon must acquire before he or she ever picks up a scalpel. Chapters
such as surgical ergonomics try to outline what generations of surgeons have only
assimilated in the course of their training rather than being taught as concepts.
The traditional surgical skills are covered in chapters on instruments, needles,
sutures, wound management and specific surgical techniques.

This book has been authored by a group with wide experience in teaching
basic surgical skills to aspiring surgeons, and their insight has allowed them to
distil what the surgeon training in the 21st century must know and be able to do
prior to engaging in surgical procedures on patients. That a surgeon should know
which end of a needle to grasp before suturing a wound is intuitive, but that he
or she should behave professionally, use evidence as a basis for good decision
making and have appropriate team membership skills is less intuitive. Trainees
who incorporate the principles outlined in this text and at the same time practice
and master the skills in appropriate settings will have the platform to undertake an
effective training programme in whichever discipline of surgery they choose.

Ian Civil
Censor in Chief
Royal Australian College of Surgeons

CONTENTS

CONTENTS

CONTENTS

CONTENTS

PREFACE

Fundamental Skills for Surgery aims to be a key reference book for doctors embarking upon a surgical career. Produced by The Royal Australasian College of Surgeons as part of an initiative to improve the teaching of generic surgical skills, it provides an excellent foundation of skills from which trainees can develop a safe, effective and efficient approach to surgical practice.

The Royal Australasian College of Surgeon's Australian and New Zealand Surgical Skills Education and Training Committee consulted widely to identify the skills to include in the book. The scope of skills presented extends beyond those of manual techniques to include interpersonal and leadership skills so often overlooked in formal surgical training.

Basic Surgical Skills, the 1997 textbook by Mr Iain Skinner, was the main platform from which *Fundamental Skills for Surgery* has evolved. Many practising surgeons from a wide range of specialties have contributed to the text and members of the Australian and New Zealand Surgical Skills Education and Training Committee undertook the compilation and editing process.

I hope this book will inspire young surgeons to master the broad base of skills essential for the practise of surgical excellence.

Richard Perry FRACS
Editor

ACKNOWLEDGMENTS

Editor

Richard Perry FRACS, Colorectal Surgeon, Christchurch

Contributors

Robert Davies FRACS, Urology, Perth

Matthew Carmody FRACS, Upper GI and Laparoscopic Surgeon, Brisbane

Matthew Clark FRACS, General Surgeon, Auckland

Matthew Lawrence FRACS, Colorectal Surgeon, Adelaide

Simon Journeaux FRACS, Orthopaedic Surgeon, Brisbane

Christine Castle FRACS, Orthopaedic Surgeon, Sydney

Francis Kimble FRACS, Plastic and Reconstructive Surgeon, Hobart

Andrew Cochrane FRACS, Cardiothoracic Surgeon, Melbourne

David Watson FRACS, General Surgeon, Adelaide

Athol Mackay FRACS, General Surgeon, Queensland

Michael Patkin FRACS, General Surgeon, Adelaide

Jenepher Martin FRACS, General Surgeon, Melbourne

Christine Cuthbertson, General Surgical Trainee, Melbourne

Iain Skinner FRACS, General Surgeon, Melbourne

Michael Solomon FRACS, Colorectal Surgeon, Sydney

Jane Young, PhD FAFPHM, Surgical Outcomes Research Centre (SOuRCe), Sydney

CHAPTER ONE
SURGICAL CONDUCT

Eminence without merit earns deference without esteem

Chamfort (1741–1794), *Maximes et pensees*, 1805

INTRODUCTION

Technical aspects of operative surgery are only one part of a surgeon's skill. Technical skill underpins safe surgical practice, but it does not guarantee it, and is not enough on its own. A competent and safe surgeon will be able to interact with patients and other members of the surgical team in an appropriate manner, make good clinical decisions, and perform complex surgical tasks to a high standard.

Most medical graduates can be trained in the technical aspects of operative surgery. However, mastery of conduct and decision making is essential to the development of a safe and effective surgical practice.

WHAT IS A SURGEON?

It is said that 'a surgeon is a physician who operates'. This statement emphasises the fact that knowing *when* to operate is at least as important as knowing *how* to operate. Hence, one of the most important surgical skills that trainees must acquire is clinical perspective. Surgeons undertake a wide range of tasks and assume many roles within their day-to-day work. Most of these are not dependent on technical skill alone. The roles and attributes required of a surgeon are defined by the Royal Australasian College of Surgeons (see Table 1.1). The definition of surgical competence is expanded on the RACS website, http://www.surgeons.org.

Table 1.1	Essential roles and key competencies for surgeons
	Professionalism
	Scholar/Teacher
	Health advocacy
	Management and leadership
	Collaboration
	Communication
	Medical expertise
	Judgement—clinical decision making
	Technical expertise

Source: Royal Australasian College of Surgeons. Originally adapted from 'Skills for the new millennium: report of the societal needs working group', Royal College of Physicians and Surgeons of Canada's Canadian Medical Education Directions for Specialists 2000 Project, September 1996.

Clinical skills

Clinical skills direct the actions of a surgeon to obtain the best clinical outcome for a patient. The clinical skills that underpin competency in the operating theatre are built on a foundation of competency in the basic skills required by all medical practitioners: history taking and physical examination. These basic skills alone are not sufficient to guarantee that the surgeon will be able to synthesise clinical information to develop an informed opinion, construct an appropriate differential diagnosis, request appropriate investigations and formulate a sound management plan. Underlying this is the assumption that a competent surgeon will have good interpersonal and communication skills which enable the surgeon to interact, communicate and work with patients from diverse social, economic and ethnic backgrounds. The surgeon should be able to use these skills to establish a 'therapeutic relationship' with the patient and their family in order to facilitate the treatment process.

In the role of a surgeon, the technical task of 'performing' in the operating theatre is actually a simpler task. It requires the integration of a series of defined technical steps. If these are performed for the right reasons, at an appropriate standard and in the correct sequence, the operation should be a success. All complex operations can be broken down into a series of simpler steps.

Behaving as a surgeon

Most surgeons in training are keen to engage their surgical mentors and become part of the surgical team. They usually model their behaviour on how they see their mentors behave towards colleagues, juniors, patients and other hospital staff. Although it is hoped that these mentors will be positive role models, there is no guarantee!

The stereotype of the senior surgeon from past decades, in particular, may be a poor example for trainees to emulate.

The modern surgeon must be an excellent communicator and treat colleagues (at all levels) courteously and with respect, while maintaining those characteristics that are essential to surgery: decisiveness, willingness to make a decision based on incomplete information, and the ability to take control of situations when appropriate. Trainees should seek to balance the practical role required for good surgical practice with responsibilities and opportunities in other areas of endeavour.

It is also important for surgeons to develop a balance between their workload and the rest of their life. Demands made of surgeons can be considerable, but it is neither appropriate nor sustainable for surgeons to allow all their time to be consumed by surgical practice. Surgeons may become overwhelmed with work-related tasks, and it is essential that reasonable limits are set so that a balance is achieved between work and life outside work.

Teaching

Teaching is an integral part of the surgical profession. It is not only students who benefit from the surgeon's teaching. Teaching requires a deeper understanding of the principles, processes, knowledge and skills that are the foundation of surgery. One of the best ways to refine one's own practice is to teach it. Surgeons have the privilege and responsibility to pass their professional knowledge and skills on to medical students and trainee surgeons to ensure that high-quality surgical services are available to future generations. All surgeons must be engaged in teaching at some level. Past and current generations of surgeons have assisted with undergraduate and postgraduate teaching, often *pro bono*. Teaching undergraduate medical students the principles of surgical disease, diagnosis and treatment is an important responsibility. If surgery as a discipline is to continue to attract the best and brightest undergraduates into its ranks, then all surgeons will need to inspire their students and give them a positive experience of surgical practice. The postgraduate teaching of basic and advanced surgical trainees is equally important. How surgeons interact with early postgraduate trainees has a profound impact on future career choices. For many surgeons, postgraduate teaching will be their principal contribution to the activities of the Royal Australasian College of Surgeons.

Keeping up to date

Surgeons have a responsibility to remain up to date with advances in surgical knowledge, and to keep abreast of new developments. Continuous professional development, clinical audit and reaccreditation all contribute to this. The body of surgical knowledge does not remain fixed in time, and it is critical that trainees develop habits and strategies that facilitate keeping abreast of new developments throughout their independent surgical practice. The ability to assess and critically appraise one's own practice will facilitate and drive ongoing learning. Support from colleagues, particularly in the area of audit and acquiring new skills, is also necessary for this. As a clinical practice evolves and changes, it will be necessary to learn new procedures and skills, and the support of colleagues who can work together will facilitate this.

Research

Through research, surgeons contribute to their profession and to the wider community. Some surgeons may become involved in laboratory science research. All surgeons engaged in clinical practice can contribute to clinical research. This might involve clinical audit (which can be presented and published as a clinical case series) or participation in clinical trials. Opportunities exist for surgeons in teaching hospitals, rural practice and in full-time private practice to engage in collaborative clinical research efforts, either led by other surgeons or instituted by the individual. Engagement in research leads to understanding of the issues, practicalities and difficulties of conducting and publishing high-quality research. This is particularly useful when appraising the strengths and limitations of published papers. For this reason, surgical trainees are required to undertake a research project within the training programmes of the Royal Australasian College of Surgeons.

Leadership

The role of a surgeon inevitably requires skills as a leader, even at the level of a junior surgical trainee. Levels of leadership and responsibility are delegated to all members of the surgical team. Leadership skills are needed in direct patient management and in managing the surgical team and environment. At times, a surgeon must take a lead in health advocacy on behalf of a patient, hospital or community. Ultimately, critical decisions and clinical responsibility rest on the attending surgeon who must have developed the leadership ability to manage the surgical environment to the best benefit of the patient. A good leader must sometimes make tough decisions and assume responsibility for them. As a leader, a good surgeon does not function in isolation, but consults with colleagues, respects and listens to other members of the team, and acts as a role model.

THE SURGICAL TEAM

Surgical trainees and 'trained' surgeons interact at different levels in a surgical department and should function as an effective team. This team also includes a variety of nursing and non-medical staff. It is essential that all of these individuals work as a team, understand and perform their roles well, and have excellent communication skills. In a teaching hospital, the surgical resident (or intern) and the surgical registrar are responsible to a consultant surgeon for the day-to-day management of patients under the consultant's care. A trainee who cannot function as part of a team is unlikely to progress within the training programme.

Surgical training is an apprenticeship of graded responsibility, progressing with maturity and experience. All team members, from junior trainee to senior consultant, must be aware of their own limitations and seek early assistance or advice. A competent, responsible surgeon will recognise when assistance is necessary and will request it. Collegial support may be needed in situations of technical, psychological, ethical or physical difficulty.

Exercising such clinical judgement is in the patient's best interest, and it will earn the surgeon the respect of his/her patients and colleagues. Failing to recognise the need for help, and proceeding regardless, will lose that respect and is an unsafe and unacceptable practice.

All surgeons have a professional and ethical obligation to respond appropriately to calls for assistance from their colleagues.

Teamwork is important in surgical practice and a close working relationship with non-surgical staff, including nurses and paramedical staff, is essential. Good and appropriate communication, respect and courtesy should be the foundation of all interactions with staff and patients.

SPECIFIC COMMUNICATION ISSUES

Communication with patients and relatives is as important as communication with members of the surgical team. It should be open and honest. Information about diagnosis, treatment and outcomes should be shared sensitively and fully with the patient. The Privacy Act requires that the surgeon has the patient's consent to talk to relatives about their condition, but in general open communication and disclosure should be encouraged. When complications and adverse outcomes occur, good communication with the patient, and their family, will minimise the risk of litigation and complaints.

Informed consent

When patients make decisions about their medical care they should be provided with correct information, preferably in written and verbal form. It is also important to ensure that the patient actually understands the information.

There are five aspects of informed consent that should be addressed:

1. The treatment or procedure should be described in appropriate detail, using language that the patient can understand.

2. The reason for recommending a specific procedure or course of treatment needs to be clearly outlined.
3. The expected benefits should be conveyed accurately and realistically, and put in context with possible suboptimal outcomes or detractors.
4. The risks associated with the procedure must be explained. In addition to common risks, it is important to explain less common but more significant (material) risks, particularly if they are likely to influence the patient's decision making.
5. Any other options to the proposed procedure should be offered and discussed, including the option of no treatment.

In some situations, including those where procedures are planned on minors, critically ill patients or patients with dementia, consent needs to be sought from another individual or from the guardianship board. For critically ill patients who are unable to provide consent because of their illness, permission should be sought from the next of kin or an appropriate relative. For elderly patients who are no longer competent to make a decision (e.g. those suffering from dementia), consent should be sought from an individual who has medical power of attorney.

Although minors are not legally allowed to give independent consent, it is still desirable that they be given information about the proposed procedure in understandable language.

The operative note

Good record keeping and communication with colleagues is important. The operative note should describe succinctly and accurately what has happened in the operating theatre. It is good surgical practice for the operative note to include the indications for performing the procedure, the operative findings, a description of the key technical elements of the procedure, and postoperative management instructions. It should also record whether the procedure was uneventful, and describe any difficulties that were encountered and any unusual aspects to the case. It should provide enough information to enable the important details to be understood by another surgeon who encounters the patient at a later date.

Adverse events

No surgical procedure is risk free. Every procedure has an inherent risk of an adverse event and unexpected events do happen. If the risk is significant, it should have been discussed as part of the informed consent process. When the event is rare or unexpected, this may not have happened. When an adverse event occurs, open and honest communication and discussion should take place between the surgeon and the patient or the surgeon and the relatives. The patient should be told what has happened, how it happened and what will be done to rectify the problem.

It is usually appropriate to offer an apology. An apology is not an assumption of blame, and is more likely to reduce than to increase the likelihood of litigation. The majority of complications are not the fault of the surgeon and are not due to negligence.

Perhaps surprisingly, an adverse outcome due to negligence will not necessarily lead to litigation if good, effective and caring communication between the surgeon, patient and their family occurs. Human nature, however, may lead a surgeon to avoid the patient, communicate poorly, or not acknowledge the event following an adverse outcome. This behaviour will make subsequent legal action more likely.

Adverse events are an opportunity for learning. This is the principle behind clinical audit, morbidity and mortality meetings, and hospital quality assurance meetings. It is appropriate to review most adverse events and outcomes in a controlled environment that is conducive to open discussion of the event. Quality improvement can follow if the contributing factors are identified. The clinical practice improvement (CPI) movement seeks to rectify system issues in the environment in which surgeons work that contribute to adverse events, so that the system can be redesigned to minimise risk.

Dealing with conflict

Conflict with patients, relatives and other staff inevitably arises from time to time. A competent surgeon has the strategies and skills to deal with this. When conflict occurs, or an angry patient or relative is encountered, it is important not to respond with anger. Often the problem is due to poor communication or misunderstanding, and an angry response only makes the situation worse. First, listen to what the other person is saying. It is very important to hear them out. This is the first step in defusing tension. When they believe they have been heard, they will be more receptive to you. After hearing their concerns, calmly and honestly explain what has happened, acknowledge issues of importance to them, outline any review process that will be undertaken, and apologise! It is important to be seen to be sympathetic and responsive.

LIFELONG SURGICAL EDUCATION

Surgical training and surgical education does not cease after passing the Part 2 Examination of the Royal Australasian College of Surgeons. It must continue throughout a surgeon's career. Attendance at courses and conferences is a good way of updating knowledge and expertise. Participation in a conference by presenting a paper is an even better way of engaging in education and peer review. As new procedures are introduced, or a surgeon's repertoire changes, it is necessary to have a strategy for acquiring new skills and knowledge. Although information can be obtained at conferences and workshops, an appropriate way to commence a new technique is to gain assistance from another surgeon who is already skilled and trained in the procedure, and to engage this colleague as a mentor. If there is no locally available expertise, then operating with another consultant surgeon is a sensible strategy. This demonstrates responsibility and integrity, and should help to reduce the risk of an adverse outcome.

SUMMARY

Surgical conduct is the mature professional behaviour that results from the accumulation of surgical skills and wisdom through a long apprenticeship and throughout a career as a surgeon. The many facets of a competent surgeon extend far beyond technical and manual surgical skills to encompass sophisticated interpersonal skills, communication, decision making, teaching, learning and leadership.

CHAPTER TWO
SURGICAL DECISION MAKING

One must attend in medical practice not primarily to plausible theories, but to experience combined with reason.

Hippocrates (460–377 BC)

INTRODUCTION

Decision making occurs when a choice must be made between a number of possible options. Decision making comprises a large part of the work of a surgeon as choices must be made at all stages of the patient's treatment pathway, from selection of preoperative tests and assessments, through choice of surgical procedure and intra-operative techniques, to decisions about postoperative management and ongoing follow up. Surgical decisions often must be made quickly, are frequently irreversible and may have major and long-lasting impact on patients' lives. Therefore, surgeons need to develop sound decision-making skills so as to achieve the best possible outcomes for their patients.

THE DECISION-MAKING PROCESS

The word 'deciding' has been defined as *'to settle something in dispute or doubt'*.[1] Decisions can only be made where there are a number of options available; it stands to reason that if there is only one possible course of action, no choice or decision is necessary. Decision making is based on a process of reasoning that involves weighing up all the likely consequences of each possible course of action and an individual's values or preferences for the likely outcomes.

There are a number of ways in which decisions can be made. 'Rational' or 'informed' decision making involves the application of knowledge in the decision-making process. This has been framed within evidence-based medicine (EBM) as the *conscientious, explicit and judicious use of current best evidence in making decisions about the care of individual patients.*[2] There is a common misconception that EBM is synonymous with randomised control trials (RCTs) but this is not the case. First, the 'best' study design depends on the type of research question. Although it is widely recognised that the RCT is the best study design for assessing whether a treatment works, other types of study are more appropriate to look at questions about the cause of disease, prognosis or the accuracy of diagnostic tests. Second, the 'best' theoretical study design may be impossible for practical or ethical reasons, and so the best *available* evidence of treatment effectiveness will come from non-randomised studies. This is particularly an issue in surgery where RCTs may not be possible if patients or surgeons are unwilling to have their choice of operation determined by a randomisation process. The ranking of research evidence creates a hierarchy of study designs including RCTs to assist decision making.[3] For surgeons and other clinicians, evidence-based clinical practice guidelines based on such hierarchies of evidence provide a ready summary of the scientific literature on a topic, often with recommendations for clinical practice based on an expert appraisal of this evidence.

DECISION MAKING UNDER UNCERTAINTY

There are many situations where there is no clear evidence of the best approach to a particular problem. This may be due to a lack of high-quality research studies or due to conflicting findings from different studies. Another common situation is where one treatment may confer a higher chance of survival or cure than an alternative approach, but with detrimental impact on aspects of quality of life. Figure 2.1 presents the example of a choice between open and laparoscopic surgery for colon cancer to demonstrate some of the various issues that must be considered in surgical decision making.

For reasons of inadequate, incomplete or conflicting evidence, there is often great uncertainty among surgeons about what constitutes the 'best' treatment approach. A state of genuine uncertainty about the relative merits of two treatments is referred to as a state of 'equipoise'.[4] This can work on a number of levels. 'Individual equipoise' occurs when an individual clinician believes that, after weighing up the relative benefits and potential harms of two different treatments, neither is superior to the other. 'Community equipoise' occurs when there is no clear consensus view of the relative merits of two treatments among the expert clinical community.[4] In this case some surgeons would favour one treatment approach, whereas other

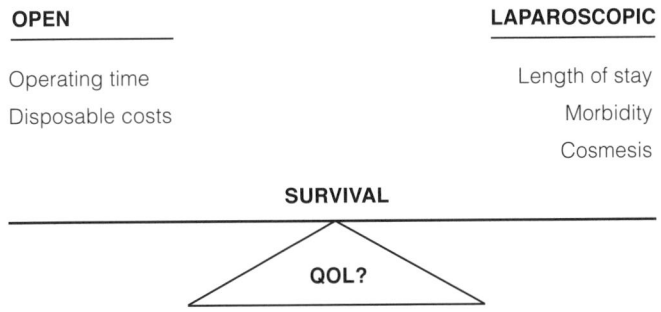

Fig. 2.1 Issues in surgical decision making around choice of surgery for colon cancer

surgeons would favour the alternative. Each surgeon may not be in a state of individual equipoise, in fact, it is common for surgeons to hold strong but opposing treatment preferences.[5]

In situations of uncertainty the values ('utilities') that people place on the likely outcomes of a treatment, as well as the probabilities of these outcomes, should determine treatment choices. While patient preferences can be measured formally,[6, 7] to date this has primarily been done for research purposes rather than within clinical consultations. However, surgeons should discuss patients' treatment preferences and the values they place on different outcomes such as functional ability and aspects of quality of life as part of routine clinical care.

Not only do surgeons need to talk to patients about the various aspects of quality of life most important to them, but they must also find out how involved patients wish to be in the decision-making process itself. Previous research has found that a large proportion of patients want to take an active role in making the decisions about their medical treatment, whereas a substantial minority (approximately one third) prefer to leave the decision making to their clinician.[8, 9] Patients who achieve their desired level of involvement in decision making are more likely to be satisfied with the treatment they receive.[9–11]

An additional consideration in the decision-making process is the implication of the decision for society as a whole. Health resources are limited and so there is always an 'opportunity cost' whereby the personnel, equipment and facilities used to treat one patient are not then available to treat others. Not only should actual costs be taken into account, but also the outcomes that can be achieved. One treatment may be considerably more resource intensive and expensive, but confer superior outcomes. Plotting the relative costs and benefits of a new treatment on a 'cost effectiveness plane' (Figure 2.2) can be a useful aid for decision making.[12, 13]

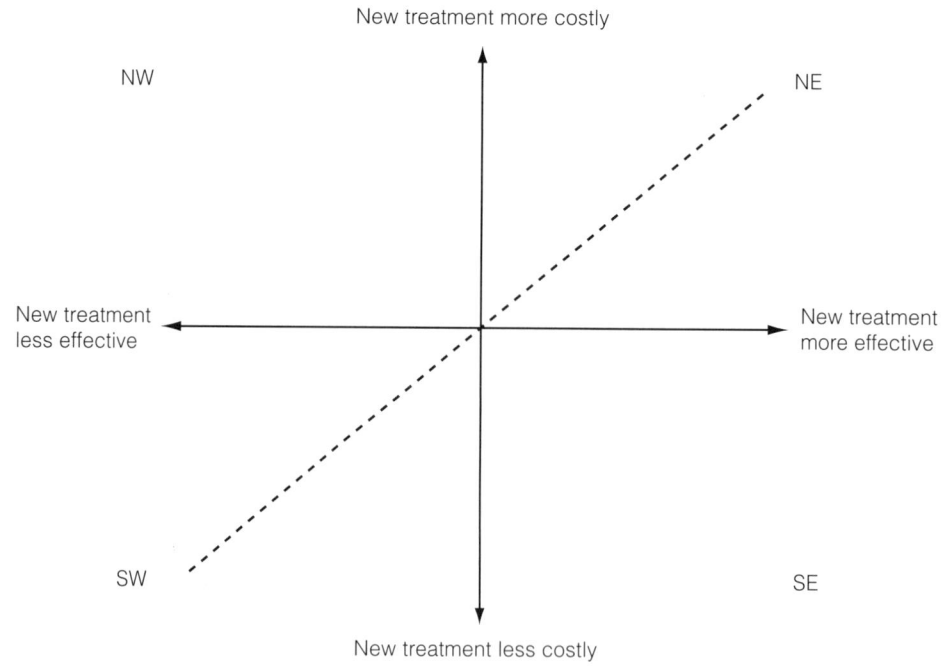

New treatment more costly

NW

NE

New treatment
less effective

New treatment
more effective

SW

SE

New treatment less costly

Fig. 2.2 Cost effectiveness plane

As shown in Figure 2.2, the plane is divided into four quadrants based on whether the new treatment is more or less effective (horizontal axis) and more or less expensive (vertical axis) than an alternative such as standard therapy. These results can be obtained from randomised trials or other comparative studies that include assessment of costs as well as outcomes. A treatment that is more effective at less cost (SE quadrant) is clearly superior, whereas a treatment that is less effective and more costly (NW quadrant) is clearly inferior and should not be supported. Decisions around treatments that fall into the remaining two quadrants are less clear-cut. For treatments that are more effective but at higher cost (NE quadrant), the decision to use this therapy depends on the availability of funding and the opportunity costs. In some situations it may be appropriate to support treatments that are less expensive but also somewhat less effective (SW quadrant) if this frees up funding for other concerns. The dashed line in Figure 2.2 represents a cut-off between treatments that would or would not be funded. The slope of this line will vary according to the context in which the decision is being made.

In this way, assessment of the relative cost effectiveness of different treatment approaches can help surgeons decide on the most efficient use of health resources.

INFORMAL DECISION MAKING—HEURISTICS

Informal processes for decision making are often used when either there is no empirical evidence on which to base a rational decision or there simply is no time to follow a formal process. Surgeons must often make very rapid decisions, for example during emergencies or intra-operatively, and do not have time to review known evidence and discuss patients' values. In these circumstances, surgeons use their prior knowledge and training to assess the situation rapidly, make a decision and act.

This more informal method of decision making often involves 'rules of thumb' or 'intuitive judgements', which are known in psychology and information science as 'heuristics'.[14] Heuristics are common in clinical education: most surgeons would be familiar with such axioms as *common things occur commonly* or *if you hear the sound of hooves, think horses not zebras*. In this case, the mental short-cut will lead clinicians to investigate common diagnoses first before considering rare conditions to explain a patient's symptoms and signs. When used to make judgements that are generally accurate, heuristics can provide a 'fast and frugal' approach to decision making.[15]

Unfortunately, heuristics can be misleading and doctors may make a number of cognitive errors when making decisions in this way. Some of the problems that have been found in studies of doctors' decision-making processes include overconfidence, having an inaccurate perception of the probabilities of good or bad outcomes, and failure to consider all the options. Over-reliance on heuristics could lead surgeons, for example, to overlook a brain lesion in someone presenting with an unsteady gait who also has the smell of alcohol on their breath (the 'representativeness heuristic'), or to overestimate the risk of a patient becoming addicted to opioids prescribed for severe pain due to widespread awareness of the problems of opioid addiction in the community as opposed to the low rate of addiction in those receiving this class of drugs for clinical reasons (the 'availability heuristic').[16] On the other hand, some commentators believe that those heuristics that result in an unacceptably high rate of error would be of no value and so would fail to become established 'wisdom'. This line of reasoning suggests that established heuristics can provide an efficient strategy for decision making, especially given the routine and repetitive nature of much of the work in clinical medicine.[17]

As noted by Hippocrates, clinical decision making requires *experience combined with reason*,[18] utilising in some cases the advice of mentors and peers as well as other medical and non-medical advisors. Ongoing audit as well as awareness of the current best evidence provides the forum for feedback to balance and guide one's own equipoise and surgical decision making.

SUMMARY

Decision making is an important part of the role of a surgeon. Assessment of the likelihood of various outcomes of a treatment based on the scientific literature together with an appraisal of the values that are placed on these outcomes is at the core of an evidence-based approach to decision making. The use of heuristics and the advice of mentors and peers are also important components of decision making in surgical practice.

REFERENCES

1. Macquarie Dictionary, 4th edn, North Ryde: The Macquarie Library Pty Ltd, 2005.

2. Sackett DL, Rosenberg WMC, Muir Gray JA, Haynes RB, Richardson WS. Evidence-based medicine: what it is and what it isn't. BMJ 1996;312:71–2.

3. National Health and Medical Research Council. How to use the evidence: assessment and application of scientific evidence. Canberra: NHMRC, 2000:8.

4. Freedman B. Equipoise and the ethics of clinical research. N Engl J Med 1987;317:141–5.

5. Young JM, Harrison J, White G, May J, Solomon MJ. Developing measures of surgeons' equipoise to assess the feasibility of randomized controlled trials in vascular surgery. Surgery 2004;136:1070–6.

6. Salkeld G, Solomon M, Butow P, Short L. Discrete-choice experiment to measure patient preferences for the surgical management of colorectal cancer. Br J Surg 2005;92:742–7.

7. Solomon MJ, Pager C, Keshava A, Findlay M, Butow P, Salkeld G, Roberts R. What Do Patients Want? Patient preferences and surrogate decision-making in the treatment of colorectal cancer. Dis Colon Rectum 2003;46:1351–7.

8. Blanchard CG, Labreque MS, Ruckdeschel JC et al. Information and decision-making preferences of hospitalized cancer patients. Soc Sci Med 1988: 27:1139–45.

9. Butow PN, Maclean M, Dunn SM et al. The dynamics of change: Cancer patients' preferences for information, involvement and support. Ann Oncol 1997;8:857–63.

10. Cassileth BR, Zupkis RV, Sutton-Smith K et al. Information and participation preferences among cancer patients. Ann Intern Med 1980;92:832–6.

11. Gattellari M, Butow P, Tattersall M. Sharing decisions in cancer care. Soc Sci Med 2001;51:1865–78.

12. Black WC. The CE plane: a graphic representation of cost effectiveness. Med Decis Making 1990;10:212–4.

13. Laupacis A, Feeny D, Detsky AS, Tugwell PX. How attractive does a new technology have to be to warrant adoption and utilization? Tentative guidelines for using clinical and economic evaluations. CMAJ 1992;146:473–81.

14. McDonald CJ. Medical heuristics: the silent adjudicators of clinical practice. Ann Int Med 1996;124:56–62.

15. Gigerenzer G, Todd PM and the ABC Research Group. Simple heuristics that make us smart. Oxford, UK: Oxford University Press, 1999.

16. Klein JG. Five pitfalls in decisions about diagnosis and treatment. BMJ 2005;330:781–3.

17. Eva KW, Norman GR. Heuristics and biases—a biased perspective on clinical reasoning. Med Educ 2005;39:870–2.

18. Jones WHS. Hippocrates, Volume 1. Loeb Classical Library: London, Harvard University Press, 1923.

CHAPTER THREE
SURGICAL SAFETY

Whenever a doctor cannot do good, he must be kept from doing harm.

Hippocrates (460–377BC)

You want a surgical team that faces each error, each mishap, straight up, names it, and takes steps to prevent its recurrence.

Francis D Moore (1913–2001)

I have made many mistakes myself . . . the best surgeon, like the best general, is he who makes the fewest mistakes.

Astley Cooper (1768–1841)

INTRODUCTION

Surgical safety refers to the minimisation of harm to a patient arising from a surgical intervention and the prevention of harm from accidental injury. For centuries, surgeons have recognised that errors do occur in surgery and that human error is inevitable and unavoidable.[1]

We now recognise the need to have systems in place that render it virtually impossible or at least extremely difficult for human error to cause harm to our patients. The airline industry has adopted a systems approach with great success.

Pivotal to surgical safety is the need for surgeons to recognise their fallibility openly, report complications of diagnostic and therapeutic interventions, and to develop processes and strategies that minimise errors.

Errors can occur at any stage, from the initial consultation through to the final discharge of a patient. Experienced surgeons often have their own strategies in place to minimise errors and complications but unfortunately this information is seldom passed on to trainees, who are more focused on acquiring surgical skills and experience.

DEFINITIONS

Error in planning: use of the wrong plan to achieve an aim.

Error in execution: failure of a planned action to be completed as intended.

Active error: operator errors committed by individual practitioners at the point of care (e.g. the surgeon in the operating theatre).

Latent error: circumstances established by policies and practises of an institution, culture or society that predispose surgeons to error (e.g. inadequate training, inadequate supervision, sleep deprivation).

Active errors are commonly recognised at the time they occur (e.g. the surgeon recognises that he/she has cut the ureter inadvertently, the pilot forgets to put down the landing gear), while unpicking latent errors can be much more difficult. Errors can be intercepted by an appropriate action that negates the threat to patient safety. A close call is an event that *almost* leads to patient harm but is avoided by chance or timely intervention (e.g. a surgeon stops a registrar from dividing the ureter during a pelvic dissection).

An *adverse event* is an unintended injury, caused by medical management rather than the disease process, which is sufficiently serious to lead to prolonged hospitalisation, to temporary or permanent disability, or which contributes to or causes death. If an adverse event is caused by error, it is preventable. Human error does not necessarily lead to adverse events, and not all adverse events are necessarily due to error.

MAGNITUDE OF THE PROBLEM

Two-thirds of adverse events in hospitals are surgical, and half of these are preventable. A Western Australian audit of surgical mortality for the period 1 January 2002 and 30 June 2004 identified deficiencies in care in 20% of 876 deaths.[5] In 5% the deficiency of care caused the death, and 2% of deaths were considered preventable. The main deficiencies identified were technical errors of surgery, delays, general complications such as aspiration and septicaemia, failure to use facilities such as DVT prophylaxis or ICU/HDU beds, and incorrect or inappropriate therapy.

A review of claims brought to the attention of the Medical Defence Union in the UK from 1990 to 2003 identified 306 cases of operations that went wrong. In 39% of these cases, the operation was carried out on the wrong side or site. Twenty per cent of cases were orthopaedics/trauma and 49% were dental.

FACTORS IN ADVERSE EVENTS

1. Organisational: These factors include resource allocation, personnel and equipment, rosters, scheduling and timing of procedures, cover, and change-over of personnel. Adverse events increase at shift changeover, at the beginning of new terms and whilst covering other units at night or weekends.

2. Situational: These factors include distractions, interruptions, environment and physical conditions, and equipment design.

3. Team: Surgeons work with other members of the health profession including anaesthetists, nurses, physiotherapists and a whole host of other professionals. Poor communication and failure to work as a team greatly increase the risk of error. *In theatre, the most important person is the patient* and the team looking after the patient needs to communicate, trust each other's abilities, and be able to deal with unexpected emergencies safely and efficiently. Antagonistic communication between surgeon and nursing staff may stifle the flow of information and lead to errors.

4. Individual: Fatigue is an important cause of error in surgery. Twenty-eight hours of sleep deprivation is equivalent to a moderate blood alcohol level in terms of cognitive and motor impairment. Psychological factors such as depression, stress, medication and other personal factors can profoundly affect performance and lead to errors. It is important to be psychologically prepared for and focussed on clinical tasks.

5. Task: Performing a surgical procedure involves the execution of a series of complex tasks, each with many possible steps. Omission of a necessary task is the most common cause of error. For example, counting swabs, instruments and needles at the end of the procedure is an important task to ensure that no foreign body is left in the patient.

6. Information: Impaired access to vital information can lead to serious errors in surgery. For example, adverse drug events due to drug allergy, renal impairment or drug–drug interactions can be avoided with easy and reliable access to the appropriate information.

7. Patient: There are many patient factors that may lead to an increase in error rate: morbid obesity, disease severity, coexisting disease and anatomical variations, for example. Patient personality and familiarity may adversely influence therapeutic decisions and responses.

THE SYSTEMS THEORY

High-risk errors are not unique to the field of surgery. Other fields where errors carry a high risk of severe consequences, such as the aviation industry and anaesthesia, have been able to reduce the rates and consequences of errors by applying well thought-out error reduction and response systems. These systems are based on the theory which contends that 'events, objects, locations and methods do not exist independently, but rather are intertwined as interdependent components of complex systems'.[3] Chaos theory indicates that the most complex systems function at the interface with chaos. A small aberration can tip a highly complex, sophisticated system into chaos. The clinical process is further complicated, by social, economic, cultural, legal and other issues that are thrown in to form the ultimate shape of the system.

The systems theory is based on three principles:
1. Human error is unavoidable.
2. Faulty systems allow human error to harm patients.
3. Systems can be designed to prevent or detect human error before a patient is harmed.

For example, while surgeons largely deny the negative effects of sleep deprivation on performance, the aviation industry recognises that fatigue leads to error and has set strict limitations on hours of work. Anaesthetists have followed suit. Often, even when safe hours policies are in place, they are not rigidly enforced. So, for surgeons, the system is faulty at present.

Complex systems have many steps and failures can be detected along the way, thereby preventing the error from harming the patient. James Reason proposed what is now referred to as the 'Swiss cheese model' to explain how failures can lead to patient harm[6]. If you think of a stack of slices of Swiss cheese, the holes represent opportunities for error to occur, and the slices are defensive layers (see Fig. 3.1).

Because of the random distribution of holes, an error passing through one layer often hits a solid bit in the next layer and is deflected (Fig. 3.1a). If, by chance, the holes in all the layers are aligned, the error gets through the system and harms the patient (Fig. 3.1b).

Detecting errors and adverse events

There are a number of methods in routine use to increase the chance of detecting errors and adverse events.

- Direct observation of clinical care is the most sensitive method. This includes attending ward rounds, reviewing clinical records and having discussions with members of the team looking after the patient.
- Retrospective studies detect fewer errors.
- Incident reports suffer from inconsistent reporting, poor follow-up and poor compliance, especially if voluntarily completed.
- Morbidity and mortality meetings are a form of voluntary reporting but they have been shown to detect only a small proportion of adverse events.
- Peer review, applied vigorously, can positively impact on patient outcomes and reduce errors.

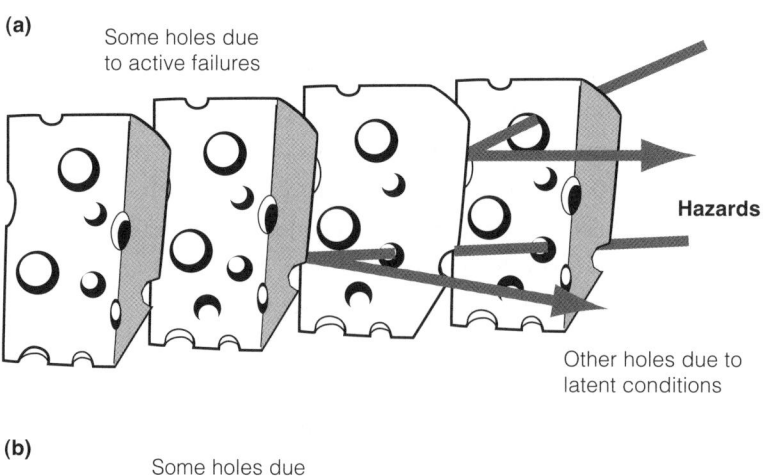

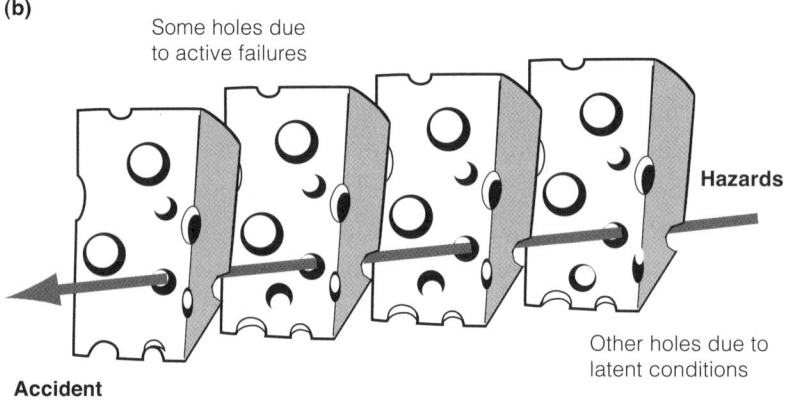

Fig. 3.1 Successive layers of defences

Steps to ensure patient safety

1. Personally see and examine all patients before surgery.
2. Make accurate notes recording the side and site of the problem, previous operations, allergies, and all other relevant information about the patient. Document the proposed procedure including an operative plan, if appropriate. Make sure that proper informed consent has been obtained. Ask the patient if they have any questions or concerns, or if they do not understand anything.
3. Ensure that the relevant investigations have been performed and that the results and films are available.
4. Communicate with the theatre if special instruments, equipment, implants or conditions are required.
5. Communicate with the anaesthetist if there are any special requirements including unusual positions or intubation routes.
6. Anticipate postoperative resources and make appropriate arrangements, for example, special nursing or intensive care.

7. See the patient before induction of anaesthesia, preferably in the preoperative area or waiting bay. Re-examine them, explaining the proposed surgery yet again, if necessary. Follow the RACS guidelines (see page 23) to ensure correct patient, correct side and correct site surgery[7]. Mark the patient and have them confirm the site and side.

8. Check that the theatre is correctly set up and instruments and implants are available and correct.

9. Re-read your patient notes and check that the relevant investigations/films are available. Re-study any imaging, if appropriate.

10. Take a 'time-out' with the theatre team to do a final check before the patient is anaesthetised.

11. Before making your incision, always check if the anaesthetist has given a prophylactic antibiotic, anticoagulant or other drugs if required.

12. Operate slowly and meticulously. The secret of the apparently fast surgeon is that to speed up, you need to slow down, and never have to take the same step twice—do it right the first time!
    a) Be meticulous with haemostasis.
    b) Be gentle with tissues: respect them and keep them moist.
    c) Communicate with the anaesthetic team from time to time: 'How is the patient doing?'
    d) Never cut if you can't see.
    e) Never be afraid to ask for assistance.
    f) Be aware of anatomical variations.

13. At the end of the procedure, ensure that the instrument, swab and needle count is correct. Ensure that appropriate dressings and splints, if required, are applied.

14. Make accurate and clear operation notes and fill out histology forms, ensuring correct labelling of specimens. Write clear postoperative instructions and include your postoperative plans.

15. The postoperative care is as important as the operation:
    a) Check your patient in the recovery room.
    b) Always do a postoperative round to check on the patient and clarify the postoperative care, if necessary.

16. See postoperative in-patients daily. Always ensure that an entry is made in the notes on a daily basis. Have a 'system' to check the results of investigations including pathology reports. Ensure that the results are noted, signed and acted upon.

17. Communicate with patients and their relatives in a kind and compassionate way. 'Nice' doctors are seldom sued! Failure to communicate can lead to litigation.

18. At discharge from hospital, ensure that the patient has been given adequate written instructions on wound care and any special requirements, a contact point if things go wrong, and a follow-up appointment if appropriate. Ensure that the GP is sent a discharge summary that includes the relevant diagnosis, results, interventions and postoperative plans.

SUMMARY

Human error is a fact of life. As surgeons, we need to acknowledge that we can and do make errors, we need to report these errors accurately and openly, and we need to have systems in place that render it impossible or extremely unlikely for human error to cause harm to our patients.

REFERENCES

1. Etchells E, O'Neill C and Bernstein M. Patient safety in surgery: Error detection and prevention. World J Surg. 2003;27(8):936–42.

2. Gawande AH, Thomas EJ, Zinner MJ et al. The incidence and nature of surgical adverse events in Colorado and Utah in 1992. Surgery 1999;126:66–75.

3. Calland JF, Guerlain S, Adams RB et al. A systems approach to surgical safety. Surg Endosc 2002;16:1005–14.

4. Krizek T. Surgical error: reflections on adverse events. Bull Am Coll Surg 2000;85:18–22.

5. Semmens JB, Aitken RJ, Sanfilippo FM et al. The Western Australian audit of surgical mortality: advanced surgical accountability. MJA 2005;183(10):504–8.

6. Reason J. Human error: models and management. BMJ 2000;320:768–70.

7. Royal Australasian College of Surgeons. Implementation guidelines for ensuring correct patient, correct side, and correct site surgery. Melbourne: RACS, 2006, viewed December 2007, <http://www.surgeons.org/AM/Template.cfm?Section=Policies3&TEMPLATE=/CM/ContentDisplay.cfm&CONTENTID=15658>

Royal Australian College of Surgeons Implementation Guidelines for Ensuring Correct Patient, Correct Side and Correct Site Surgery

Correct Patient, Side and Site

The Royal Australasian College of Surgeons recognises the paramount importance of patient safety and expects hospitals and surgeons to adopt protocols utilising multiple, complementary strategies. To the extent possible, the patient or their designated representative should be involved in the process. Adopting a "team approach" in the theatre will reduce risk but the operating surgeon is ultimately responsible. Every member of the operating theatre team has a duty to be aware that the correct patient, side and site are operated on. If any member of the team believes the incorrect patient, side or site is being prepared for surgery, they should immediately voice their concerns. There should be no criticism of persons raising concerns even if their concerns prove to be unfounded. Surgeons should be aware of the level of risk for wrong site or side surgery for a particular procedure.

Consent and Documentation

Verification of the patient must be made with the patient or the patient's designated representative (if the patient is legally a child or unable to answer for him or herself). Appropriate legal requirements in this matter must be attended to.

Patient consent must be obtained.

The consent form must include and the patient or representative must verify:

- Patient's full name
- Name of procedure
- Site of procedure
- Side of procedure

The site and side of the operation must be recorded in full (i.e. RIGHT or LEFT) and not abbreviated to R or L, whenever the side is recorded. All documentation must include the side and site. This includes patient notes, hospital forms and operating theatre lists.

Marking the Site of the Procedure

- The surgeon should be satisfied on which side and site the procedure is to be performed. This should occur in consultation with the patient.
- An indelible pen is used to unambiguously mark the side/site of the procedure. This is done or checked by the surgeon in consultation with the patient (where possible) and medical record. The patient (who should not have been sedated) is informed that the pen mark indicates the site of the operation. The mark should be within the operative field and should be initialled by the person making the mark. Multiple operation sites must be individually marked.

- The pen mark is checked by the nurse as the patient leaves the ward or holding area for the operating theatre.
- The pen mark is checked by the scout nurse prior to the patient entering the operating theatre. This mark must then be verified by the scrub nurse.
- The surgeon visibly checks the pen mark prior to commencing surgery and ensures this is in accord with his or her intended operation before induction of anaesthesia.

Implants

The surgeon and the operating nurse must check the presence of the appropriate implants in the operating theatre before the anaesthetic commences.

Imaging

The surgeon and his/her team must confer that the appropriate images are available, and confirm the site and side of the proposed surgery.

Final Verification

The surgeon, anaesthetist and nursing team must confer and concur to ensure the correct patient, procedure, site and side. Marking of the operative site must be confirmed. A "time out" or "final check" should be part of this procedure. This should preferably occur before induction of anaesthesia.

Emergencies

In emergency (life or limb threatening situations) some of these steps may be omitted.

At all stages of this process, there should be consistency of documentation of side/site. If any inconsistency arises, progress towards operation should be suspended, the incorrect documentation should be changed and signed, and an explanation of the inconsistency recorded in the patient's medical history and signed by the surgeon. The surgeon should satisfy him/herself of the appropriate side/site of surgery and record this in the patient's medical notes before proceeding with surgery. An incident form should be completed. If the surgeon remains uncertain of the side/site of surgery or the side/site differs from that previously discussed with the patient, the procedure should be postponed or cancelled.

CHAPTER FOUR

STERILE TECHNIQUE AND STANDARD PRECAUTIONS

In safety, do not forget danger; in peace, do not forget disorder.

Chinese proverb

INTRODUCTION

One of the greatest advances in surgical science was the introduction of an antiseptic environment for surgery by Lord Lister. Influenced greatly by the germ theory of infection and work by Pasteur and others, Lister found that the use of carbolic acid spray in the theatre and on wounds significantly reduced the rate of infective complications. Unfortunately, carbolic had its own problems, but Lister's concepts led to the development of the principles of sterile technique.

The practical aspects of modern sterile technique have evolved significantly since Lister's time. A range of active measures, now employed routinely, help prevent patient-borne infections during an invasive procedure. Conversely (and no less importantly) are measures designed to minimise the risk of reverse contamination and prevention of infection of clinical staff by the patient.

Sterile technique refers to the steps taken to minimise microbiological contamination of patients. It embodies four main principles, which are strictly adhered to in the operating theatre (see Table 4.1). Failure to do so may compromise the patient, the surgeon or other personnel, and is unacceptable in modern surgical practice. The principles of sterile technique are less rigorously applied outside the operating theatre, and may be less important for procedures that do not involve an open wound.

Table 4.1	The four basic elements of sterile technique
1.	Reduction in contamination of the immediate environment
2.	Disinfection of the surgical site
3.	Isolation of the surgical site
	Barriers between:
	• the clinical team and the patient
	• the patient and the environment
4.	Sterilisation of surgical equipment

Standard precautions are rules of conduct in the operating theatre designed to minimise risks to patient and staff from the many hazards present in the operating theatre, including micro-organisms, sharp instruments, flammable liquids and gases, toxic smoke, and intense energy sources such as high voltage electrical currents and lasers.

THE PRINCIPLES AND PRACTICE OF STERILE TECHNIQUE

This section examines the principles of sterile technique, and highlights the specific practices and situations required for each. While this is by no means the final word in sterile practices, the aim is to provide a practical guide for all junior theatre personnel.

Principle 1: Reduction of environmental contamination

This involves providing clean air, clean surfaces and equipment, and clean staff. Environmental decontamination is relatively easy to achieve within the theatre suite, but it becomes progressively more difficult in the procedure rooms, wards, emergency departments and surgeries where sterile technique is also practised. For some procedures, such as joint replacement, it is a vital point of practice, whereas in other situations, such as suturing a clean minor laceration, it is less critical.

Clean air

Traffic in and out of theatre and movement of personnel within theatre during a procedure create air flow. Air currents can carry microbes into the operating theatre. Minimising draughts is thought to reduce the airborne contamination of wounds. This concept has led to 'closed' theatres for joint surgery.

Creating a positive air pressure in the operating theatre also reduces the chance of outside air entering the operating theatre. This is achieved by laminar airflow units, whereby incoming filtered air is directed down over the patient and exhaust air is removed at or beyond the theatre doors (Fig. 4.1).

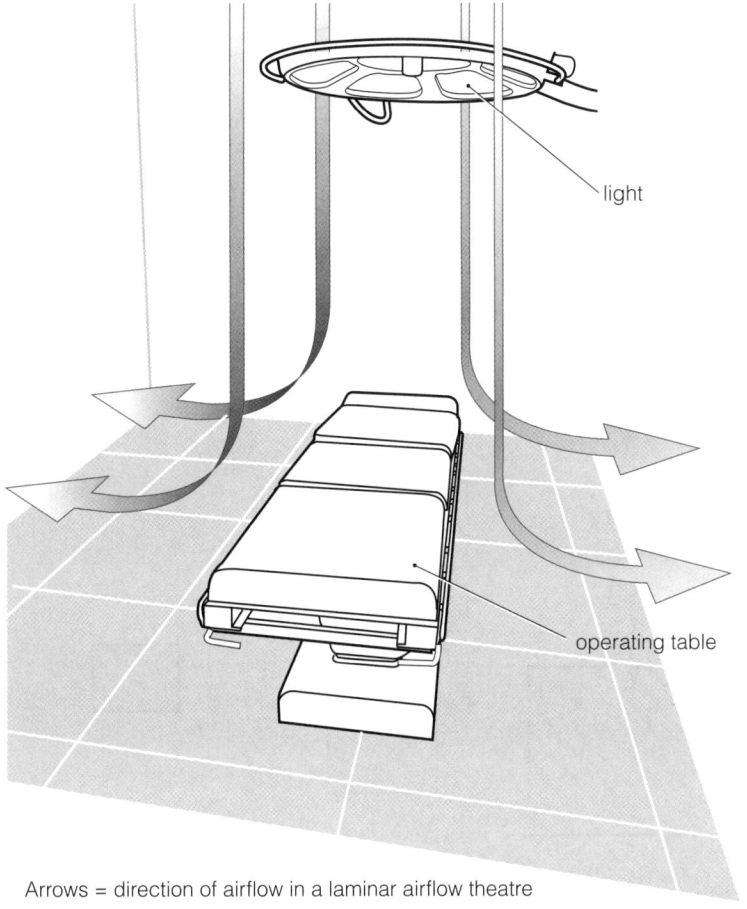

light

operating table

Arrows = direction of airflow in a laminar airflow theatre

- filtered air is blown down from above the table
- pushes particles away from patient
- air is extracted at the sides of the theatre.

Fig. 4.1 Laminar airflow

Clean surfaces and equipment

Everything in the operating theatre should be cleaned and disinfected to a very high standard, and all surfaces should be free of debris and dust. All personnel have a responsibility to help maintain this environment. Food should not be taken into the operating theatre. All staff should remain at least one metre from anything covered with sterile drapes, including draped patients, instrument trays and sterile trolleys (Fig 4.2). Be aware that it is easy to contaminate the sterile field by leaning or reaching over sterile instruments and fields while not gowned and gloved, by touching sterile personnel and trolleys, or by dropping non-sterile items onto the operative field or sterile trays. In general, it is best policy not to touch any equipment in theatre unless you are required to. If in doubt, ask for permission to touch an object or move into

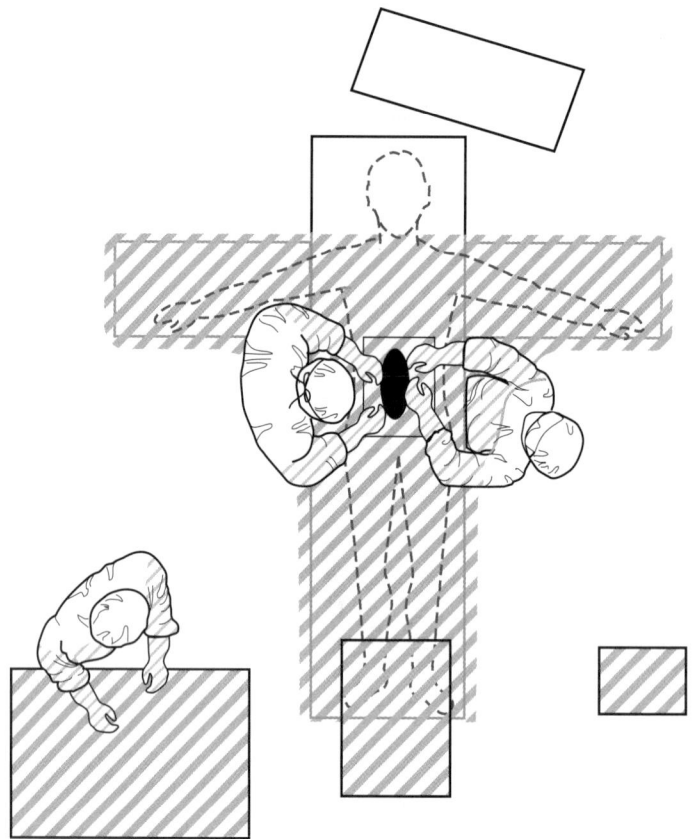

All blue or green drapes, sterile trolleys, and the gloves, arms and thorax regions of sterile personnel are regarded as being sterile. Backs, shoulders and the fronts of gowns below the waist are *not* considered sterile.

Fig. 4.2 Sterile areas on the operative field

a specific spot. It is much better to be overly cautious than to contaminate a sterile field and incur the wrath of the scrub nurse and surgeon, potentially putting the patient's life at risk with a single ill-considered act! Novices such as student nurses and medical students, who have not yet developed the instinctive response required to avoid inappropriate contact, are a particular risk in the operating theatre. Inadvertent contact with a sterile field is probably the most common cause of a break in sterile technique by inexperienced personnel.

Clean staff

To maintain the clean theatre environment, external dirt and contamination should be excluded as much as possible. To this end, staff are required to wash and change into clean theatre clothing before entering the suite. Hair and beards must be fully covered to prevent hair and debris falling in theatre. To prevent walked-in contamination, street shoes must be covered with over-boots, or special theatre footwear used. If the latter is preferred, these must be cleaned (no need for sterilisation) regularly as contamination will build up over time and lead to unacceptable soiling of the theatre environment. Masks are required in most theatres when sterile instruments are open to prevent droplet contamination. Masks also play a very important role in protecting staff from inadvertent oral contamination.

Clean hands

The importance of hand washing cannot be overemphasised. It is the single most important factor in reducing nosocomial infection. All theatre staff should wash their hands frequently to prevent cross-transfer of bacteria, and wear gloves during patient handling. Before each case, every member of the scrub team should wash their hands and forearms with antibacterial solutions such as povidone-iodine or chlorhexidine. The objective is to reduce the resident bacterial flora present on the hand and upper limb prior to gloving. Guidelines are based on skin surface bacteria counts. There is actually no evidence that the surgical scrub reduces the incidence of postoperative infection. The first scrub of the day should be for five minutes and the rest for three. This should encompass all the hand and forearm to elbow. Care needs to be taken to avoid dripping excess fluid from arms, in particular, the elbows on to the sterile gown as the hand towel is picked up to commence drying. Low-irritant antiseptics (such as triclosan) or normal soap are acceptable alternatives for those with allergies to scrub solutions. A summary of the Australian Confederation of Operating Room Nurses (ACORN) guidelines for the sterile surgical scrub is found in Table 4.2.

Movement of staff

While gowned and gloved, members of the scrub team should keep their movement around the operating theatre to a minimum. All movements should be made with great care to avoid contamination. Contact with non-sterile areas must be avoided. Gloved hands are held against the chest in the 'safe' area as indicated in Figure 4.3 (page 31). Constant concentration is necessary to avoid succumbing to the temptation to scratch an itchy nose or eye, or to touch a non-sterile item such as a light handle. Passing another person should be done 'back-to-back'.

Principle 2: Disinfection of the procedural site

This refers to the process of cleaning, depilating (removing hair) and decontaminating the site of operation. It involves cleaning the surgical site, removing hair and applying disinfectant solution. The objective is to reduce the bacterial population in the vicinity of the surgical site in order to minimise the risk of bacterial contamination of the wound. In spite of virtually universal implementation of preoperative

Table 4.2	Summary of ACORN guidelines for the surgical scrub
Preparation	1. Wear proper attire, cover hair, jewellery off, keep nails short, don mask and plastic apron.
	2. Ensure presence of a sterile scrub sponge and anti-microbial wash solution.
The scrub	1. Time scrub for 5 minutes (first for the day) or 3 minutes (all subsequent scrubs).
	2. Wet arms to elbow under running water.
	3. Wash with 2 mL of solution for 30 seconds with a circular motion, clean the nails then rinse.
	4. Wash again with 2 mL—between fingers up to elbow and rinse
	5. Wash arms with 2 mL and rinse.
	6. Wash hands with 2 mL and rinse.
	7. Keep hands above elbows, turn off water and enter theatre with hands above elbows still.
Pre-gowning	1. Dry hands and arms with a sterile towel—use a quarter for each hand and forearm.
	2. Gown and glove as appropriate.

Source: Australian College of Operating Room Nurses (ACORN) Standards Manual, 2006.

skin preparation, surgical wound infection rates are still as high as 15% for clean wounds and 30% for 'dirty' wounds. A 2004 Cochrane review found that there is insufficient evidence to conclude that cleaning patients' skin with antiseptic before clean surgery reduces wound infections after surgery[1].

Gross cleaning should preferably take place before the patient arrives in the operating theatre. A shower in the ward using chlorhexidine or triclosan reduces the skin bacteria count. Grossly contaminated wounds may be washed with normal saline to remove macroscopic contamination prior to preparation of the surrounding skin. Depilation should be achieved using electric clippers immediately before surgery. Shaving the day before is associated with higher wound infection rates.

Preoperative skin preparation solutions should kill all bacteria, including tubercle bacilli, fungi, spores, viruses and protozoa, and must be safe for patient and staff. The three main antiseptic agents are iodine (either free or bound to surfactants as Iodophor), alcohol and chlorhexidine gluconate. Common preparation solutions include chlorhexidine (0.5%) in alcohol (70%), chlorhexidine (0.5%) and cetrimide (2%), 10% povidone–iodine solution (aqueous or in alcohol), alcoholic iodine solution, and aqueous chlorhexidine (0.5%) (Table 4.3, page 32). Note that cetrimide has very limited antiseptic properties and is used mainly for its detergent action on skin grease.

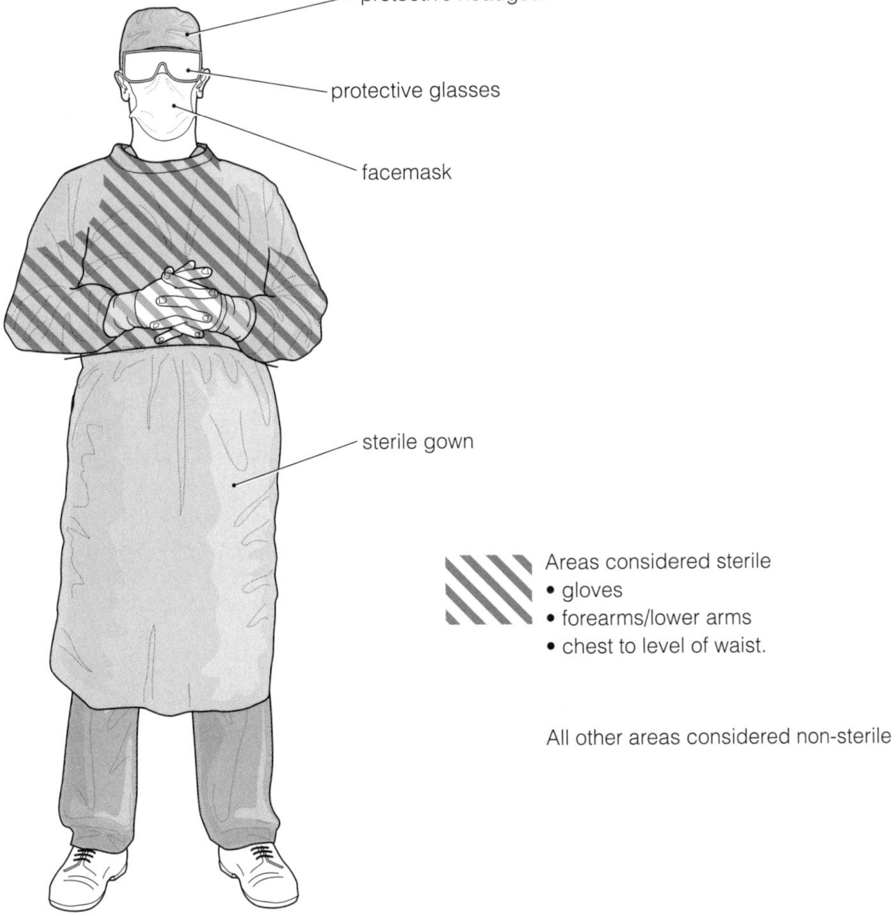

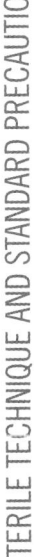

protective headgear

protective glasses

facemask

sterile gown

Areas considered sterile
• gloves
• forearms/lower arms
• chest to level of waist.

All other areas considered non-sterile

Theatre staff member in sterile gown and gloves. Note the protective glasses, some form of which should always be worn.

Fig. 4.3 Sterile areas on scrubbed personnel

All these preparations have some degree of bactericidal action and all but the aqueous chlorhexidine overcome the skin's natural oils to 'stick' to the patient. Alcohol-based preparations are flammable, and several cases of patient burns from skin preparation are reported in Australia and New Zealand each year. All pools of preparation solution should be blotted dry before using diathermy or other surgical energy sources.

Chemical burns may occur if pools of preparation solution remain in prolonged contact with patient's skin. Skin preparation solutions containing alcohol should not be used on mucous membranes, such as in the mouth or vagina, and should not be used on sensitive skin, such as eyelids, scrotum and vulva. Only normal saline should be used to clean or prepare open or infected wounds. Antiseptic solutions have a detrimental effect on tissues other than skin.

Table 4.3 Skin preparation solutions

Name	Contents	Uses	Precautions
Aqueous chlorhexidine	Chlorhexidine gluconate 0.05% w/v	General antiseptic and preoperative skin preparation	Should not contact eye, brain or middle ear Not for injection
Alcoholic chlorhexidine	Chlorhexidine gluconate 0.5% w/v in 70% w/w isopropyl alcohol BP	Hand rinse preoperatively or a preoperative skin preparation	Flammable should not contact mucous membranes or brain, eye and middle ear Not for injection
Chlorhexidine and cetrimide	Chlorhexidine gluconate 0.015% w/v in cetrimide PhEur 0.15% w/v	General antiseptic and preoperative skin preparation May be mixed with aqu. chlorhexidine to reduce cetrimide concentration	As for aqueous chlorhexidine
Povidone–iodine (aqueous)	Povidone–iodine 10%w/v (iodine and polyvinylpyrrolidone complex bound for slow release of iodine)	General preoperative skin preparation	Iodine hypersensitivity Long-term use in thyroid disease and lithium therapy Do not allow to pool on skin (burns) Not for injection
Povidone–iodine (alcohol base)	Povidone–iodine 10%w/v in ethanol	Preoperative skin preparation for keratinised skin only	Do not use on mucous membranes Do not allow to pool anywhere (risk of fire) Allow time for preparation to dry Iodine hypersensitivity Long-term use in thyroid disease and lithium therapy
Alcoholic iodine	Iodine 0.5% in isopropyl alcohol 70%	General preoperative skin preparation	Flammable Iodine hypersensitivity Do not allow to pool on skin (burns) Not for injection

Source: Compilation assisted by information from data sheets contained in Compendium of Data Sheets and Summaries of Product Characteristics, Great Britain: Datapharm Publications Ltd, 1998.

Once gowned and gloved, a member of the scrub team will paint the operative site with the antibacterial solution (prep). This should start at the site of incision and go outwards in circles of ever-increasing diameter. Swabs for prepping should be discarded when dry and new ones used. The old swab should not be re-dipped in the solution. The area prepped should be much wider than required to allow for potential wound extension in unforeseen circumstances (Fig. 4.4).

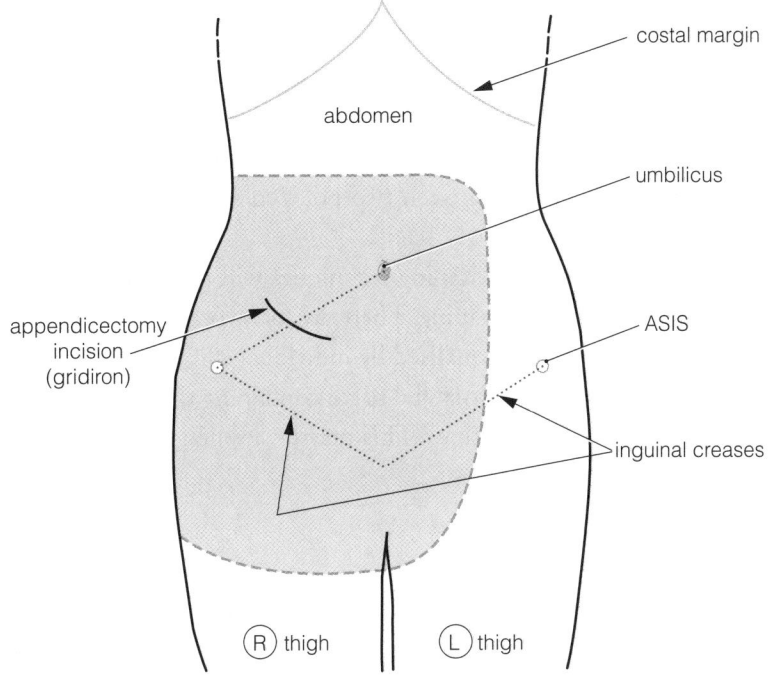

Despite the usually small nature of an appendicectomy incision, a wider area has been prepared in case extension of the incision is required to deal with unexpected findings.

Fig. 4.4 Example of wide skin preparation

Principle 3: Isolation of the procedural site

Barriers are placed between the patient, the clinical team and the environment to prevent direct contamination of the patient from outside and contamination of the outside by the patient.

Draping the procedural site

Exclusion of the operative site with sterile towels or sheets to protect the patient from environmental contamination is called draping. Sterile drapes may be made of cotton, polyester, paper, woven polypropylene or plastic and are held in place by a combination of gravity, friction, clips and adhesives.

Additional site isolation measures are sometimes used, including placement of a sterile or iodophor-impregnated polythene adhesive film over the prepared area, or painting the area with a layer of cyanoacrylate-based paint to create an impervious adherent film on the skin surface. There is no evidence that these methods affect the wound infection rate. Perhaps more importantly, adhesive film does have a role in maintaining the drapes in place throughout the operation.

Drapes should be impervious. If waterproof drapes are not available, a plastic sheet should be placed between the first layer of drapes and the patient to prevent fluid soaking through to the patient below. Saturated drapes break the sterile barrier by allowing diffusion of bacteria from the non-sterile underside.

In general, the whole patient is covered with impervious drapes. Where possible, a raised sterile curtain is placed between two poles to separate the anaesthetist and the surgeon.

Only the two most common draping techniques will be dealt with in this book —square draping and shut-out draping. There are many other techniques specific to specialties, and often further personalised by individual surgeons.

Square draping creates a quadrilateral space containing the operative field within a combination of four or more drapes. This may be applied to the head, trunk and larger diameters of the limbs (Fig. 4.5).

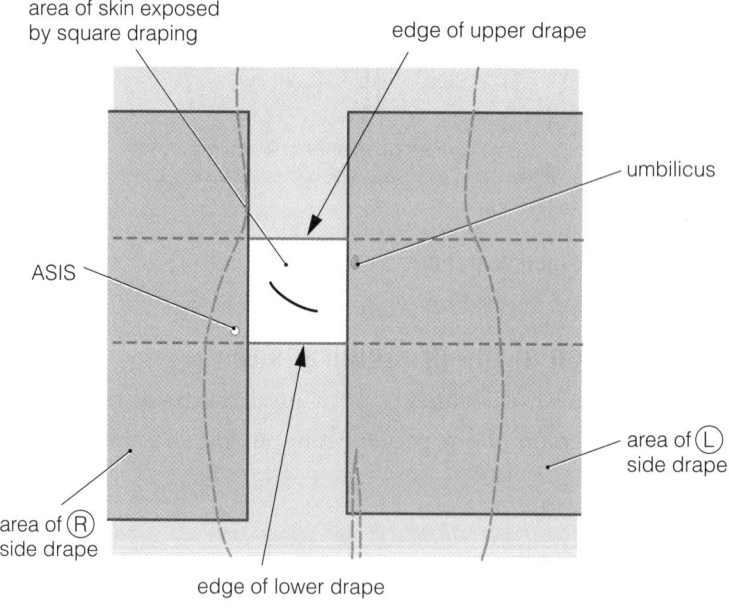

Notice that the drapes expose a wide area but there is still much more prepared skin available (see Fig.4.4).

Fig. 4.5 Square draping for an open appendicectomy

Shut-out draping is used to expose the distal part of a limb and involves a sterile base sheet, full preparation of the distal limb and application of a drape around the proximal limb to shut out the non-sterile segment (Fig. 4.6). A combination of the two methods may be required for the middle segment of a limb.

Once draping is complete, only the top of the trolley and/or the patient is considered to be sterile. Anything that drops below the level of the trolley or patient is assumed to be no longer sterile, and must be allowed to drop to the floor and be discarded.

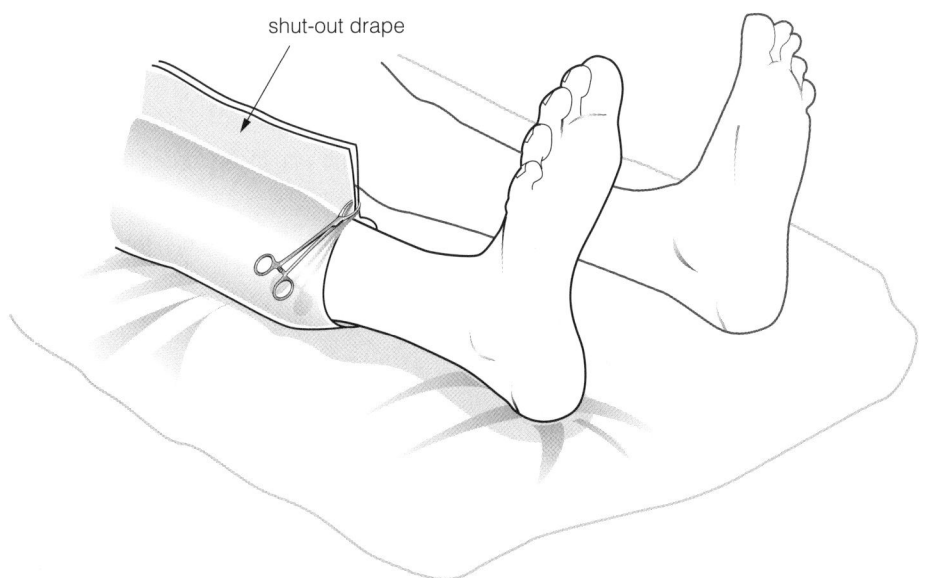

Fig. 4.6 A shut-out drap positioned around the right calf

Gowning and gloving

Gowns and gloves come in contact with the patient but masks, protective eyewear and 'space-suit helmets' do not. The entire surface of every gown and glove is fully sterilised prior to use, although the forearms, hands and chest region are the only parts of the theatre attire that are considered truly sterile (see Fig 4.3). Contact, then, between other parts of the body and the operative field should be avoided as it creates a theoretical break in technique.

A summary of the ACORN guidelines for gowning and gloving is given in Table 4.4 (over), with a visual guide in Figure 4.7 on pages 37 to 38.

Historically, gloves were usually made of natural latex, but modern surgical gloves are more often made from a variety of other materials, including deproteinised latex, neoprene, bonded polyurethane, vinyl and silicone. They come in sizes 5½ to 9, with different patterns and thicknesses to suit individual needs and the type

Table 4.4	Summary of ACORN guidelines for gowning and gloving
Gowning	1. Remove the gown from the sterile field and allow it to fall open in front of you.
	2. Locate the sleeves and work the arms into them.
	3. Keep hands within the sleeves unless the scrub nurse is to put on your gloves.
	4. Allow the back of the gown to be tied.
	5. Once gloved, spin the wrap-around tie, with other sterile personnel, to cover the back of the gown.
Gloving (closed method)	1. Pick up the left glove with the right hand, through the sleeve material.
	2. Place it palm-to-palm and thumb-to-thumb with the upturned left hand.
	3. Grasp the lower fold of the glove, with the left hand, through the sleeve material.
	4. Lift the upper fold of the glove over the open sleeve end.
	5. Slide the hand into the glove.
	6. Repeat on the right hand.
Removing gowns and gloves	1. Undo the wrap-around tie.
	2. Allow the back ties to be undone by other staff.
	3. Pull down the gown and remove it first, bundle it and deposit in the linen skip.
	4. Remove the gloves by grasping the cuffs and turning inside out.
	5. Deposit gloves in contamination disposal bin.

Source: Australian College of Operating Room Nurses (ACORN) Standards Manual, 2006.

of surgery. In the past, gloves were powdered with starch for easy donning. With the awareness that glove powder acts as a vehicle for latex allergens, and increases the risk of adhesions and delayed wound healing, use of powdered gloves is strongly discouraged. 'Washing' powder off gloves is ineffective. Hypoallergenic gloves are available for personnel with allergies to glove material (usually the latex).

Many personnel also choose to double glove for all procedures. A Cochrane Collaboration Review in 2006 concluded that there is no direct evidence that additional glove protection worn by the surgical team reduces surgical site infections in patients[2]. However, the addition of a second pair of surgical gloves significantly reduces perforations to innermost gloves. Wearing inner gloves that contain a perforation indicator dye results in significantly more glove perforations being detected during surgery. Double

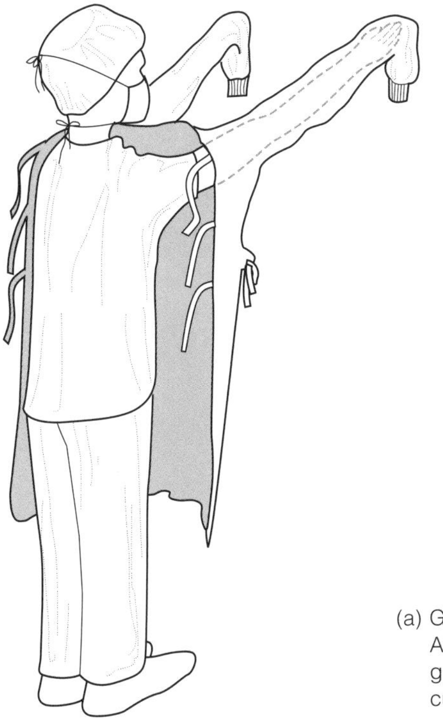

(a) Gowning: Step 1
After drying the hands and forearms the gown is slipped on until the hands are at cuff level.

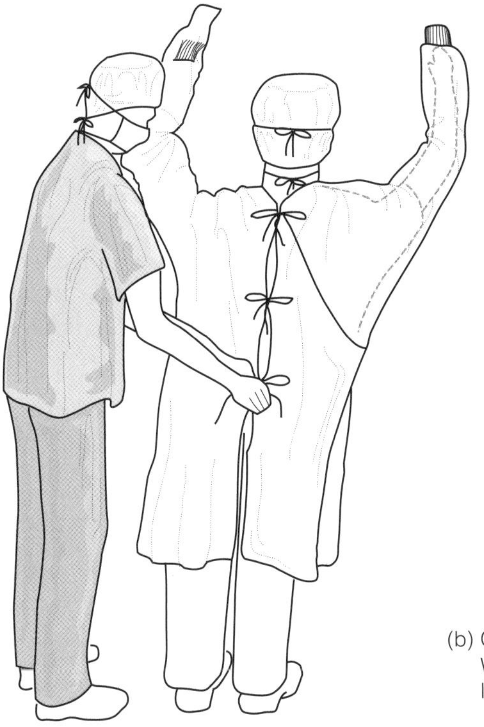

(b) Gowning: Step 2
With the hands still in the sleeves at cuff level the gown is tied.

Fig. 4.7 Gowning and gloving

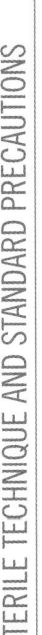

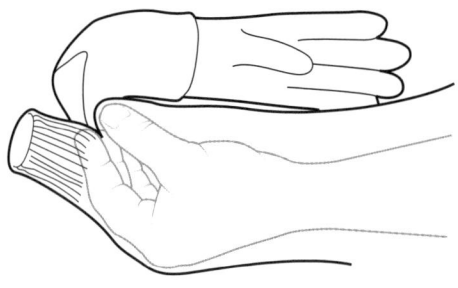

(c) Gloving: Step 1

The glove is laid thumb down on the forearm with the
glove cuff gripped through the gown cuff.

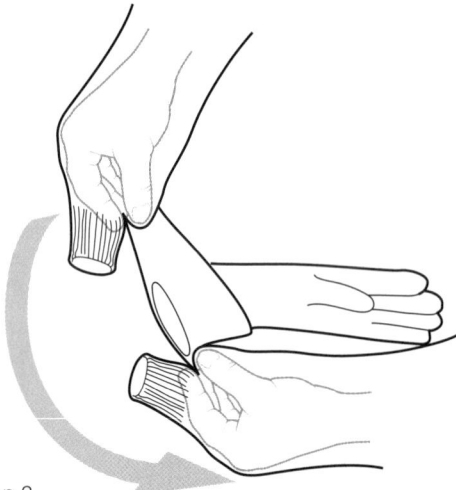

(d) Gloving: Step 2

The uppermost glove cuff is grasped through the cuff on the other arm.
It is lifted over the open cuff end to effectively 'seal' the open cuff.

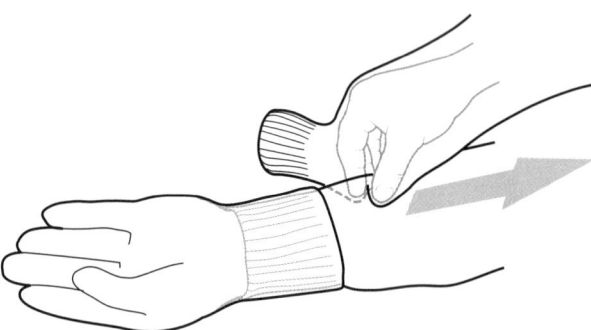

(e) Gloving: Step 3

Once the glove cuff is fully over the gown cuff, the other hand grips both
and the hand slips into the glove against gentle counter-traction. Gloving
is completed by performing the same steps on the other hand.

Fig. 4.7 Gowning and gloving *(cont.)*

gloving may also increase the amount of contaminant blood removed from a solid needle passing through two layers compared with the same needle passing through just one.

Double gloving does not prevent needle-stick injuries in itself, and the potentially reduced sensitivity and increased tightness with double gloves may impair dexterity, mitigating against their protective effect. What double gloving does achieve is to provide a second, impervious protective layer over the skin. If a breach then occurs in the outer glove, and body fluid leaks through it, there is still protection for the skin. Double gloving probably reduces the chance of acquiring a blood-borne infection from glove perforation or needle stick. Irrespective of the type and number of gloves worn, the single most important factor preventing injury is the avoidance of direct handling of sharps.

Non-sterile protective equipment, such as masks and eyewear, should be used during procedures and at times of risk from spills, splashes and airborne hazards. The wide variety of masks available are either simple or incorporate a shield. From a philosophical point of view, the facemask is protection for the surgeon as much as for the patient. Some studies have suggested that certain types of facemask become saturated within minutes and do not prevent droplets from being blown onto the patient. Despite this, the physical presence of a mask prevents contact between the individual's face and mucous membranes, and powder, aerosols or droplets of body fluids. It is important to emphasise that gloves should never be brought anywhere near the mask, as it cannot be considered to be at all sterile.

Eye protection is an equally important barrier for members of the scrub team. This may be as simple as a shield fitted to a mask, non-prescription glasses (with or without side shields), over-glasses to fit over prescription glasses, or even protective frames fitted with prescription lenses.

No-touch technique

This method of operating, used frequently in orthopaedics, involves the use of instruments alone to manipulate and handle tissues, sutures and prostheses. The gloved hand never touches the tissues or any prosthesis inserted into the body. 'No-touch' operating is believed to prevent infections by eliminating the possibility of tissue contact with a glove-borne contamination. Possible sources of this contamination include microscopic breaches in glove material and contact, by the gloves, with the patient's skin or other external source of bacteria. While possible in some specialties, the necessity for tactile impressions and hand dissection makes this technique impractical in others. There is no evidence to suggest that these measures improve patient outcomes in general surgery.

Principle 4: Sterilisation of instruments and equipment

Sterilisation is the process by which all forms of microbial life (viruses, bacteria, spores, fungi and prions) are completely destroyed. Of these, prions and spores (such as *Cl. difficile*) are the most difficult. Disinfection, on the other hand, is a process that destroys most harmful organisms, but only reduces the population of spores or prions, rendering the instrument clean but not sterile.

The level of sterilisation required for equipment, instruments and implants is determined by the intended use. Sterile instruments and equipment are critical for procedures involving open wounds, sterile tissue or the vascular system. In other conditions, such as urinary catheterisation and endoscopic procedures that involve mucous membranes, high level disinfection, rather than sterility, is adequate.

Appropriately sterilised instruments and equipment must be used for every case to prevent the spread of infection. It is essential that all members of theatre staff actively pursue the maintenance of an appropriately clean or sterile environment. Any instrument whose sterility cannot be guaranteed for any reason must be discarded, resterilised or replaced. Single-use items come prepacked and sterile. Before opening, it is important to check that the packaging is intact and the shelf-life expiry date has not been exceeded.

Most reusable instruments are sterilised in a hospital-based, or regional, sterile supply department (SSD). This is usually performed in bulk in a high-pressure, high-temperature steam autoclave. All items should be double wrapped prior to autoclaving to avoid subsequent contamination. Short cycle 'flash' sterilisation is less reliable and should be reserved for unwrapped items that must be used immediately. It is mandatory that all sterilisation processes, whether in hospitals or consulting rooms, have quality control documentation and use chemical and biological indicator strips to confirm efficacy.

Methods of sterilisation

The first important step in the sterilisation process is always the macroscopic removal of debris, protein and salts from the surface of the instrument. This is carried out manually, with the assistance of enzymatic agents and ultrasonic cleaning machines. After cleaning, the item is double wrapped for sterilisation.

Sterilisation can be achieved by steam, dry heat, chemical processes or radiation (Table 4.5, pages 42–3). Each method has its own applications. Steam can be used for all wrapped articles (including gowns and drapes) and unwrapped instruments, but cannot be used for paper, inks, oils and heat-sensitive items. Dry heat can only be used on anhydrous items that can withstand 160 °C for at least one hour. Chemical methods, such as ethylene oxide, peracetic acid, ortho-phthaldehyde and glutaraldehyde, can be used for items that cannot tolerate steam or dry methods.

Use of glutaraldehyde has been largely discontinued due to staff hypersensitivity issues, particularly skin and respiratory. Ionising radiation is used industrially by manufacturers to sterilise certain medical devices, equipment and supplies.

Steam sterilisation

Steam is used for the sterilisation of most surgical equipment. The underlying principle of this method is that all micro-organisms can be destroyed if their intracellular enzyme and protein systems are denatured and coagulated. Steam, especially when present without other gases, will permeate the packaging of supplies and come into contact with the micro-organisms present. Water catalyses these processes and, as the steam condenses to liquid water on the organisms, latent heat is released, fuelling the denaturation and coagulation process. Even spores are destroyed by steam.

At atmospheric pressure, steam exists at a temperature of 100 °C. At this temperature, steam sterilisation is a very slow process. Higher temperatures decrease the time taken for sterilisation, but to achieve this, the pressure must be increased. Air acts as a barrier to water molecules, and removing air from the chamber allows a greater increase in temperature.

Three types of steam steriliser are in common use. The traditional autoclave pumps steam into a sealed chamber. The lighter water vapour displaces the heavier air from the chamber, and prevents its mixing with the steam (gravity displacement method). The temperature and pressure are increased by the continued addition of steam to the sealed chamber. The steam cycle typically maintains 121 °C at 103 kPa for at least 15 minutes. Steam is then exhausted and a drying cycle is completed. All steam and temperature stable material can be processed in an autoclave.

Flash (high-speed) sterilisers are usually gravity displacement in type and are set at 186 kPa and 134 °C. Due to the high temperature and pressure, the cycle lasts only for 3–10 minutes. Flash units can be used for most items except implantable prostheses, as the reliability of sterilisation may be somewhat reduced due to the speed of the cycle. In most theatre suites, urgently required instruments that are not sterile are the only items to be flash sterilised.

Pre-vacuum, high-temperature sterilisers are much faster for routine sterilisation. The air is removed by a pump prior to steam injection into the unit. This means rapid heating occurs and sterilisation time is reduced. Filtered hot air is pumped in at the end of the cycle to dry the contents. In all, this may take as little as 12 minutes to complete.

Dry heat sterilisation

Dry heat sterilisers work on the principle that mechanical convection of dry, hot air at temperatures of around 160 °C can destroy micro-organisms. The cycle

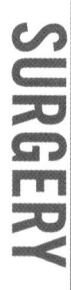

Table 4.5 Summary of common sterilisation methods

Method	Description	Main application	Precautions
Steam—autoclave	Air elimination by downward displacement Pressure and temperature dictate cycle Drying component of cycle	Preferred method for all items that are not temperature or steam sensitive	Pressure vessel precautions, training required Burns risk
Steam—flash	Air elimination by downward displacement High pressure and temperature (27 psi, 134 °C) Fast cycle (3 min)	Emergency resterilisation of dropped instruments	As for 'autoclave' Items should not be wrapped because of unreliable drying Does not destroy prions
Steam—vacuum	Rapid air elimination by vacuum extraction Rapid heating to pressure and temperature Drying cycle Speed intermediate between autoclave and flash	As for 'autoclave'	As for 'autoclave'
Dry heat	Fan-forced hot air Long cycle with heating, sterilising (160 °C for 60 min) and cooling stages	For anhydrous, steam sensitive but heat resistant articles	Burns risk
Chemical—gas	Ethylene oxide–CO_2 mixture with > 400 mg ethylene oxide per litre, at between 36 and 60 °C and 40–100% humidity Shorter cycle times with higher temperatures and gas concentrations (3–7 h)	Temperature and steam sensitive articles, prostheses and devices	Major risk of toxicity and flammability of gas requiring environmental monitoring (< 0.5 ppm) Plastic corrosion

Chemical—liquid	Peracetic acid 0.2% solution	Endoscopes, anaesthesia equipment	Minimal toxicity. Damages aluminium anodised Coatings
Chemical—liquid	Ortho-phthaldehyde (OPA) 0.5% solution. Glutaraldehyde 2% solution (now largely discontinued)	Endoscopes, anaesthesia equipment	Patient toxicity with inadequate rinsing. Staff hypersensitivity—respiratory and skin reactions
Chemical—plasma	Vaporised hydrogen peroxide in a vacuum, which is ionised by a radiofrequency field	Most items except paper, linen and liquids. Limited by small chamber size	No toxic effects known. Synthetic packaging required

STERILE TECHNIQUE AND STANDARD PRECAUTIONS

CHAPTER 4

must be maintained for one hour at that temperature with extra time required for heating and cooling. Only anhydrous items that cannot be steam sterilised require this method.

Chemical sterilisation

The use of chemical sterilisation techniques at low temperatures is a viable alternative to heat-based sterilisation. Gas, liquid and plasma media are in routine use.

Gas sterilisation with ethylene oxide takes place at 54–60 °C. Carbon dioxide is added to reduce the risk of ignition. Sterilisation requires the presence of some water and is thought to occur by alkylation of cell constituents and prevention of cell replication. Ethylene oxide penetrates most materials, is broadly active, non-corrosive, and does not require heat or pressure. However, it is expensive, highly flammable, severely toxic, may be retained in tubular equipment (e.g. tubing) and may damage some plastics. This method should not be used on items that can be steam sterilised.

A number of liquid solutions offer effective sterilisation. Currently, peracetic acid 0.2% and ortho-phthaldehyde (OPA) 0.5% are the most commonly used. Earlier systems used a solution of 2% glutaraldehyde, but this frequently caused skin and respiratory reactions in staff, and its use has largely been discontinued.

Peracetic acid is the safest, with no toxicity and environmentally friendly by-products (acetic acid, oxygen and water). Its main disadvantage is that it can cause oxidative damage to some materials, shortening the life of sensitive instruments such as endoscopes. It requires a 30–45 minute cycle, and can only process a small number of instruments (e.g. one endoscope) in a cycle.

Orthophthaldehyde is a derivative of glutaraldehyde but rather less toxic. It can process a higher volume of instruments in a 20 minute cycle without significant material damage. Copious irrigation is required to ensure removal of all toxic chemicals at the end of the cycle.

Plasma sterilisation utilises a low-temperature hydrogen peroxide plasma. The sterilising chamber is evacuated. Hydrogen peroxide liquid is introduced, vaporised and then ionised by a magnetic or radiofrequency field. The reactive cloud of ions, electrons and neutral particles then collides with and destroys, micro-organisms.

Plasma sterilisation requires a cycle time of 28–52 minutes and the small chamber limits the number of instruments that can be processed. It cannot be used for devices with small internal luminal diameters, liquids or materials such as paper and linen. Synthetic (polypropylene) wraps are required.

It is very effective against all viruses, bacteria, fungi and spores. There is also no toxicity, as the ions recombine as oxygen and water. This method may eventually supersede steam sterilisation.

STANDARD PRECAUTIONS

This section deals with protection of the operating theatre staff from the hazards present in the operating theatre, particularly with the prevention of contamination from patients with infectious diseases.

All patients are potentially infectious, and it must always be considered that there is a risk of spreading infectious organisms from the patient to members of the theatre team. Surgeons are particularly vulnerable to contamination from body fluids, and precautions should always be taken.

Standard precautions are a set of guidelines designed to reduce the chance of contamination. Although the likelihood of contamination of unbroken skin or intact mucosal surfaces leading to infection from the contamination is very small, the accumulated risk over a long operating life is high. Standard precautions cover eye protection, mouth protection and skin protection, including the use of gloves and problems associated with gloves. They also cover rules of conduct in the operating theatre such as how to transfer sharp instruments, and how to handle and dispose of sharp needles.

Eye protection

It is very easy for fluids of all types to splash into the eyes during surgical procedures. This becomes very obvious when protective eyewear is worn and then inspected after a long case. There are always many obvious marks on the eyewear that could well have gone in to the eyes had the protection not been in place.

For those with normal vision there are now a number of types of disposable and non-disposable eyewear available that provide protection. Those surgeons requiring glasses when operating will need to decide whether their glasses provide enough protection particularly from the side, as most prescription glasses do not have wrap-around lenses.

Mouth protection

The mucous membranes of the mouth and nose can provide a portal of entry for contamination. In the past a face mask was worn to protect the patient from contamination from the surgeon and there has been a great deal of debate as to whether this was of any benefit. However we now have an additional reason to cover our mouth and nose as a protection from the patient as well as for the patient. The usual precautions concerning the regular changing of masks and the inadvisability of wearing a mask down around the neck still apply.

Skin protection

The types and manufacture of gloves are dealt with earlier. If all the skin surfaces of an operator are intact there is little or no chance of contaminants entering the body. It is however very difficult to ensure that all skin surfaces are intact, so the routine wearing of skin protection by way of gloves is a very wise one and a practice that is used in the majority of situations where there is possible exposure to patient body fluids.

Another important skin protection strategy is to avoid the chance of being wounded with 'sharps' such as scalpels, needles, bone, or any other sharp instrument or object that has been contaminated during the procedure. Correct handling and disposal of sharps is of critical importance during surgical procedures. Protocols should be in place for transfer of instruments between staff members but important aspects to remember include the following:

- Scalpels and needles should never be passed directly from person to person on the surgical team. They should be stored and transferred on a tray or dish that is colour coded for the purpose.
- Sharps should be disposed of in a secure sharps receptacle when they are no longer required.
- Needles should not be held in the fingers. Always hold and manipulate suture needles with appropriate thumb-forceps (preferably with a tungsten needle platform).
- Ideally, hypodermic needles should not be removed from syringes. When absolutely necessary, they should be removed by holding in forceps or using the dedicated slots on sharps containers. Hypodermic needles should never be re-capped.

Medical waste management

The disposal of waste from the operating theatre after an operation, although not the direct responsibility of the surgeon, is of such importance and involves the surgeon to such a degree that it is imperative to understand the principles involved. Most operating theatres have different coloured containers for the different categories of waste, such as clinical or contaminated waste, general waste and recyclable waste. It is essential that the defined segregation is adhered to, as outside agencies monitor the waste and heavy penalties are applied if breaches are detected. Each surgeon must understand the disposal regime and adhere to it.

CONCLUSIONS

Sterile technique is the basis for the operative field. Creation and maintenance of this field is one of the skills that must be developed as part of broader surgical training. Intra-operatively, the responsibility for maintaining the field lies with all members of the scrub team. Standard precautions protect all the staff from the risk of contracting an infectious disease from the patient.

An understanding of all the concepts contained in this chapter, including sterilisation procedures, is also essential for the success of the practitioner undertaking any minor surgical procedures.

REFERENCES

1. Edwards PS, Lipp A, Holmes A. Preoperative skin antiseptics for preventing surgical wound infections after clean surgery. Cochrane Database of Systematic Reviews 2004, Issue 4. Art. No.: CD003949.pub2. DOI: 10.1002/14651858.CD003949.pub2.
2. Tanner J, Parkinson H. Double gloving to reduce surgical cross-infection. Cochrane Database of Systematic Reviews 2006, Issue 3. Art. No.: CD003087. DOI: 10.1002/14651858. CD003087.pub2.

FURTHER READING

Australian College of Operating Room Nurses. 2006 ACORN Standards for Perioperative Nursing. ACORN Pty Ltd, 2006.

Mangram A, Horan T, Pearson M, Silver L, Jarvis W. Guidelines for Prevention of Surgical Site Infection. Infection Control and Hospital Epidemiology 1999;20(4):247–78.

Standards Association of Australia. AS/NZS 4187: Cleaning, disinfecting and sterilizing reusable medical and surgical instruments and equipment, and maintenance of associated environments in health care facilities. Sydney: Standards Association of Australia, 2003.

CHAPTER FIVE
SURGICAL INSTRUMENTS

Call that a knife? This *is a knife!*

John Cornell and Paul Hogan, *Crocodile Dundee*

INTRODUCTION

The aim of this chapter is to provide an easily understood classification of surgical instruments, a visual guide to some basic instruments and a description of their common uses. After reading this chapter, you should have a basic understanding of common surgical instruments, and know how to select an appropriate instrument, use it, and care for it correctly and safely.

CARE OF INSTRUMENTS

Surgical instruments are precision pieces of equipment that should be treated with care and respect. Instruments should be stored and transported in such a manner that they do not damage each other. They should be cleaned with appropriate agents and methods, taking particular care of moving parts and hinges, sharp edges and serrations. Special attention is required where bone, tissue or blood can sequester. At the same time, their function should be checked, and any faults repaired before use. While these responsibilities usually fall primarily on the operating room nursing and technical staff, it is important that the surgeon maintains some oversight of the management of instruments that are fundamental to the surgical profession. The surgeon should know the specific purpose for which every instrument is designed. In some situations, a number of different instruments could be used to perform the same task. Whenever possible, it is important to select the best instrument available for the job. Using a large instrument to perform a delicate task is more likely to result in unintended tissue damage. Conversely, using a fine instrument for a coarse task is likely to result in damage to the instrument. The surgeon has a key responsibility for correct use of an instrument. He or she should avoid using an instrument inappropriately or in a manner that could result in its damage. Damaged instruments do not work reliably. They slow down an operation and cause frustration. Their use risks unintended tissue damage and increases the risk of complications.

ERGONOMICS AND HANDLING INSTRUMENTS

Some general principles apply to the handling of surgical instruments. The surgeon should maintain a comfortable posture throughout a procedure, without tension in any muscle group. Head and neck should be in a neutral position, avoiding uncomfortable bending or twisting. Patient positioning, optimal placement of assistants and retractors, sitting down when possible, use of a foot stool and use of a wrist or elbow rest can contribute to reducing fatigue and optimising surgical performance. It is usually better to move from one side of the operating table to the other rather than work at an awkward or uncomfortable angle. The flexors and extensors of the fingers have their maximum efficiency when the wrist is straight (watch any good musician!). These fine quick-twitch muscles, together with the intrinsic muscles of the hand, are the primary muscles used to manipulate instruments. The coarser, slower-twitch muscles of the arm and shoulder should be kept relaxed (e.g. elbow by the side) whenever possible. Prolonged active arm abduction is not only tiring but impairs fine motor movement at the finger tips. Ergonomics in surgery is discussed in detail in Chapter 8.

CLASSIFICATION OF SURGICAL INSTRUMENTS

Surgical instruments are tools to facilitate four basic functions:
- cutting
- grasping
- clamping
- exposing.

Nomenclature for surgical instruments is inconsistent and eponyms abound. Unfortunately different centres and manufacturers often use different names for the same instrument. This may lead to a long and fruitless search in theatre for an item when an acceptable 'generic' alternative is already present in the instrument set-up.

In this book, generic names have been used whenever possible, but common eponyms are also given as they can be useful in identifying a specific instrument (see Table 5.1, page 94–6). In each subsection, representative examples of instruments are illustrated.

Most instrument catalogues list many thousands of instruments. This chapter is not an instrument catalogue. In deciding which instruments to present, the most commonly used instruments were selected to illustrate the basic principles of surgical instrumentation.

CUTTING INSTRUMENTS

The instruments used for cutting tissues can be divided into three groups:
1. scalpels
2. scissors
3. other cutting instruments.

Scalpels

The scalpel is the surgeon's oldest and most basic tool. In the mid-20th century, a disposable blade mounted on a reusable handle replaced the single piece knife that required regular sharpening. The scalpel is used for the deliberate and precise division of structures with the minimum trauma to surrounding tissue. The blade is always sharp (it should be replaced whenever it seems blunt). Scalpels can be used to incise skin, connective tissue, muscle, cartilage and viscera. They should not be used on metal or bone.

Scalpel handles

The two most common handles are the Bard Parker style sizes 3 and 4. The numbers refer to the size of the attachment point for the blade as well as handle dimensions. Standard handles are straight and flat (Fig. 5.1), but long, curved and octagonal profile handles are available for special situations.

Scalpel blades

Blades come in various sizes and shapes designated by a number. The larger ones are used for long incisions in thick skin (e.g. on the trunk), while the smaller and finer blades are used for small, thin skin incisions, dissecting viscera or incising vessels (Figs. 5.2 and 5.3). Special blades are also available for specific areas such as ophthalmology and microsurgery.

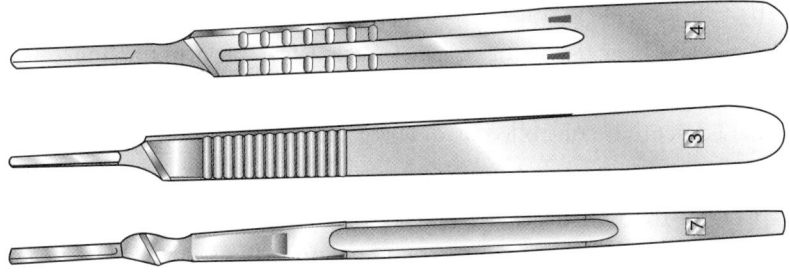

Note the different size heads for attaching the blades to.

Fig. 5.1 Scalpel handles, sizes 3, 4 and 7

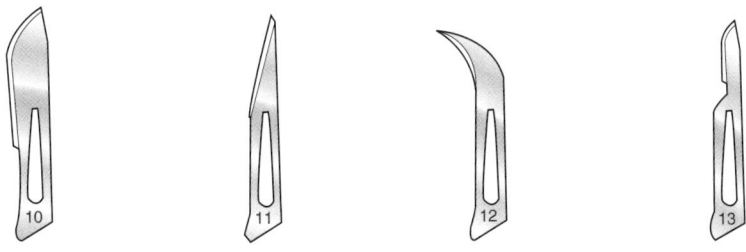

Small scapel blades for fine work are used on a size 3 or 7 handle. Note the hooked 12 blade which can also be used by hand and is designed as a stitch cutter.

Fig. 5.2 Small scalpel blades

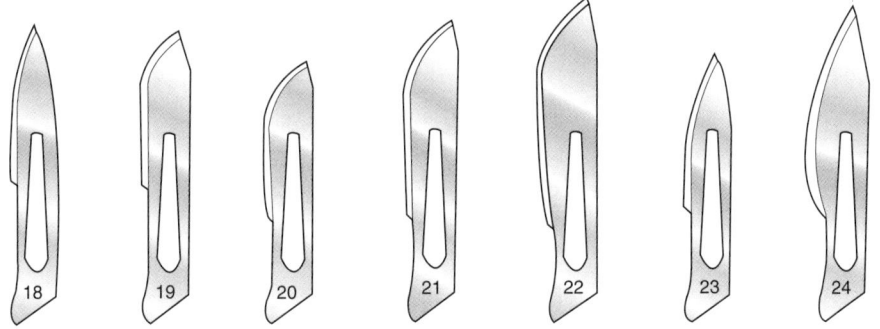

These larger blades are used for major incisions on a size 4 scalpel handle.

Fig. 5.3 Large scalpel blades

Using a scalpel

The scalpel should be held with the index finger along the dorsum of the blade. The preferred grip uses the thumb along one side of the handle, apposed to the last three fingers on the other side (Fig. 5.4a). This hold allows optimum dexterity with free movement of wrist and fingers. Alternative holds include the 'carving knife'

(Fig. 5.4b), which can be useful when cutting through thick, tough tissue, or the 'pencil' (Fig. 5.4c), which can be useful for very fine work. With this grip the surgeon's wrist can be placed against the patient, an instrument or another hand to steady the blade while cutting. Incised depth is controlled by drawing the blade smoothly over the tissues with a constant, firm, downward pressure being exerted on the blade by the forearm.

The whole length of the blade, not just the tip, should be employed in cutting (Fig. 5.5). Skin should be incised perpendicularly to ensure the minimum surface area of incised edge. For long skin incisions, such as in a laparotomy, a large handle and blade (e.g. size 4 handle and #22 blade) are employed. For smaller incisions or fine dissection work, such as excising small lesions or dirty wound edges, a small handle and blade (e.g. size 3 handle and #10 or #15 blade) should be used.

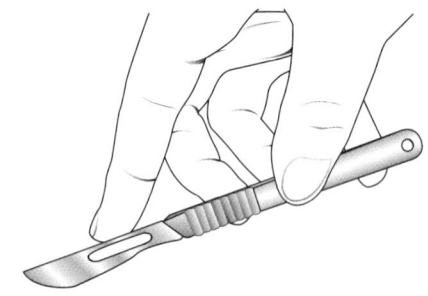

(a) Holding a scalpel handle for optimum control and dexterity.

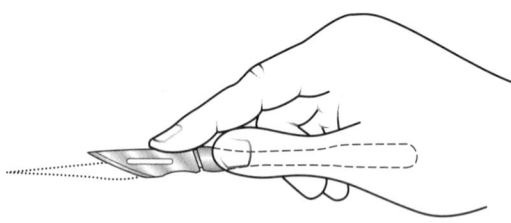

(b) The carving knife or underhand grip, used for long incisions.

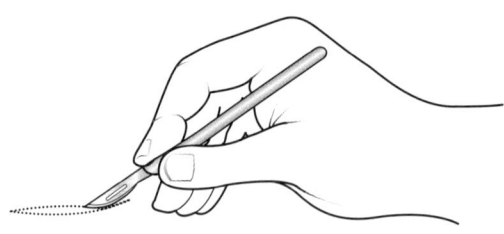

(c) The pencil grip is used for fine incisions or excisions and for dissection with the scalpel.

Fig. 5.4 Holding a scalpel

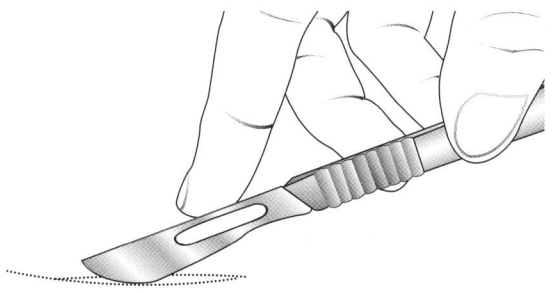

Fig. 5.5 Using the whole length of the blade

The scalpel is traditionally used for incising mesothelium, such as peritoneum or pleura, while it is tented between two artery forceps. The rationale is that a light touch with the scalpel will make a tiny hole, allow air into the cavity and so allow viscera or lung to drop away from the parietal surface. Using scissors, on the other hand, risks cutting subjacent structures.

The ease of cutting with a scalpel is one of its great dangers. Inappropriate assessment of a situation may lead to the incision or division of a vital structure (e.g. a peripheral nerve). Some simple rules will minimise this risk.

1. Do not cut anything that is not clearly in view.
2. If the tissue to be divided is adjacent to a vital structure, insert an instrument or cutting guide between the tissue and that structure.
3. When dissecting near a known vital structure (e.g. nerve or vessel) cut parallel to or in the line of the structure to prevent dividing it accidentally.
4. Plan (and mark) your incisions and practise the cut in the air first.
5. Support your wrist to prevent 'overshoot' cutting too deeply.

In principle, time spent improving the access and exposure equates to time saved repairing an error and reduces risk of complications such as occult bowel perforation. 'Cut once and cut well': a well-executed clean incision is easier to close and effects a better repair that one made by a rabid dog.

Scissors

Scissors employ a pair of sharp parallel blades hinged to allow them to shear over each other in close apposition, severing tissue between the blades. Most scissors have a 'right-handed' construction, so that when held in the right hand, the blade held in the fingers is on the palmar side of that held by the thumb. This mechanic is important, because torque on the hinge created by flexion of the fingers in opposition to the thumb results in the blades being forced more firmly together for a 'cleaner' cut. To grip a pair of scissors properly, the tip of the thumb is inserted into the upper ring and the tip of the ring finger is inserted into the lower ring. The middle finger supports one shaft of the instrument, with the index finger positioned on or near the hinge to steady it. Gentle torque pressure on the hinge keeps the cutting edges closely applied to each other (Fig. 5.6). When the scissors are held in the left hand, the natural torque on the blades applied by inexperienced fingers drives the blades apart, and tissue can pass between them uncut. Therefore the reverse torque action must be applied by drawing the thumb towards the palm while the ring finger maintains extension pressure to push its blade away from the palm (Fig. 5.7).

Optimum manoeuvrability of the scissors is obtained when the wrist is held straight, so that the scissors function as an extension of the forearm. When dissecting scissors are held correctly, the curve of the tip is in line with the forearm and extended index finger (Fig. 5.8).

When using fine scissors, the wrist should be braced for improved accuracy of dissection. This practice is also useful when cutting sutures whereby the scissor hand is rested on the other hand (Fig. 5.9).

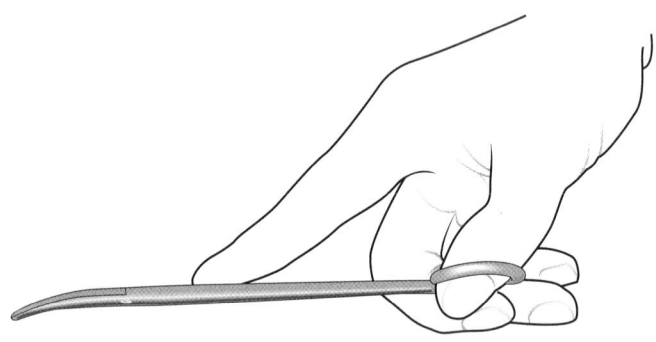

Holding a pair of dissecting scissors.

Fig. 5.6 Holding scissors with right hand

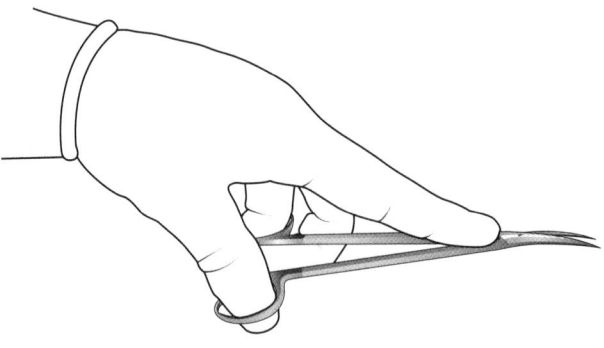

Fig. 5.7 Applying torque while holding scissors with left hand

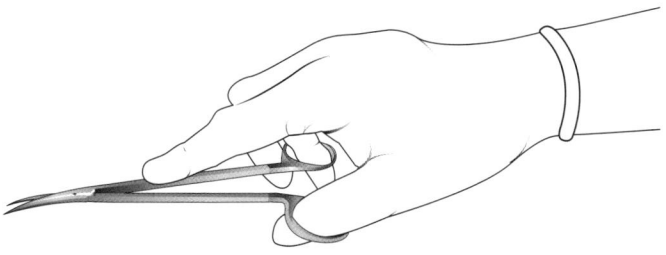

Fig. 5.8 Holding scissors in line of forearm

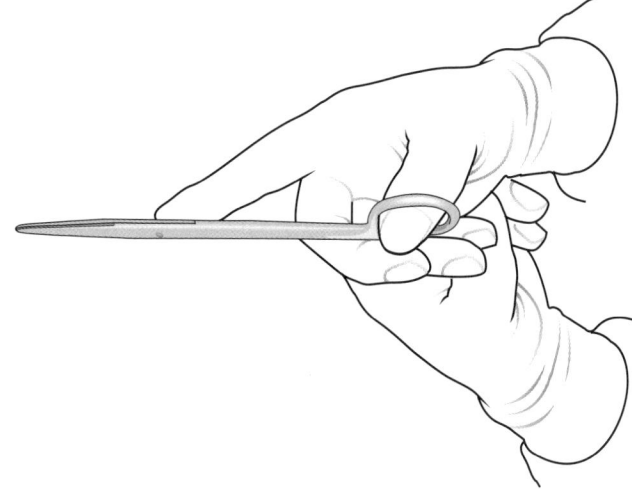

Fig. 5.9 Supporting scissors by bracing the scissor-holding hand against the other hand for stability

Scissors will not function properly if the blades do not meet accurately to shear through the tissue. This may occur if:

- an incorrect torsion is applied to the blades (e.g. novice using left hand)
- an incorrect weight of scissor is selected for the bulk of tissue
- the scissors' hinge is loose or damaged
- the scissors' edges are blunt or burred.

Poor scissors function will result in tissue being torn and crushed by the 'chewing' action of jamming tissue between the flat surfaces of the blades. This frequently leads to unexpected tearing of adjacent tissues and bleeding, and is fundamentally incompatible with good surgical technique.

When not being used, the scissors may be swung on the ring finger to face back along the forearm. They are held in place by the little finger thereby leaving the thumb, index and middle free to manipulate threads, instruments or other structures (Fig. 5.10).

STERILE INSTRUMENTS   CHAPTER 5

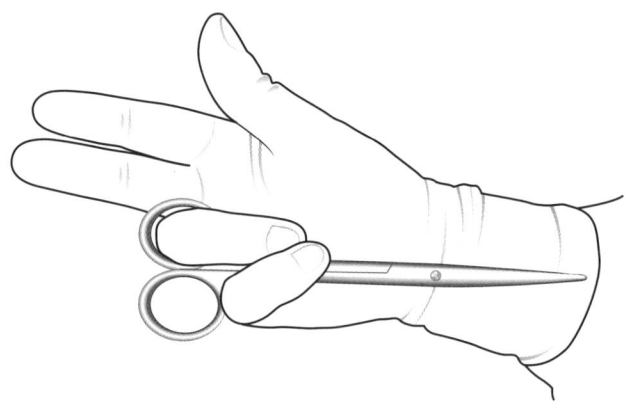

This hold frees up the thumb, index and middle fingers for other functions.

Fig. 5.10 Palming scissors

Scissors are used to cut and dissect tissues. Basic variations include sharp-pointed and blunt-ended scissors, straight, angled or curved blades, long or short bodies, and light, medium or heavy gauge material. Each variant has its own particular use. Curved scissors are ideal for dissection and division of tissues. Curved blunt-tipped scissors are used to dissect by inserting the tips into a plane and spreading tissues apart by opening the blades, or by sliding the slightly opened blades along the line of tissue fibres. For most surgeons, scissors 160–180 mm long are the most ergonomic and comfortable, but longer or shorter models are necessary for dissecting fine superficial structures or dissecting down in deep body cavities such as the pelvis or thorax. Sharp-pointed or angled scissors are often used for precision work such as opening small blood vessels or for fine dissection. Heavier angled scissors are used to cut sutures. In general, straight scissors are not recommended for cutting living tissue and are usually reserved for cutting dressings.

Dissecting scissors

Curved, blunt-tipped dissecting scissors are the most commonly used scissors in general surgery (Figs 5.11 to 5.13). Finer patterns, such as Metzenbaum or McIndoe scissors, in long or short, or the long Nelson scissors are some of the most commonly used scissors for basic dissection of soft tissues and intra-abdominal structures (e.g. adhesion division or bowel mobilisation). These invariably have curved blades. The heavier curved dissecting scissors, such as Mayo scissors in the short variety and the longer Dubois or Goligher scissors, may be used in similar instances to those mentioned above. They come into their own, however, when cutting through thick fascia (e.g. joint capsule, ligaments, rectus sheath) or when dissecting deep in the pelvis.

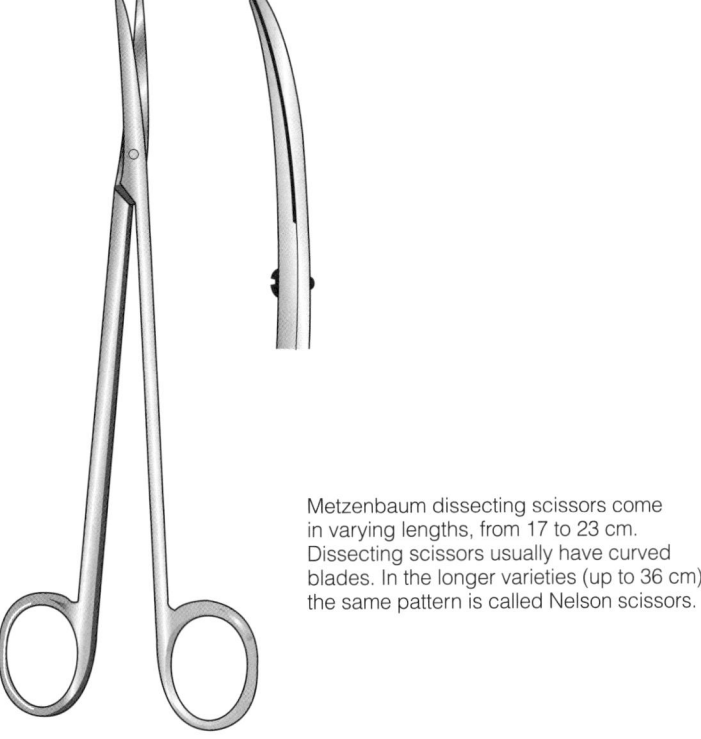

Metzenbaum dissecting scissors come in varying lengths, from 17 to 23 cm. Dissecting scissors usually have curved blades. In the longer varieties (up to 36 cm) the same pattern is called Nelson scissors.

Fig. 5.11 Metzenbaum dissecting scissors

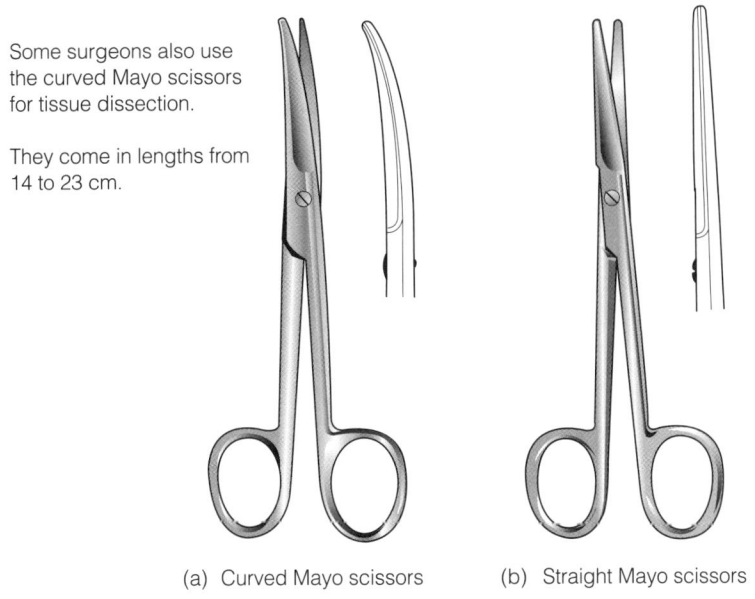

Some surgeons also use the curved Mayo scissors for tissue dissection.

They come in lengths from 14 to 23 cm.

(a) Curved Mayo scissors   (b) Straight Mayo scissors

Fig. 5.12 Mayo scissors

Suture scissors

Angled or curved medium-weight scissors, such as Ferguson angled (Fig. 5.13) or curved Mayo scissors (Fig 5.12a), are best for cutting sutures. Straight Mayo scissors, nurses scissors or other straight-bladed scissors are also acceptable. Fine, expensive dissecting scissors will become blunt or burred if used to cut sutures.

Dressing and general purpose scissors

Straight-bladed Mayo scissors (Fig. 5.12) are popular for cutting dressings, stomal appliances, mesh or other materials but any heavy, straight-bladed, non-dissecting scissor is acceptable. Nurses scissors, with one sharp pointed blade and one rounded blade are also designed for cutting dressings (Fig. 5.14).

Vascular scissors

Vascular scissors differ from dissecting scissors in having sharp pointed blades angled at anything up to 110° from the handles. The most common vascular scissors are Pott angled scissors, which are used exclusively to open blood vessels (Fig. 5.15).

Other cutting instruments

There are several other cutting instruments that are used for special purposes.

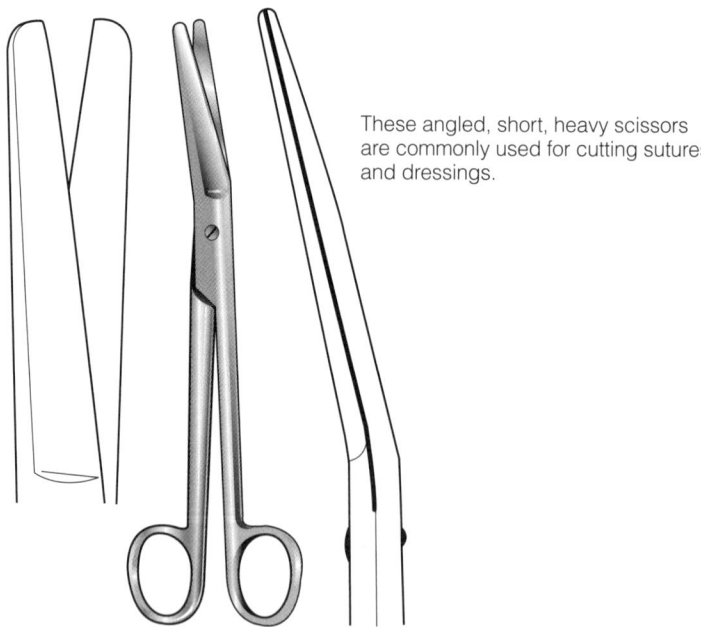

These angled, short, heavy scissors are commonly used for cutting sutures and dressings.

Fig. 5.13 Ferguson scissors

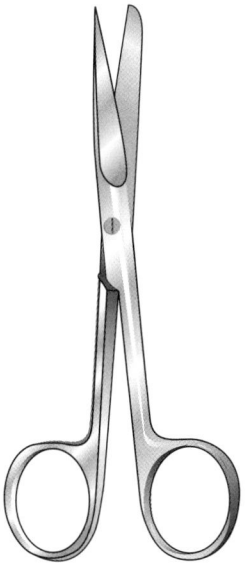

Fig. 5.14 Nurses surgical scissors

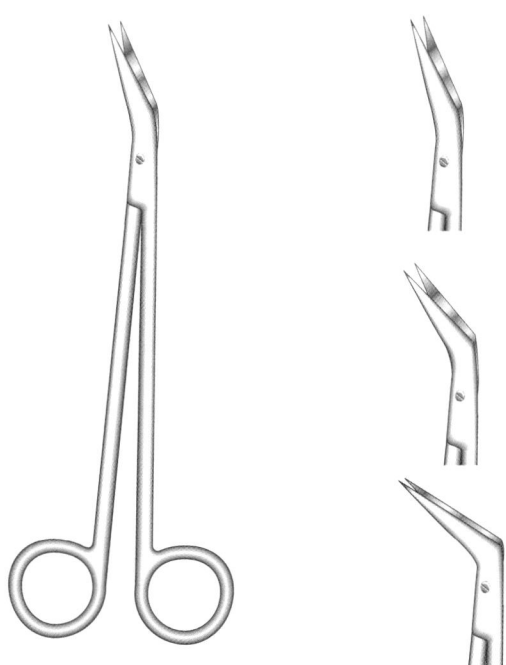

Pott angled vascular scissors, with three differently angled blades. They are used for precision opening of blood vessels for surgery. The differently angled blades are used to reach vessels in deep or awkward positions.

Fig. 5.15 Pott scissors

Skin graft knife

This instrument has several variations in size, shape and complexity, ranging from a small knife utilising a single-edged razor blade to a large electric skin graft harvester (dermatome). Skin graft knives are designed for harvesting flat sheets of skin with a uniform thickness containing the epidermis and part of the dermis. This leaves the lower dermis, with its epidermal lined structures such as hair follicles, to heal by regenerating protective epidermis over its reduced thickness.

The illustrated instrument (Fig. 5.16) bears the eponymous title of the Watson modification of the Humby knife. A long razor blade is inserted over the three lugs. Knobs on the end of the roller allow adjustment of the aperture between blade and roller to control the thickness of skin harvested. The skin is first lubricated and then flattened and stretched tightly between two small boards held by an assistant. The split skin is cut with a gentle sawing motion of the blade held at an acute angle to the skin.

The smaller silver knife is useful for small grafts. An excellent dissertation on skin grafting can be found in McGregor's book *Fundamental Techniques of Plastic Surgery*.

Bone cutters and nibblers

These instruments are used in any situation requiring resection or trimming of bone. They are shaped like scissors and have either heavy scissor-like blades (cutters) (Fig. 5.17) or a pair of scalloped cups (nibblers) (Fig. 5.18).

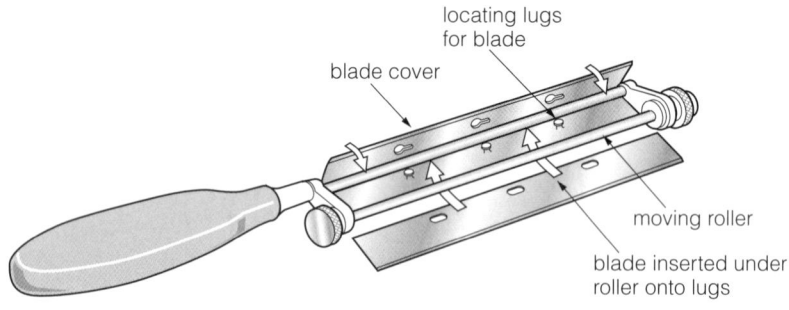

(a) Watson modification of the Humby kife

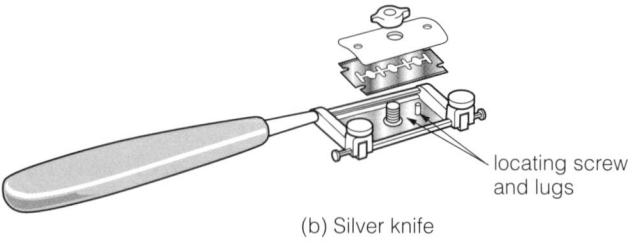

(b) Silver knife

Fig. 5.16 Skin graft knives (left-handed versions shown)

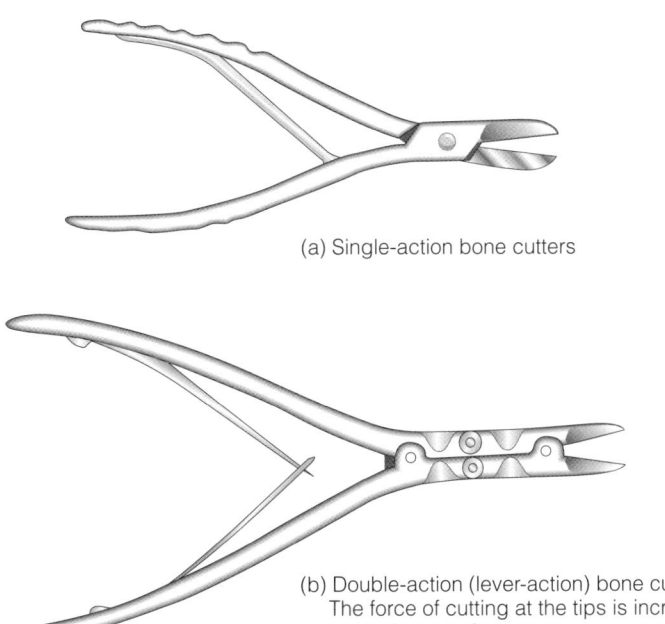

(a) Single-action bone cutters

(b) Double-action (lever-action) bone cutters
The force of cutting at the tips is increased
by the lever action.

Fig. 5.17 Bone cutters

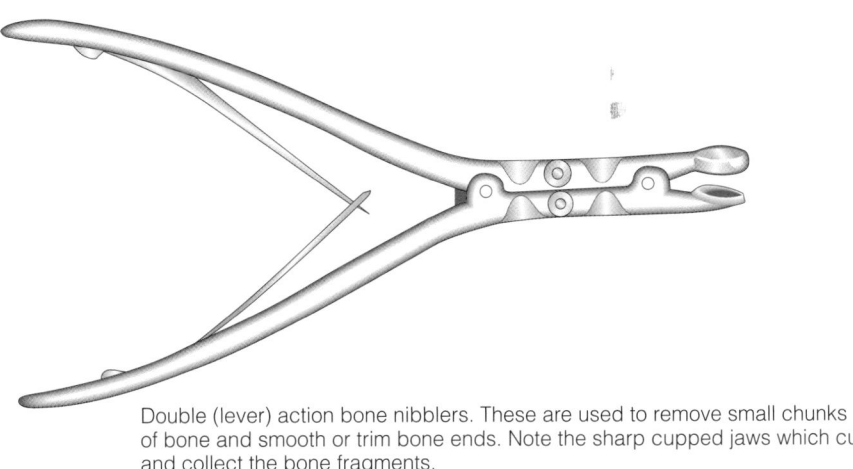

Double (lever) action bone nibblers. These are used to remove small chunks
of bone and smooth or trim bone ends. Note the sharp cupped jaws which cut
and collect the bone fragments.

Fig. 5.18 Bone nibblers

Periosteal elevator

The blunt, broad blade of the periosteal elevator (Fig. 5.19) is used to lift periosteum off bone before it is resected (e.g. ribs in thoracic surgery). Preservation of the periosteum, which contains osteocytes and their precursors, allows some bony regeneration and aids bony healing.

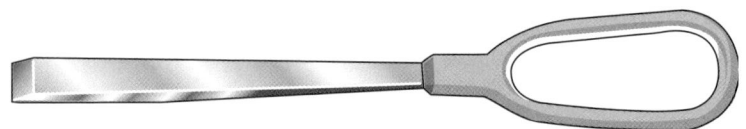

A periosteal elevator is used to lift the periosteum from bones before cutting them. The tip is sharp and angles down to a broad point.

Fig. 5.19 Periosteal elevator

Curette

The sharp edge of the spoon-shaped curette is used to scrape debris from the wall of a cavity such as an abscess, the uterus or an infected bone (Fig. 5.20).

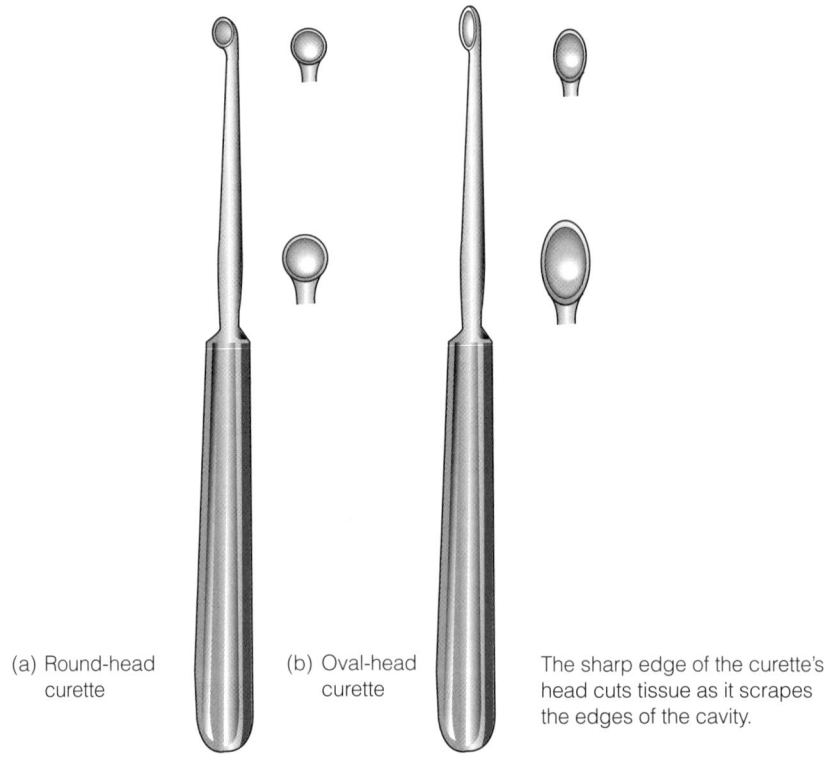

(a) Round-head curette

(b) Oval-head curette

The sharp edge of the curette's head cuts tissue as it scrapes the edges of the cavity.

Fig. 5.20 Curettes

GRASPING INSTRUMENTS

'Forceps' is the generic name for any instrument with a pair of jaws used to grasp or hold. Forceps may be used to grasp tissues, needles, sutures or even other instruments. In this chapter grasping instruments are classified as:

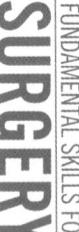

1. tissue forceps
2. clamping forceps
3. needle-holding forceps
4. other grasping forceps.

Tissue forceps

The basic purpose of tissue forceps is to grasp tissue with minimum trauma, to stabilise or retract it while performing another action such as suturing or dissecting. There are two basic designs of tissue forceps: thumb forceps, and ratcheted ring-handle forceps. Distinction is made in this chapter between tissue forceps, which are designed to grasp tissue, and clamping forceps (including artery forceps), which are designed to occlude hollow structures or crush tissue.

Thumb forceps

Thumb forceps comprise two jaws sprung from a fixed apical joint (like tweezers). The forceps' tips usually bear teeth or a variety of corrugation patterns that become apposed when the two blades are squeezed together between the fingers and thumb. They come in a range of lengths and weights, and are used for manipulation of soft tissues or viscera during dissection or suturing.

Thumb forceps are held in a 'chopstick' or 'pen' grip, and balanced by resting it in the V between the thumb and index finger (Fig. 5.21). They are generally used in the non-dominant hand to steady and display tissues, or to apply counter-traction against which to dissect. Heavy, toothed forceps are used for fascia and skin while finer non-toothed variants are used on viscera, vessels and other delicate structures.

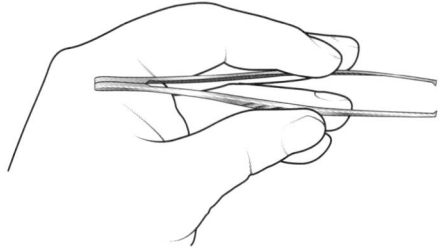

Holding a pair of dissecting forceps in the V between the thumb and index finger. In this position they act like chopsticks and therefore as an extension of the fingers.

Fig. 5.21 Holding thumb forceps

Toothed thumb forceps

Toothed thumb forceps have teeth that interlock on opposing tips (Fig. 5.22). It is said that the presence of teeth on these forceps makes the grip required to hold the structures less forceful, resulting in less trauma than if there were no teeth. Fine or

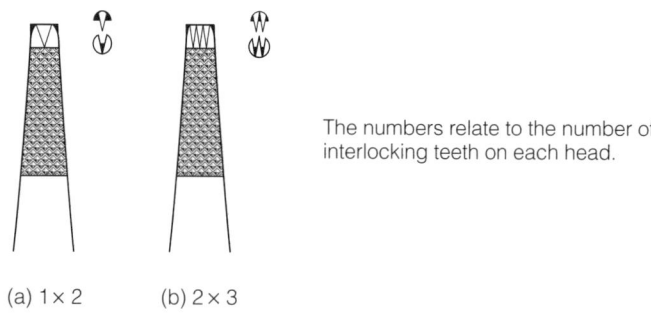

The numbers relate to the number of interlocking teeth on each head.

(a) 1 × 2   (b) 2 × 3

Fig. 5.22 Toothed forceps jaws

medium toothed forceps are commonly used for handling skin, and heavy forceps for fascia and muscle. Some toothed thumb forceps have a tungsten needle-holding platform just proximal to the teeth. These are strongly recommended (in an appropriate weight) for use during suturing. Forceps without a needle platform should not generally be used for suturing, as they do not grasp a needle reliably and encourage excessive force resulting in damage to the forceps.

Examples of toothed forceps are shown in Figures 5.23 and 5.24.

- Fine Adson forceps (1 × 2 teeth) (Fig. 5.23a) are fine-toothed forceps used mainly for dissection in plastic surgery or in the repair of minor traumatic or surgical wounds. They are delicate and should only be used in areas of thin skin (i.e. not in the trunk or scalp, which are thick-skin areas).
- Adson forceps with needle-holding platform (Fig. 5.23b) are ideal for general skin suturing.
- Gillies forceps (1 × 2 teeth) (Fig. 5.24) are longer and slightly heavier than Adson forceps. They also have a post in the middle of one shaft that fits into a small hole in the opposing shaft to ensure tip alignment. They can be used for any type of skin and are useful for dissection and suturing. Their jaws are easily bent by inappropriate use on fascia or by heavy needles.
- Medium Jarit general toothed needle-holding thumb forceps (Fig. 5.25a) have a tungsten needle-holding platform to grasp a heavy needle and are ideal for general fascia closure.
- Large thumb forceps such as Lane (1 × 2 or 2 × 3) (Fig. 5.25b) or Ferris–Smith forceps are used mainly for the grasping of bulky tissue during suturing (e.g. leg muscles in orthopaedic surgery or linea alba in abdominal closure). It is rare to use them on skin but they are excellent for heavy fascia, bone and cartilage.

Non-toothed thumb forceps

There are two basic patterns of 'non-toothed' forceps with a range of lengths and weights (Fig. 5.26). The first, such as dressing forceps (Fig. 5.26a) and McIndoe

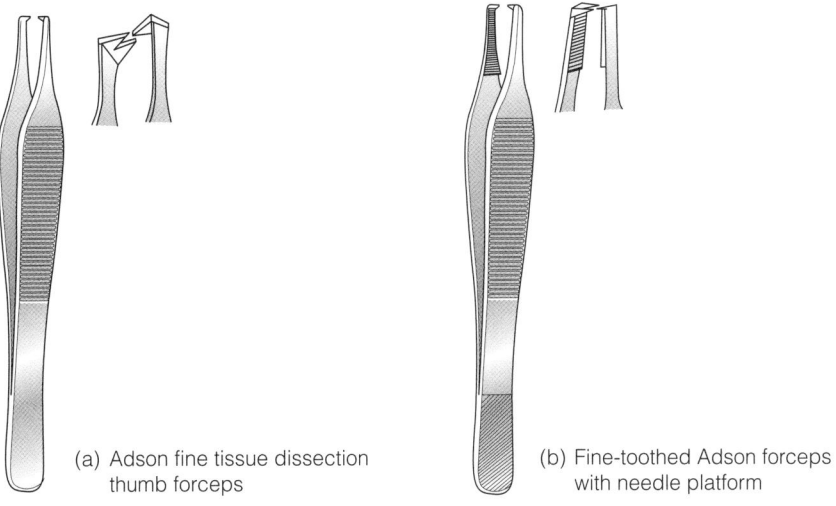

(a) Adson fine tissue dissection
thumb forceps

(b) Fine-toothed Adson forceps
with needle platform

Fig. 5.23 Adson forceps

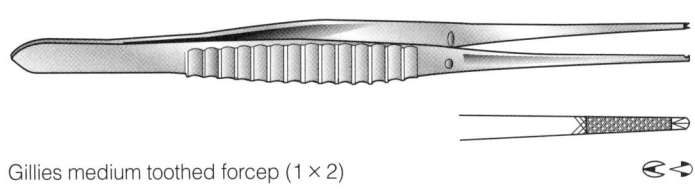

Gillies medium toothed forcep (1 × 2)

Fig. 5.24 Gillies toothed thumb forceps

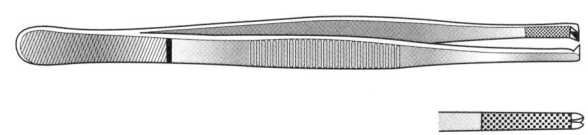

Fig. 5.25a Jarit medium thumb forceps

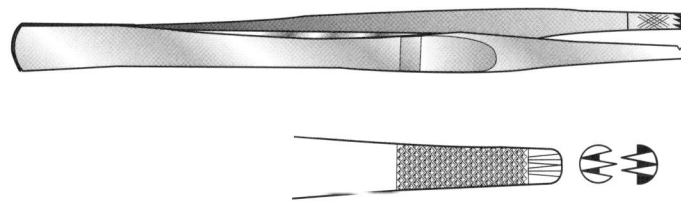

Lane heavy toothed forcep (2 × 3)

Fig. 5.25b Lane heavy toothed forceps

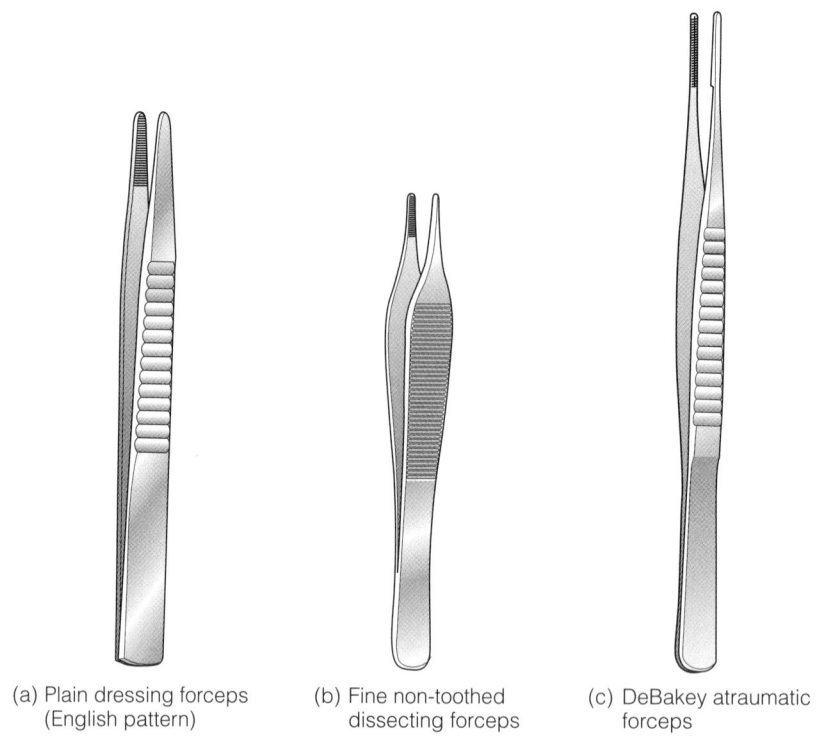

(a) Plain dressing forceps
(English pattern)

(b) Fine non-toothed
dissecting forceps

(c) DeBakey atraumatic
forceps

Fig. 5.26 Non-toothed thumb forceps

forceps genuinely have no teeth, only ridges or grooves on the surface of the tip (Fig. 5.27a). The second actually has interlocking longitudinal rows of teeth that are so small they are not easily discernible and are described as 'atraumatic' (Fig. 5.27b). One such pattern is known as the DeBakey forceps (Fig. 5.26c) (Fig. 5.27c, d), named after the American cardiovascular surgeon who designed it. Several other variants are not described here.

It is important to select the appropriate forceps for the task required. Non-toothed forceps of the grooved-jaw variety are used for manipulating packs and dressings both in theatre and on the wards. Either variety may be used for grasping viscera and serosal or adventitial surfaces, as the lack of teeth greatly lessens the likelihood of puncture. DeBakey forceps were designed as a vascular forceps but are commonly used for bowel and pulmonary work. Their design also allows secure handling of small suture needles such as those used in vascular, genitourinary and bowel work.

Ring-handled grasping forceps

The second type of tissue forceps has a variety of hinged-jaw configurations and a ratchet lock. Jaws usually have a bi-concave or ring shape to minimise tissue trauma, when closed, by allowing tissue to bulge between the jaws. These forceps can be

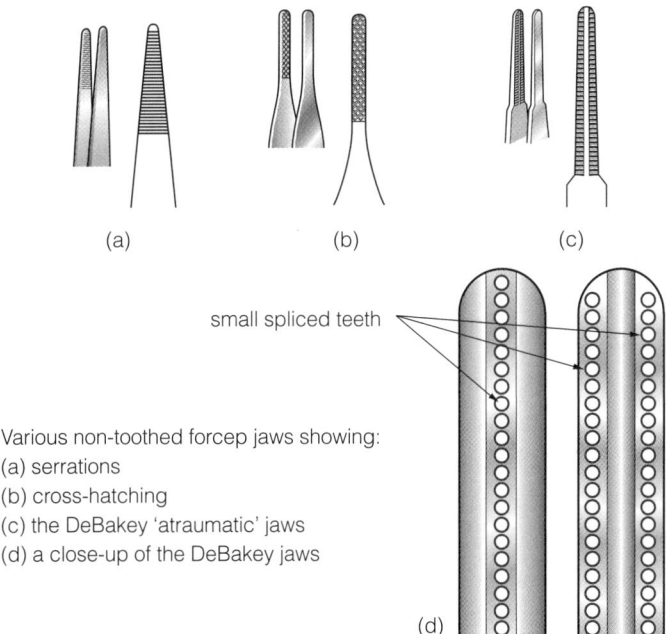

Various non-toothed forcep jaws showing:
(a) serrations
(b) cross-hatching
(c) the DeBakey 'atraumatic' jaws
(d) a close-up of the DeBakey jaws

small spliced teeth

Fig. 5.27 Non-toothed forcep jaws

used on any tissue appropriate for the instrument's weight, tip pattern (toothed or non-toothed) and jaw configuration. Weight, or 'heaviness', refers to both the gauge of metal from which the instrument is made and the force created at the instrument tips upon closure. Longer distances from the hinge to the tip of the jaws and more flexible shafts mean that less pressure is created between the tips of the jaws. This concept is evident when comparing the force exerted at the tip of a long, fine bladed Babcock forceps with the force of the short, heavy bladed Lane's forceps.

Ring-handled ratcheted forceps are held like scissors when applied, but the fingers may be withdrawn to hold the forceps by the shaft below the finger rings while retracting. Their main use is to stabilise or retract tissues, especially when a strong grip is required for a long time, where a stay suture or hook may pull out or damage the tissue, when the tissues are too slippery to hold by hand or where the direction of retraction needs to be changed frequently. Heavy and toothed varieties are used on fascia and finer, 'atraumatic' forceps are used on viscera.

Toothed grasping forceps

Toothed ratcheted forceps are used predominantly for grasping, heavy tough tissue such as fascia or bone. The actual tissue on which they are used depends on the size, strength and the tooth pattern on the instrument head, as detailed above.

- *Fine*: Allis forceps are the most common forceps in this category (Fig. 5.28a). As their head contains a row of short interlocking teeth and long fine bows (arms), they may be used for grasping bowel during suturing or for grasping dermis during subcutaneous dissection (e.g. in a mastectomy or thyroidectomy).
- *Heavy*: Lane, Littlewood and Rutherford–Morrison forceps are some common variants of this category (Fig. 5.28b, c). They have heavy, short bows, few long teeth and are commonly used to grasp heavy fascia or dermis.

Non-toothed grasping forceps

- *Fine*: Babcock forceps have a rounded head and grooved tips (Fig. 5.29a). They are commonly used for grasping bowel or other viscera because of their softness. They cannot be used for heavy or bulky tissue as they inevitably slip.
- *Heavy*: Duvall forceps have a large triangular head with grooves or tiny teeth (Fig. 5.29b). Again their grip is quite soft but as they have a large gripping area, they hold bulky viscera such as lung and stomach well.

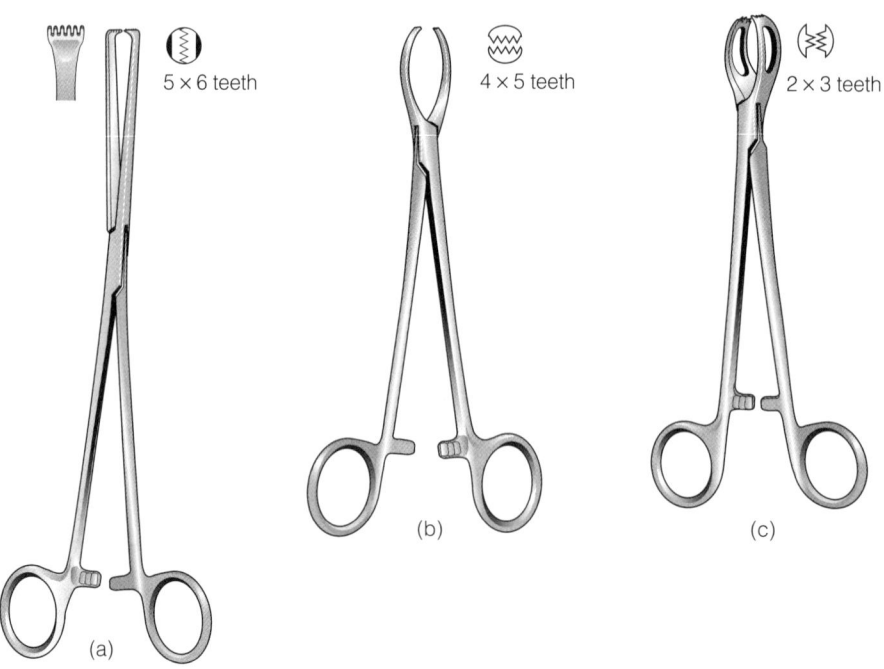

5 × 6 teeth   4 × 5 teeth   2 × 3 teeth

(b)   (c)

(a)

(a) Allis forcep showing long, fine arms and a 5 x 6 tooth configuration
(b) Rutherford-Morrison forcep showing shorter, stronger arms and a 4 x 5 tooth configuration
(c) Lane forcep showing very short, heavy arms and a 2 x 3 tooth configuration

Fig. 5.28 Toothed ratcheted tissue forceps

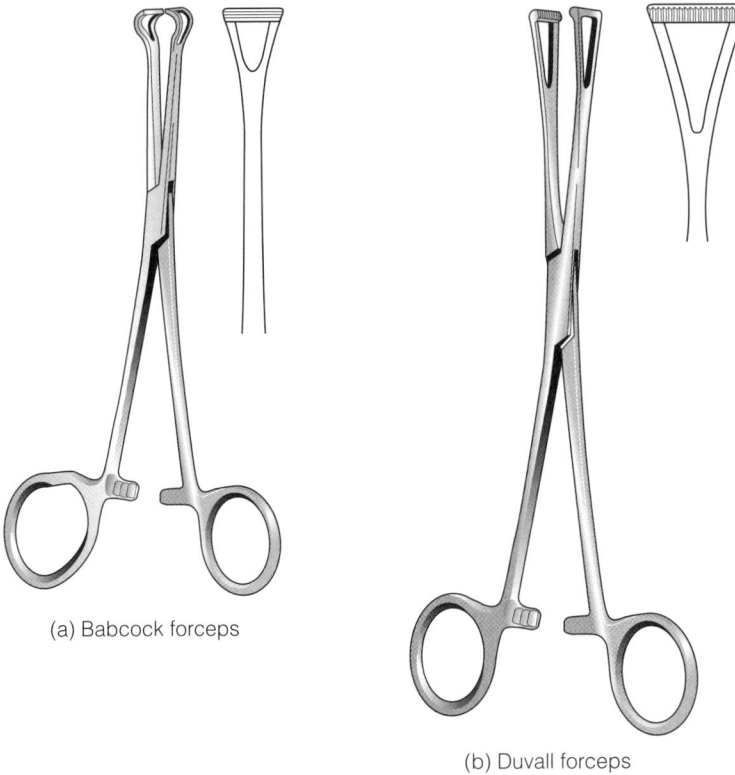

(a) Babcock forceps

(b) Duvall forceps

Fig. 5.29 Non-toothed ratcheted tissue forceps

Needle holders

Needle-holding forceps are used to drive a needle and thread through tissues. Because a needle holder must provide a strong grip on the needle, the jaws are usually relatively short compared with the handles. Premium instruments have a box-hinge joint for strength and stability and a scored tungsten carbide needle-holding platform on both jaws (Fig. 5.32, 5.33). Most have ring handles, and the majority have a locking ratchet. Needle holders with long curved shafts with no finger rings are now obsolete except for microsurgery.

Using a needle holder

Selection of an appropriate needle-holding forceps for the task is most important. The jaws should be of an appropriate weight for the needle. Fine needle holders are easily damaged by being used to drive large or heavy needles through firm tissue. The weight of the instrument does not necessarily equate to the length of the handles or jaws; for example, long fine vascular needle holders should never be used to drive a heavy fascial closure needle. In general, the length of the needle holder should be such that the hand using it is out of the operative field and does not obstruct the operator's view.

Curved needles are designed to be driven through tissue in the arc of their curve. This is achieved by rotating the tip of the needle holders by either pronation or supination of the forearm. The instrument must be held, therefore, with its long axis in the line of the forearm, with the index finger directed along the shaft. The thumb may be placed in or on the upper finger ring of the needle holder, the index finger placed on the joint and the other three fingers curled around the lower finger ring. The fourth finger may be placed in the lower finger ring if this is more comfortable (Fig. 5.30a). If correctly held, the tip of the forceps should remain at the same point in space and merely rotate along the long axis of the instrument and forearm when the arm is pronated and supinated. To achieve this, the wrist is in slight ulnar deviation. If the tip itself describes an arc of movement, the alignment is not quite correct.

Many surgeons prefer not to use the rings, holding the needle holder in the palm of the hand with the upper ring against the thenar eminence, the length of the holder along the index finger and the other three fingers wrapped around the lower finger ring (Fig. 5.30b). The axial grip achieves more accurate rotation without the need for ulnar deviation of the wrist, and is useful for accurate suture placement. However, release of the ratchet is more difficult without the fingers in the rings, and requires practice to perform smoothly.

The needle holder may also be used to tie sutures, especially in the subcutaneous tissue or skin.

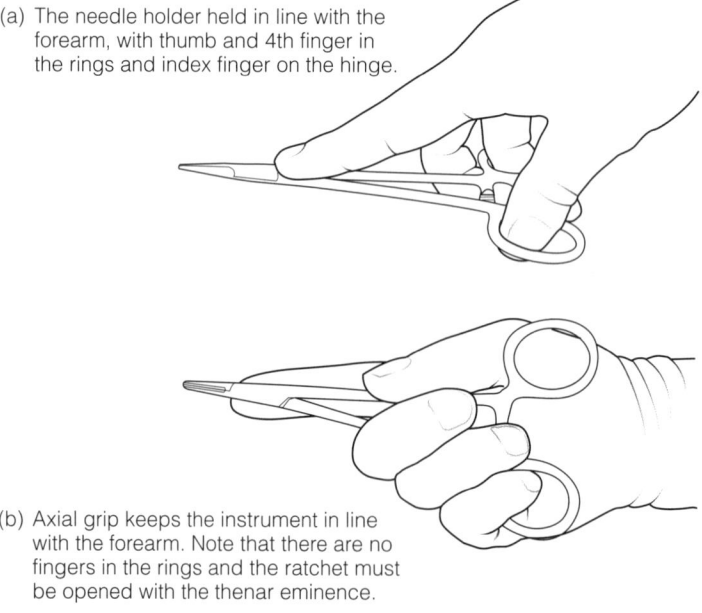

(a) The needle holder held in line with the forearm, with thumb and 4th finger in the rings and index finger on the hinge.

(b) Axial grip keeps the instrument in line with the forearm. Note that there are no fingers in the rings and the ratchet must be opened with the thenar eminence.

Fig. 5.30 Two methods of holding a needle holder

Once again, all these forceps may be palmed by swinging them back into the palm of the hand with the fourth finger inserted through the lower finger ring, similar to the position used for scissors (Fig. 5.10). Palming is especially useful during suturing as it means that the needle-holding forceps does not have to be put down and then retrieved during hand tying. Palming techniques should only be used if the needle is not in the holder. Techniques to 'protect' the needle point in the jaws of the needle holder should be discouraged as they are unreliable, do not prevent needlestick injury, and are likely to damage the point of the needle (Fig. 5.31).

Locking needle-holding forceps

The most common pattern of general purpose needle holder in general surgical use is the Mayo–Hegar (Fig. 5.32). This is a ratcheted ring-handled forceps with a short, reasonably heavy cross-hatched jaw. Mayo–Hegars come in virtually any length, from 125 mm to 300 mm. They will generally cope with heavy fascia needles. Finer needle holders for bowel, vascular or plastic surgical work include the Crile–Wood, the Gillies and the fine-jawed Ryder patterns. These should generally not be used on anything larger than a 3/0 gauge 26 mm needle. The Olsen–Hegar has scissor blades between the tungsten carbide inserts and the hinge. Curved needle holders such as the Heaney compromise ergonomics and should be reserved for specialised suturing in awkward places.

Non-locking needle-holding forceps

The most common non-locking needle holder is the Gillies pattern. It has a shorter upper shaft and large thumb ring angled away from the axis of the instrument. A pair of scissors is incorporated in the blades and the jaws are slightly curved. They are used almost exclusively by plastic surgeons.

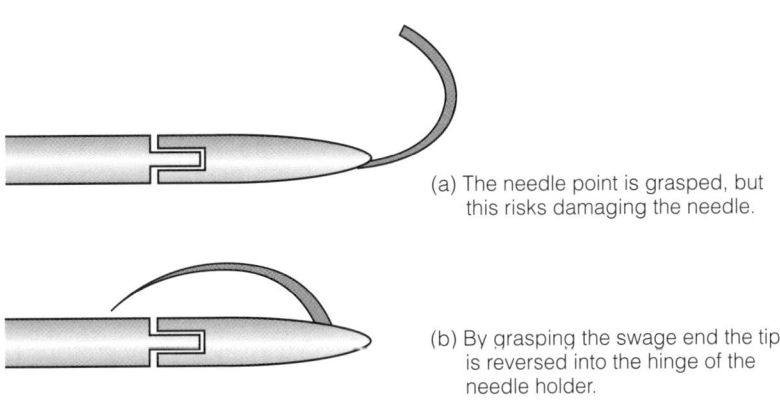

(a) The needle point is grasped, but this risks damaging the needle.

(b) By grasping the swage end the tip is reversed into the hinge of the needle holder.

Fig. 5.31 Techniques to 'protect' the needle when not in use should be discouraged

The Gillies needle holder is significantly more difficult to use than a conventional, ratcheted needle holder, as constant pressure must be applied to the blades to retain a grip on the needle. In its favour the size, shape and features of this needle holder allow for easy handling and tying (there is no ratchet) and cutting of one's own sutures, thereby improving ergonomics (Fig. 5.32).

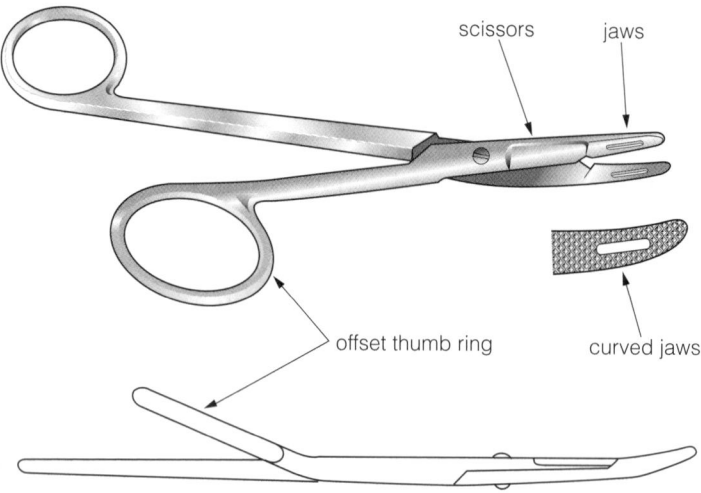

Fig. 5.32 Gillies needle holder

Other types of forceps

A variety of specialised forceps fall into the general categories discussed above but they rate a mention on an individual basis because of their frequent use and special functions.

Sponge-holding forceps

The Rampley sponge-holding forceps are long, ring-handled, ratcheted forceps with long, grooved ring-shaped jaws. They are used to hold the swabs with which the skin is prepared preoperatively and to hold gauzes for blotting tissues dry during dissection. They may also be used as a tissue forceps for the gall bladder or lung (Fig. 5.33).

Gall-bladder forceps

A variety of forceps may be used to hold the gall bladder during an open procedure, including Rampley sponge-holding forceps (Fig. 5.33) and Pennington or Lovelace forceps, which have triangular jaws specifically designed for this purpose. Many surgeons employ Moynihan forceps to hold the gall bladder, although they were originally designed to secure the cystic duct (Fig. 5.34).

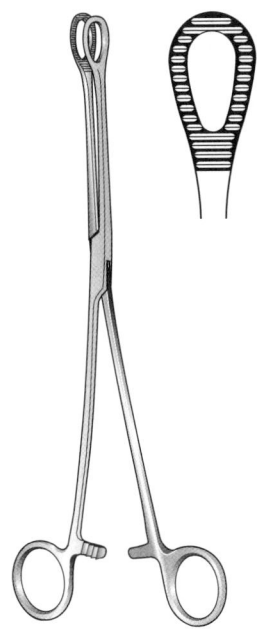

Fig. 5.33 Rampley sponge-holding forceps

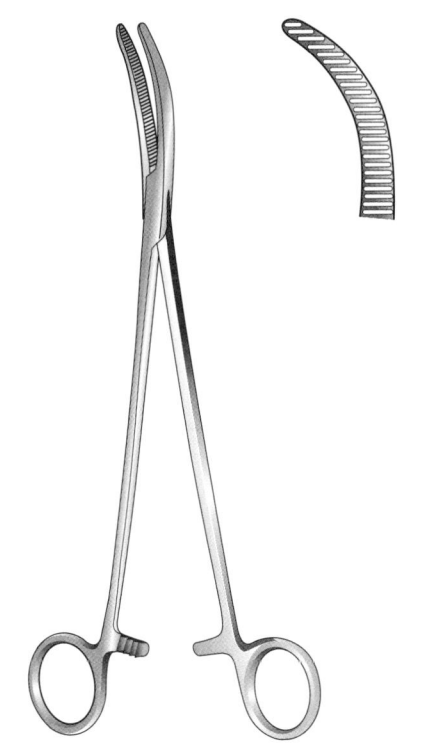

Fig. 5.34 Moynihan gall-bladder forceps

CLAMPING INSTRUMENTS

Clamps are locking devices designed to occlude or close a lumen or cavity to prevent flow or leakage of its contents. Most are ring-handle ratchet design, but some are sprung and others screwed.

Haemostatic (occluding) forceps

Haemostatic forceps consist of hinged jaws with ring handles and a ratchet to maintain closure (Fig. 5.35). During closure, the tips come together first and then the jaws come together, crushing all tissue between them. As with tissue-holding forceps, the gauge of material, length of shafts and design of the tip dictate the function. In general, the curved variety of artery forceps is used on tissues and vessels, and the straight form used to hold sutures.

In broad terms haemostatic forceps are used to control bleeding by gripping vessels, or tissues containing them, and presenting them for ligation. They can also function as dissecting instruments, spreading the blunt tips to separate tissue planes and to dissect out structures such as vessels, nerves and cystic duct. They should not be used as tissue holding forceps, in the manner described in the previous section, because tissue grasped by them is crushed and will usually necrose.

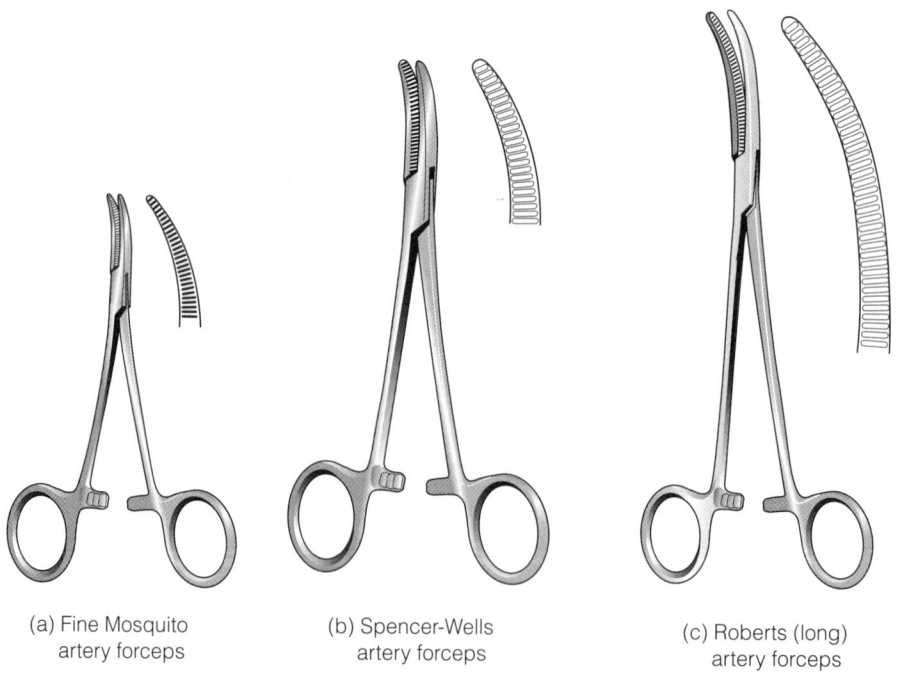

(a) Fine Mosquito
artery forceps

(b) Spencer-Wells
artery forceps

(c) Roberts (long)
artery forceps

Fig. 5.35 Haemostatic vascular (artery) forceps

Using haemostatic forceps

Haemostatic forceps are usually applied using a scissor grip (see above). When an artery forceps is applied across a vessel the tips should protrude beyond the grasped tissue so that a ligature can be slipped below them. It is most important that both jaws can be seen before closing to ensure that another key structure or extraneous tissue is not caught between them. If excessive tissue is grasped, blood vessels may retract and bleed. One click of the ratchet should be enough to ensure crushing of the tissues and a secure grip. Over-tightening damages the forceps, and may cut through thick or oedematous tissue or cause the forceps to spring apart in an uncontrolled fashion when released.

Traditionally, curved haemostatic forceps are applied with their convexity downward, facing the more critical vessel, in order to facilitate placement of a ligature (Fig. 5.36).

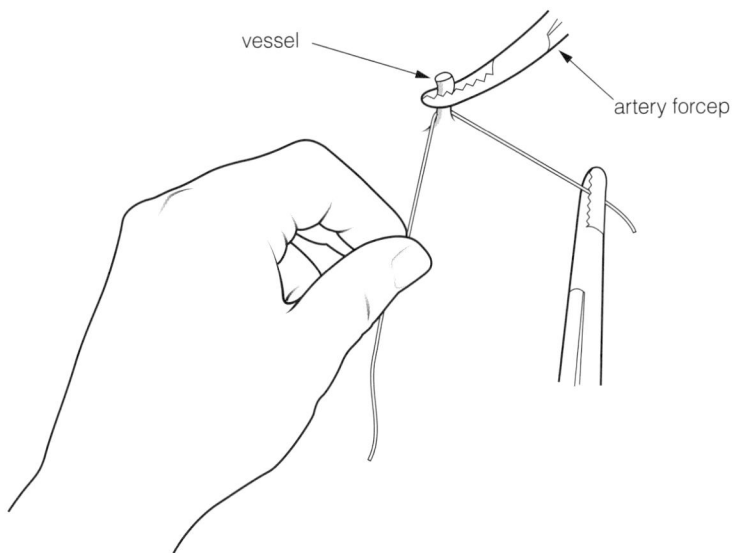

vessel

artery forcep

The tips of the artery forcep are beyond the edge of the vessel giving a 'lip' around which a tie may be placed and retained while the knot is completed.

Fig. 5.36 Positioning an artery forceps on a vessel

To remove a vascular forceps, controlled torque must be applied to the handles to disengage the ratchet. This may be achieved with the fingers inserted into the rings but if the angle is awkward for this, the thumb can be applied to the proximal ring of the forceps and the next two fingers to the distal ring. The fingers apply pressure to disengage the ratchet and the forceps are removed in one smooth action (Fig. 5.37).

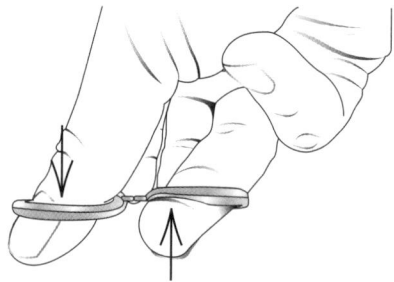

Fig. 5.37 Opening an artery forceps—correct torque

Types of haemostatic forceps

Non-toothed ring-handled ratcheted forceps

Usually just called 'artery forceps', a wide variety have eponymous names based on their length, weight, shape and local custom. The most commonly used forceps are 12–16 cm long with gently curved jaws and transverse grooves. Short, fine variants are often known as Mosquito forceps, and the medium style may be called Spencer–Wells or Halsted forceps. Longer and heavier styles are commonly known as Robert forceps. Another medium and heavy variety, such as Carmalt, uses longitudinal grooves with the theory that tissue is less likely to retract between the jaws. Forceps with a near 90° curve on the jaws, such as O'Shaughnessey, Mixter, or Lahey (Fig. 5.38), are useful for securing vessels at depth, or for passing sutures or slings around structures deep in a wound. Long, heavy Rochester–Carmalt forceps are useful deep in the pelvis or chest.

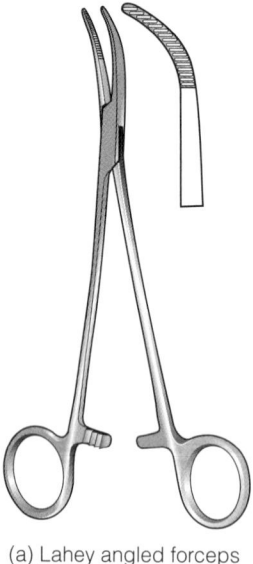
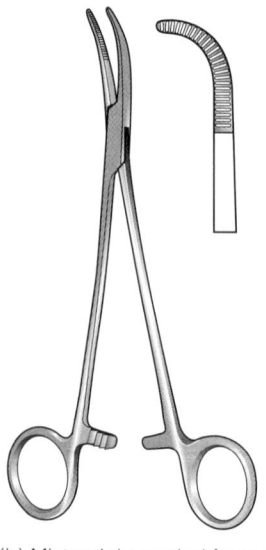

(a) Lahey angled forceps   (b) Mixter right-angled forcep

Fig. 5.38 Various ratcheted haemostatic forceps

Toothed artery forceps

Toothed artery forceps come in small and large varieties. Kocher forceps are a common straight variety (Fig. 5.39a). They are generally heavier than non-toothed forceps and the tooth at the tip aids both in gripping tissue and preventing it from squeezing out of the open end of the jaws. Heaney's (Fig. 5.39b) have heavy curved jaws with large teeth spaced along them. They are excellent for secure clamping of bulky tissue (e.g. uterine or ovarian pedicles) before division and suture ligation.

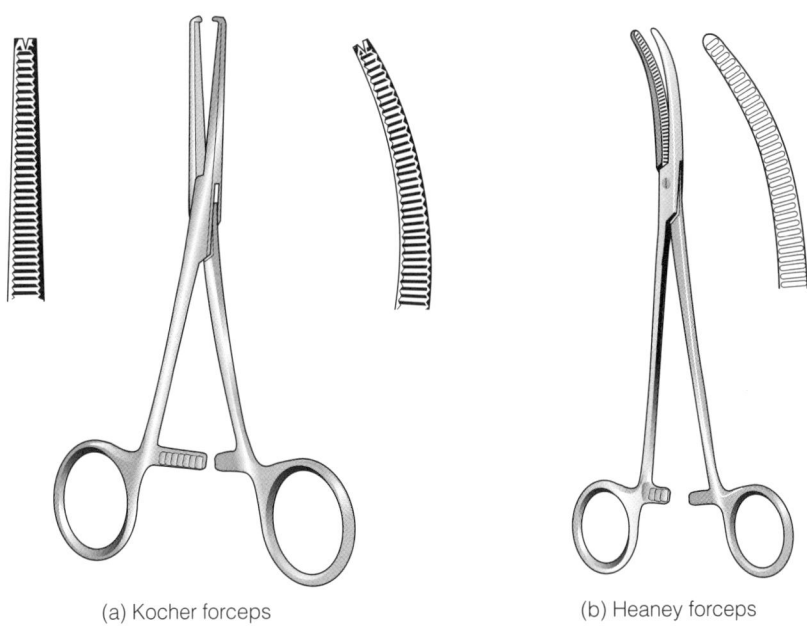

(a) Kocher forceps   (b) Heaney forceps

Fig. 5.39 Heavy toothed haemostatic forceps

Non-crushing 'clamps'

Non-crushing 'clamps' are used for the temporary occlusion of a hollow structure such as bowel, blood vessel, ureter, etc, while a surgical procedure is being performed upon it (e.g. anastomosis, endarterectomy or arterial bypass). They exert an even pressure across the jaws that is sufficient to prevent flow through the occluded lumen or leakage of other contained fluid, but not enough to damage the tissues of the structure. Non-crushing forceps typically have long, relatively flexible jaws to minimise the pressure produced between them.

Vascular clamps (non-crushing)

Atraumatic vascular clamps are either hinged and held closed with a ratchet, or are sprung like a clothes peg (Fig. 5.40). These clamps are designed to prevent the flow of blood through a vessel while it is being operated upon. Blades close

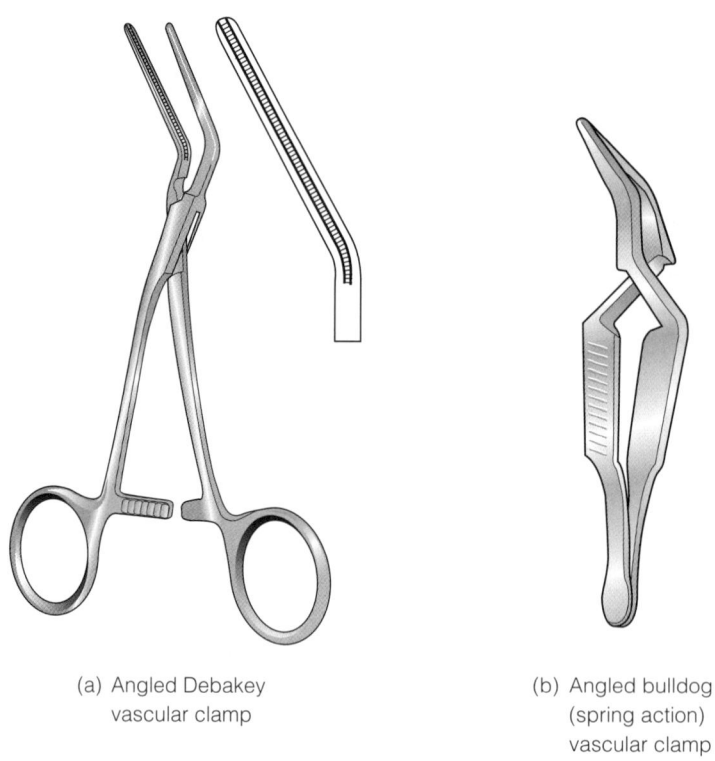

(a) Angled Debakey
    vascular clamp

(b) Angled bulldog
    (spring action)
    vascular clamp

Fig. 5.40 Non-crushing vascular clamps

parallel to each other to apply pressure evenly along their length, in contrast to the tip-first closure of artery forceps. Importantly, their design incorporates features that prevent crushing and intimal damage, which could lead to intravascular thrombosis.

Vascular clamps have a pattern of atraumatic serrations along their jaws. Different angles, curves and jaw-grip patterns are based on the type of vessel on which they will be used and on whether all, or only some, of the vessel lumen requires occlusion (Fig. 5.41). Some vascular clamps have fabric or gel-filled cushions on the grasping side of the jaw to spread the pressure and help prevent trauma. They are also produced in different lengths and weights (fine, medium and heavy varieties) for different vessel types.

The bulldog style rests in the closed position and requires squeezing to open the jaws. The occlusion pressure is predetermined by the spring tension. Ratcheted forceps should be tightened only enough to occlude, not damage, the vessel to which they are applied. Generally this means just one click on the ratchet. The forceps' tips should only just protrude beyond the vessel so as not to present an obstacle that must be avoided. Extraneous tissue must not be included within a vascular clamp, as it will compromise clamp efficacy.

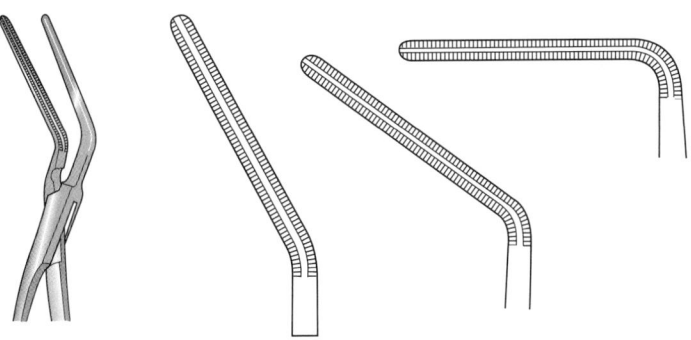

(a) A variety of angled blades for the DeBakey angled vascular clamp

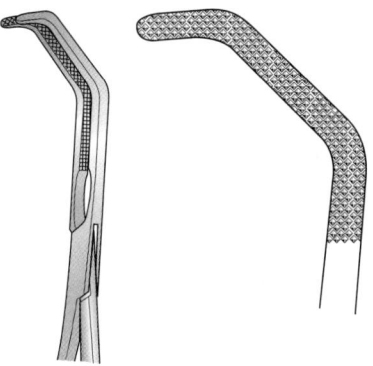

(b) The Satinsky vascular clamp, used to occlude part of the lumen of a vessel for operation

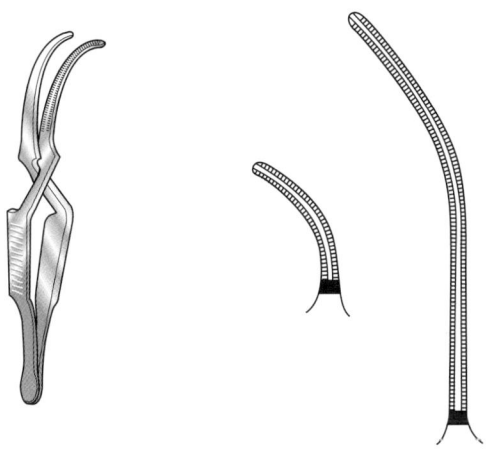

(c) Long and short blades for the curved bulldog vascular clamp

Fig. 5.41 Vascular clamp jaw patterns

Bowel clamps

When dealing with bowel there are situations where it is desirable to occlude the lumen without damaging the bowel, or to crush the bowel to ensure a watertight seal before it is divided. Specialised non-crushing and crushing clamps have been designed for these purposes. There are multiple patterns of both and many will not be dealt with here.

Non-crushing bowel clamps

Doyen non-crushing bowel clamps are ring-handled, ratcheted clamps with a pair of long, very flexible blades. These blades are significantly longer than the handles above the instrument's joint, thereby ensuring lower pressures at the tip. The flexibility and width of the blades further lessen the pressure. Non-crushing bowel clamps may be either straight or curved and the blades usually have longitudinal grooves and micro-teeth, similar to DeBakey forceps. The tips meet first and the long blades then come gently together to occlude the lumen of the bowel without interrupting the blood supply. When applying these clamps, care must be taken not to crush the mesentery between the tips as this may cause vessel damage and ischaemia (Fig. 5.42).

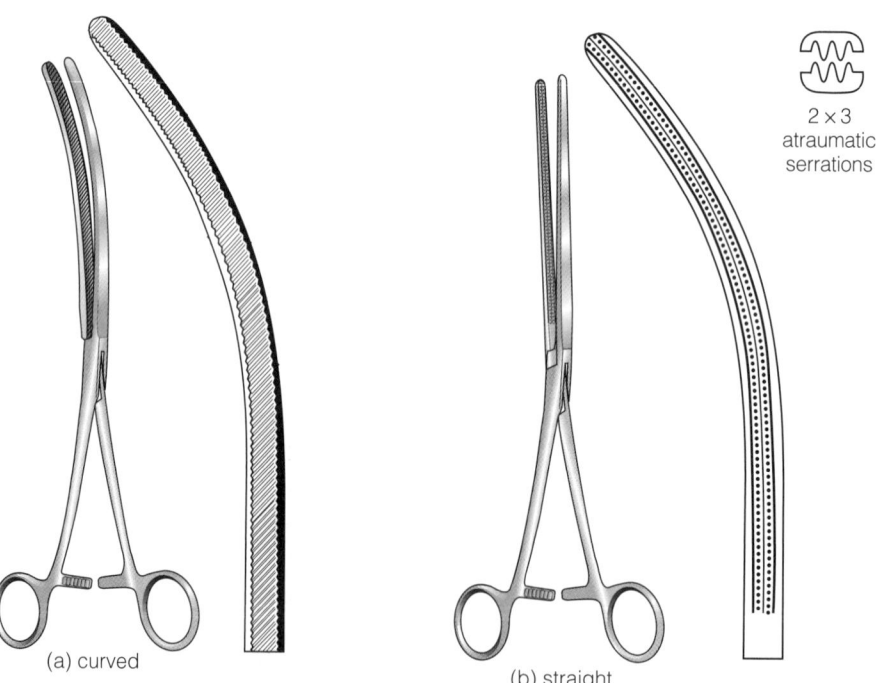

2 × 3
atraumatic
serrations

(a) curved

(b) straight

Doyen soft bowel clamps with different jaw patterns: DeBakey and cross-hatched

Fig. 5.42 Non-crushing bowel clamps

Crushing bowel clamps

Lang–Stevenson crushing bowel clamps are just one variety of these. This ratcheted ring-handled clamp has longitudinally grooved blades that are strong and virtually rigid (Fig. 5.43). The bowel is crushed between the jaws before it is divided along the edge of the instrument. In general, crushing bowel clamps are used on the specimen side of the bowel with non-crushing clamps placed on the side to be retained and anastomosed. Other similar clamps include Parker–Kerr clamps, Kocher forceps and various angled rectal clamps.

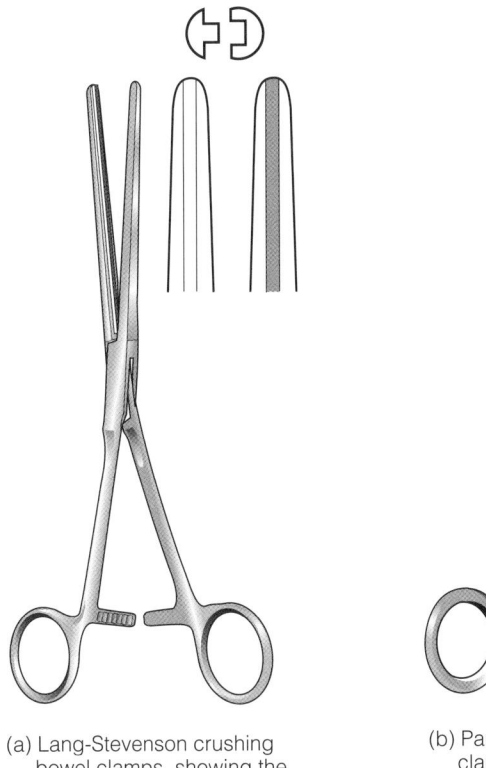

(a) Lang-Stevenson crushing bowel clamps, showing the grooved keyed blades

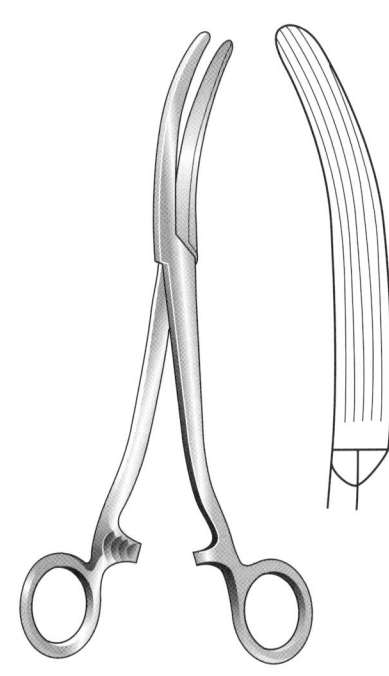

(b) Parker-Kerr curved crushing bowel clamp, showing the longitudinally ridged blades

Fig. 5.43 Crushing bowel clamps

RETRACTING INSTRUMENTS

Retractors are an essential tool for the display of tissues during an operation. They are usually held by the assistant's hand, but may be self-retaining with a spring, ratchet or screw mechanism.

The essential principle of retraction is the placement of a blade in front of tissue that would otherwise obscure the operative field. The blade may be used passively to prevent tissue falling into the wound or actively to retract tissues out of the wound. Great care must be taken not to damage the structures being retracted. This is the art of retraction. Unfortunately this role is often assigned to the most junior member of the scrub team; paradoxically it is one of the most difficult aspects to master.

There are retractors designed for every surgical purpose. There is a wide range of specialised orifice retractors for access to nose, mouth, vagina and anus. General purpose retractors will be discussed here.

Hand-held retractors

Hand-held retractors are held in position by one of the assistants to displace or prevent ingress of tissues to the operative field. If properly handled they are minimally traumatic, as pressure on the underlying structures can be varied as the need for exposure alters. All retractors have a 'blade' of some description, usually set at approximately right angles to a long handle. Exposure is achieved by a combination of judicious placement, careful pull and 'toe in' rotation of the blade. 'Toe in' movement is achieved by lifting the retractor handle away from the skin surface and keeping the bend of the retractor fixed, thus angling the toe of the retractor further into the patient (Fig. 5.44).

There are many sizes and patterns of retractor for specific retraction tasks and we deal with a few of the common ones in this section.

Small hand-held retractors

Toothed small hand-held retractors

The common small, toothed retractors include the skin hook, the cats-paw retractor and the rake retractor. These instruments are used predominantly for the retraction of skin edges during minor skin surgery. They grip well because their pointed teeth penetrate the tissue being retracted while causing minimal trauma. The cats-paw retractor also has a small right-angled blade at the opposite end from the points (Fig. 5.45). Toothed retractors must be handled with great care because of the risk of glove perforation and injury to surgeon or assistant.

Non-toothed small hand-held retractors

These include the Langenbeck, Durham–Barr and Czerny (sometimes called 'army-navy') retractors. They have a deeper blade that has specific usefulness in retracting subcutaneous tissue for minor skin surgery and body wall hernia surgery, and for subcutaneous fat retraction during deep wound closure (Fig. 5.46).

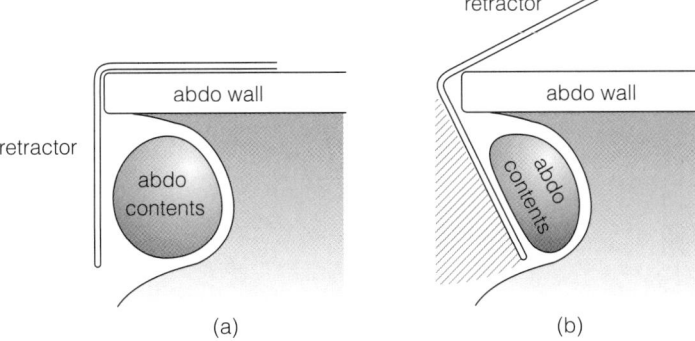

(a) (b)

As the retractor handle is lifted from (a) to (b) the toe of the retractor rotates 'into' the patient. This increases the exposure (as shown by the hatched area) but puts the underlying structures at risk from pressure exerted by the retractor.

Fig. 5.44 'Toe in' as applied to retractors

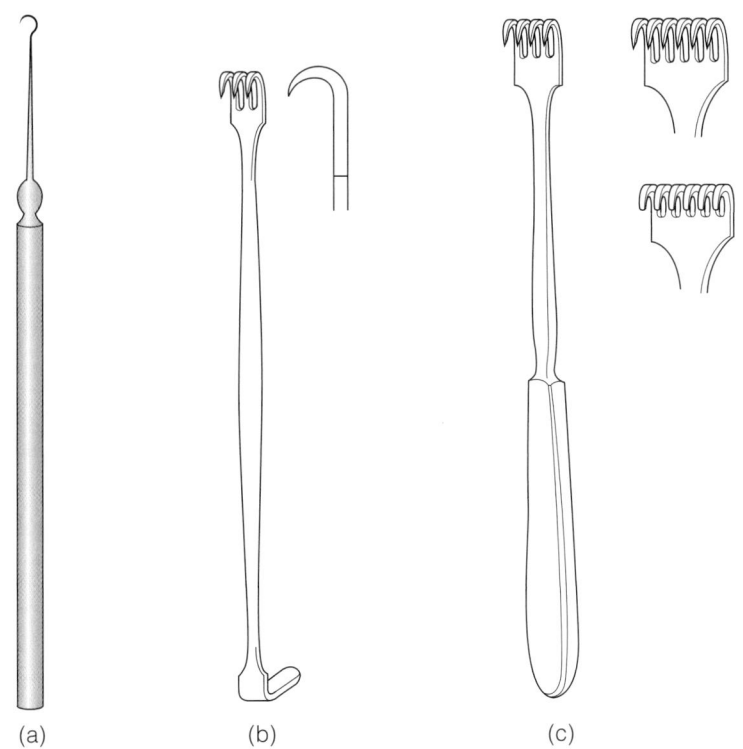

(a) (b) (c)

(a) Skin-hook retractor for the edges and corners of fine wounds
(b) Cats-paw retractor which also has a small flat blade
(c) A rake retractor which can have up to six sharp or blunt prongs

Fig. 5.45 Small toothed retractors, hand held

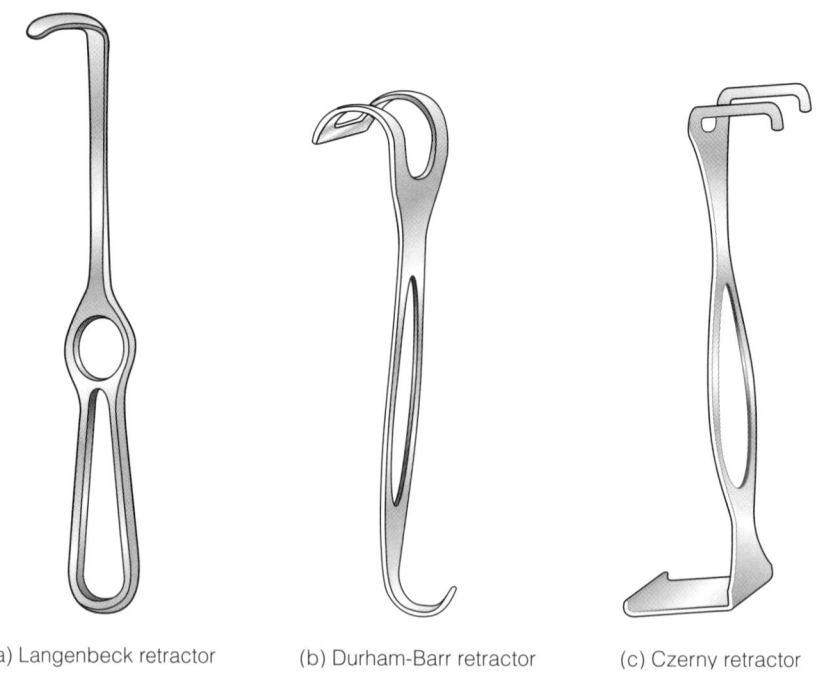

(a) Langenbeck retractor   (b) Durham-Barr retractor   (c) Czerny retractor

Fig. 5.46 Small non-toothed (bladed) retractors, hand held

Large hand-held retractors

Superficial retractors

Superficial hand-held retractors are often quite wide with short blades. They may come with a curve (Fritsch or Kocher retractors) or a backward-pointing lip (Morris retractors) (Fig. 5.47). These patterns are used to great effect in retracting and lifting the anterior abdominal wall for better access into the superior, inferior and lateral recesses of the abdominal cavity. They are also used in axillary surgery and may sometimes be fixed to a self-retaining retractor for abdominal surgery (Fig. 5.54, page 89).

Deep retractors

Long, wide-bladed, hand-held retractors, of varying lengths, are excellent for retracting structures deep within the abdominal or thoracic cavities. The Deaver (Fig. 5.48a) and Kelly (Fig. 5.48b) retractors are commonly used but other patterns include the St Mark's pelvic retractor (which may also have a light on it) (Fig. 5.48c). Great care must be exercised when using these retractors as their depth of penetration places adjacent structures, such as mesentery, liver or spleen, at risk of inadvertent damage. A gauze pack may be inserted as a protective buffer between the retractor and the structure to be retracted.

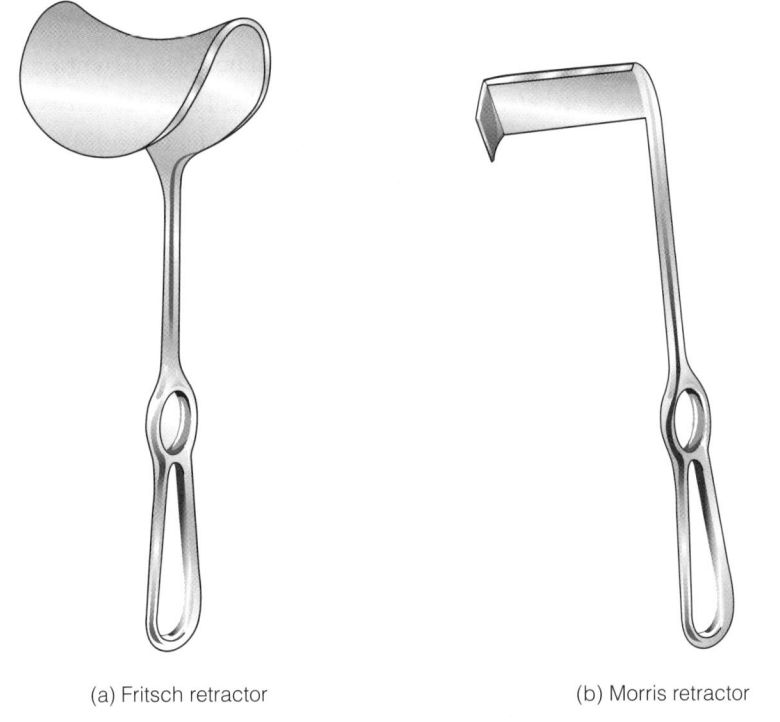

(a) Fritsch retractor

(b) Morris retractor

Fig. 5.47 Large superficial retractors

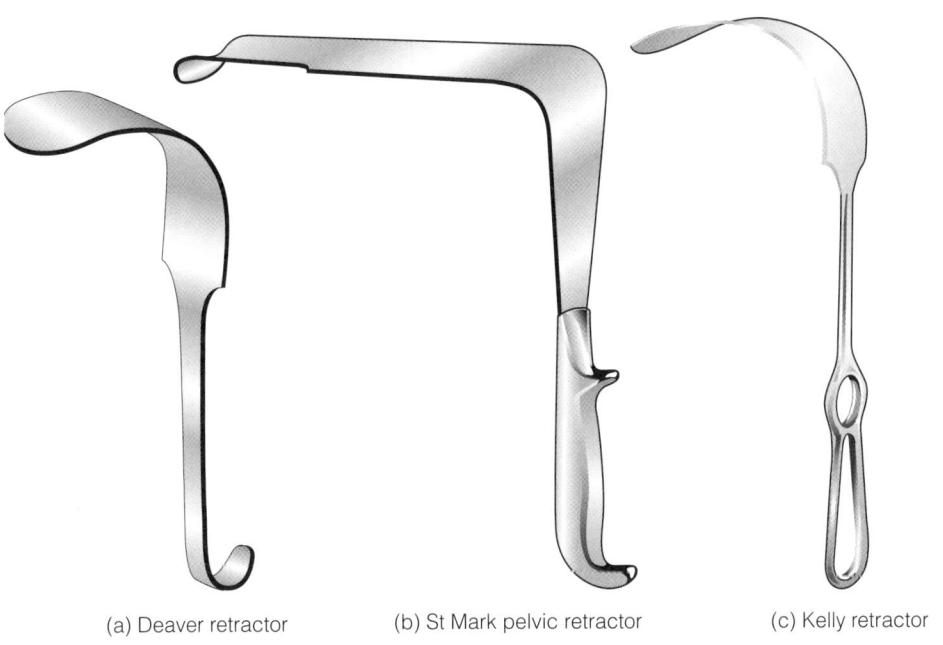

(a) Deaver retractor

(b) St Mark pelvic retractor

(c) Kelly retractor

Fig. 5.48 Deep retractors.

Self-retaining retractors

Self-retaining retractors are designed to lock into a fixed position. Retention is achieved by a system of springs, ratchets, screws, cranks or hooks. These retractors come in all sizes with toothed, flat or curved blades, which may themselves be solid or fenestrated. Self-retaining retractors can be used in virtually any operative site but care needs to be taken as they provide a constant and potentially damaging pressure when applied. In some cases, a protective pack should be inserted between the retractor and tissues.

This category of retractor also incorporates the fixed position, multi-blade abdominal ring retractor systems.

Small self-retaining retractors

The smaller self-retaining retractors are generally used for cutaneous, superficial body wall or cavity (anal, vaginal and nasal) surgery. They come in several different patterns, most notably spring retractors, ratcheted retractors and screw-thread retractors.

Spring retractors

These are usually a thick wire-bodied retractor with teeth. The spring is a circle of wire at the base of the retractor that 'springs' the retractor out to a set distance. This type of retractor is only useful on fairly small wounds. The most common spring retractors have sharp teeth that are bent at right angles and embed within the tissues. This means that they should be used only on structures such as fat and muscle (Fig. 5.49).

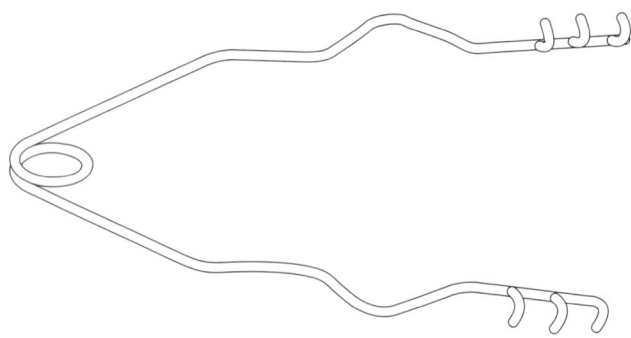

Fig. 5.49 Spring retractor

Ratcheted retractors

These retractors are usually ring-handled and may have a single hook, multiple teeth, flat blades or a combination of these with which to retract the tissues. One common pattern is the Weitlaner retractor (Fig. 5.50). They are of particular use in surgery on soft tissues, bones and fairly superficial structures including the anterior abdominal wall.

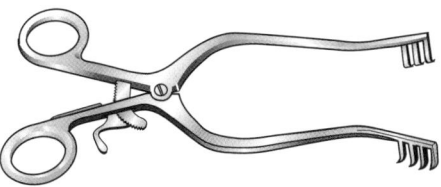

Fig. 5.50 Weitlaner retractor

Screw retractors

The most notable of this pattern is the Joll thyroid retractor (Fig. 5.51). Two clips, like towel clip heads, are used to grip the dermis of the neck skin and the retractor is then wound out to retract the edges. The duck-billed vaginal speculum and some types of anal retractor also have screw mechanisms that open the blades and retain the position. The screw mechanism allows a great deal of force to be applied between the blades, and great care must be taken not to over-retract. This is particularly important for anal retractors, where excessive retraction can damage the anal sphincter leading to incontinence.

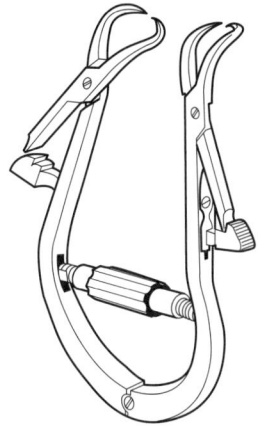

Fig. 5.51 Joll thyroid retractor

Large self-retaining retractors

The larger self-retaining retractors are used predominantly in deep-cavity surgery (abdomen and thorax), orthopaedics and various specific surgical procedures.

Screw retractors

In larger retractors, the screw describes the clamping mechanism for retaining the retractor's position, while the actual opening and positioning is done by hand. Take, for example, the Balfour–Doyen self-retaining retractor (Fig. 5.52). Two long shafts with interchangeable fenestrated blades lie parallel, one of them sliding away from the other on a double rail system. The distance between the two arms is

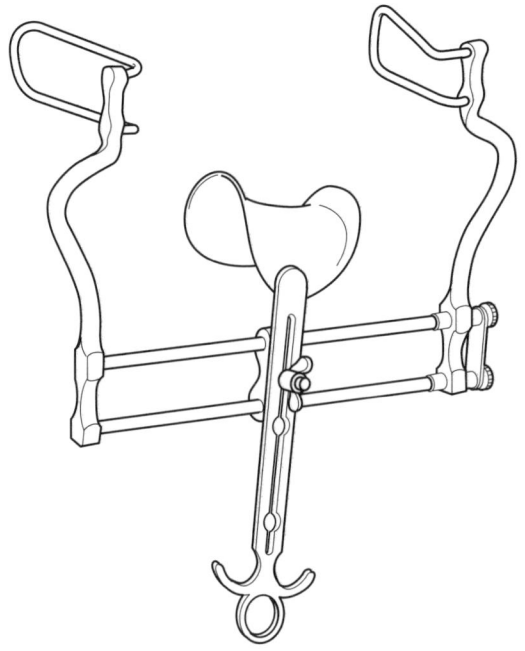

Fig. 5.52 Balfour–Doyen retractor

retained by a screw system or sometimes by friction alone. In between these blades a short body-wall retractor can be inserted to add pull at 90° to the major blades. This is also retained by a screw clamp system.

Crank retractors

Similar to the Balfour–Doyen, but without the extra blade, a Finichetto retractor has almost solid blades on the end of two heavy arms. A non-reverse rotating ratchet that must be actively cranked out to length, and actively reversed to release the tension, controls the distance between the two (Fig. 5.53). Because of its strength this retractor is used predominantly to spread ribs in thoracic surgery but may also be used in the abdomen. This type of retractor can cause considerable tissue damage if used without due care.

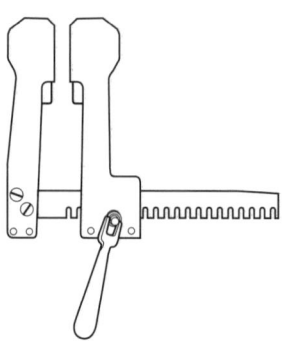

Fig. 5.53 Finichetto retractor

Ring-and-hook retractors

These retractors are usually part of a complete abdominal retractor system in which a solid 'ring' is placed around the abdominal incision and retractors are hooked onto this ring to provide exposure. The retractor blades may be of any type.

There are two distinct types. In the first, the ring is freestanding and so the direction of pull exerted by each retractor attachment must counterbalance an opposing one in order to keep the system centralised (Fig. 5.54). The Lonestar retractor employs a hinged ring of various dimensions to which tissue-holding hooks are anchored by elastic tubes. Variants of this system are also used in neurosurgery. In the second type, the apparatus is anchored to the operating table (Fig. 5.55). The ring (which may be complete or incomplete) is secured to a sterile attachment that in turn is fixed to the table but enters the sterile field. In this type, retractor attachments may be placed in any position.

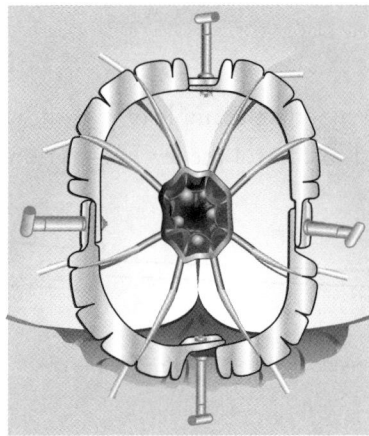

Fig. 5.54 Lonestar ring retractor system

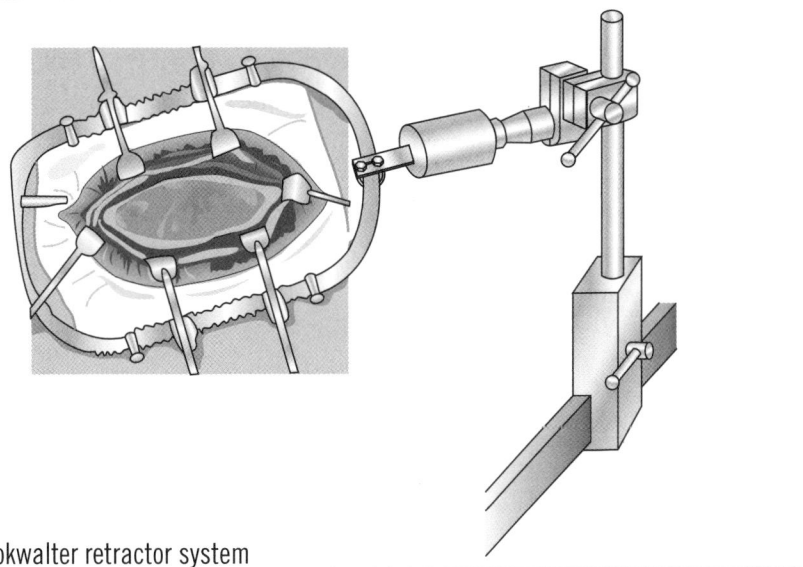

Fig. 5.55 Bookwalter retractor system

OTHER INSTRUMENTS

There are several instruments that fit into no particular category but are important requirements of many operative procedures. These include various designs of sucker, towel clips to hold the sterile drapes in place, and bowls in which to place fluids and objects.

Suckers

This group can be divided into the simple suckers in which all the material is sucked through a hole at the end of the single tube, and sump suckers in which air is mixed with the fluid to aid suction and prevent debris clogging the instrument.

Simple suckers

Small suckers

The typical ENT sucker is a perfect example of this. It has a small-calibre tube and a side hole that can be used to control the level of suction (Fig. 5.56).

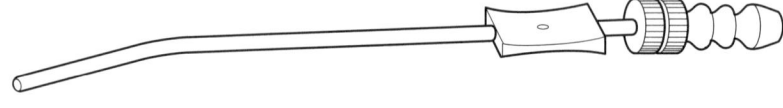

The American-pattern fine ENT-type sucker

Fig. 5.56 ENT sucker

Large suckers

The Yankauer sucker is longer and heavier than the ENT type, has an angled shaft and no side hole with which to control flow. The tip has a small screw-piece with four holes that limits what is sucked into the system. This is the most commonly used sucker in general surgery and comes in both metal and disposable plastic varieties (Fig. 5.57).

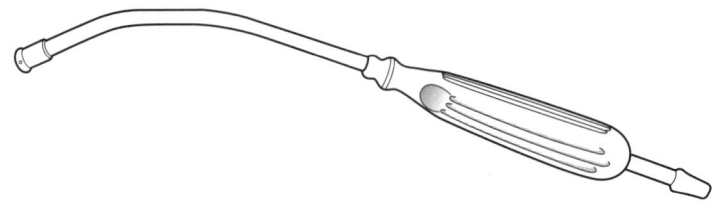

Fig. 5.57 Yankauer sucker

Sump suckers

This style of sucker has a simple central tube with a single end hole over that is screwed a sheath with multiple small perforations. This allows both fluid and air to be sucked into the gap between the two but prevents soft tissue or debris from occluding the system. Some variants have a button that turns the suction on and off as required. The Poole and Simpson–Smith suckers are two examples of this type (Fig. 5.58).

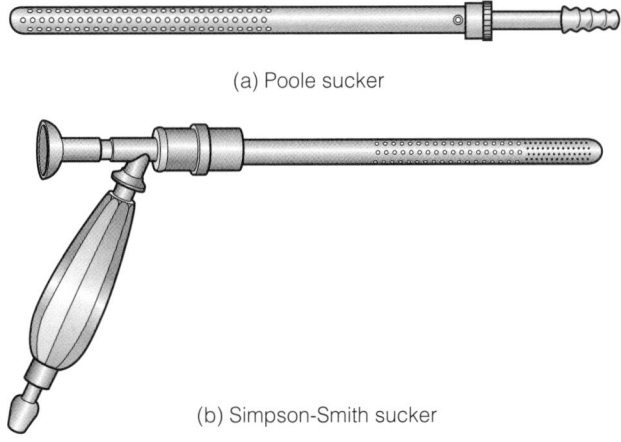

(a) Poole sucker

(b) Simpson-Smith sucker

Fig. 5.58 Sump suckers

Towel clips

These are used to hold drapes, instrument scabbards, equipment leads and tubing in place. The two commonly used towel clips are a ratcheted ring-handled instrument, and a spring type that needs to be squeezed open and then returns passively to the closed position. Either type may have sharp, pointed or blunt and flat tips (Fig. 5.59).

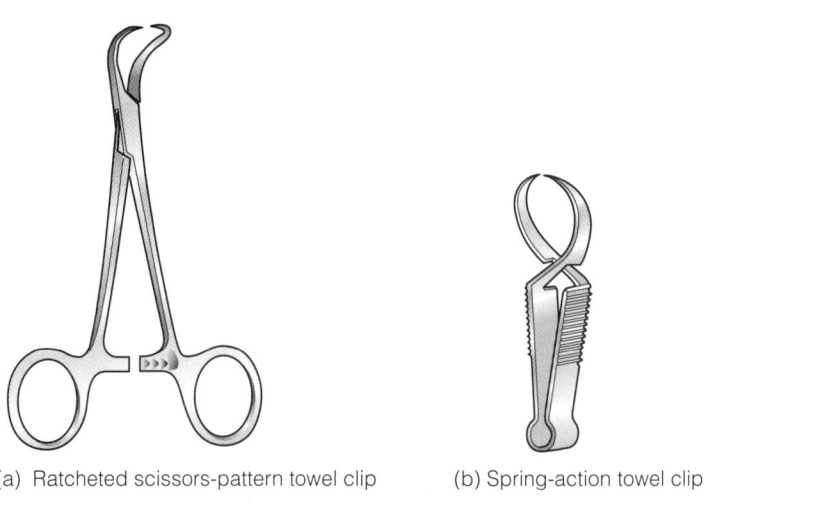

(a) Ratcheted scissors-pattern towel clip   (b) Spring-action towel clip

Fig. 5.59 Towel clips

Bowls

Every sterile set needs bowls and kidney dishes of various sizes. Their many uses include holding preparation solutions, passing sharps, holding wash or irrigation solutions, receiving specimens and collecting wound drainage (Fig. 5.60).

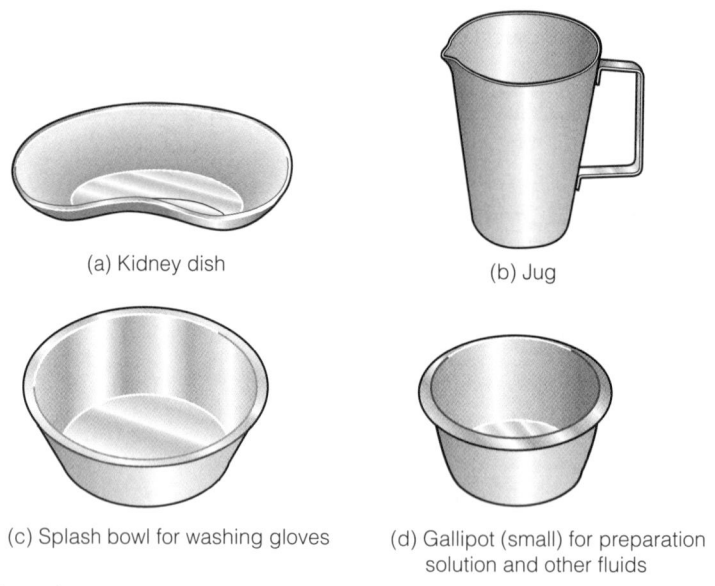

(a) Kidney dish

(b) Jug

(c) Splash bowl for washing gloves

(d) Gallipot (small) for preparation solution and other fluids

Fig. 5.60 Containers

ANCILLARY MECHANICAL DEVICES

A number of instruments are available to facilitate or automate tasks that surgeons previously performed manually. Most notable amongst these are haemostatic clip applicators, suturing devices, staplers and anastomotic devices.

Clip applicators

Titanium or polydioxanone clips ranging from 5 to 12 mm long can be used to secure small and medium blood vessels or other structures such as the cystic duct. They are placed, open, around the structure, and then crimped closed or locked with the applicator jaws. Manual loading applicators must be reloaded for each clip application. Automatic devices carry a cartridge of up to 20 clips and reload automatically after each application.

Filschie® Clip

The Fischie® Clip is a specialised clip designed to occlude the fallopian tube for female sterilisation. A sprung metal clasp locks a pair of silastic pads together on either side of the tube.

SUTURING DEVICES

Skin clip applicator

Sharp wire staples can be used instead of sutures to close a skin wound. Early versions of these included the Michel clip, which was placed using a manually loaded forceps. These are now obsolete, having been replaced by single-use multiple staple devices. Skin apposition and eversion must be achieved using thumb forceps prior to application of the staples.

Purse-string devices

The Furness clamp is a specialised bowel clamp with corrugated jaws that allows placement of a purse-string suture using a straight needle. A single-use purse-string applicator device is available that secures a purse-string suture around an open end of bowel, using staples to hold the thread in place.

STAPLERS

Linear staplers

Originally designed to divide bowel without spillage of luminal contents, staplers are finding an increasing range of application, limited only by access and imagination.

Transverse staplers place 2–4 rows of staples perpendicular to the axis of the device, and are used primarily for closing bowel. Linear cutting staplers place 4–6 rows of staples along a 30–90 mm line and cut between the two central rows. They are very useful for dividing bowel or bulky tissue pedicles (such as the uterine pedicle), securing haemostasis and tissue division rapidly. A wide range of models is available for open and laparoscopic use.

Anastomotic (circular cutting) staplers

Originally developed in the 1970s by a Russian surgeon for rectal anastomosis, the 'SPTU' has spawned a generation of circular staplers, which have found wide application in colorectal and gastrointestinal surgery. They are designed for intraluminal use, to construct a circular anastomosis between two ends of bowel. Open bowel ends are secured around the shaft, and a circle of staples 2–3 rows deep is applied between the bowel ends. A circular knife cuts out the centre of the tissue secured around the shaft, inside the staple line, to create a new aperture. A modified circular stapler is used to perform a haemorrhoidectomy. Devices are produced in diameters ranging from 25 to 33 mm.

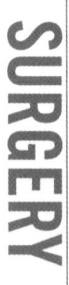

Table 5.1 Names behind the instruments

Instrument	Name and description
Adson dissecting forceps	Alfred Washington Adson, 1887–1951 Pioneer in neurosurgery at the Mayo Clinic, Rochester Minnesota. He described the sign (Adson's sign) in the thoracic syndrome where the radial pulse becomes obliterated when the head is turned to the affected side.
Allis tissue forceps	Oscar Huntingdon Allis, 1836–1931 Graduated from Jefferson Medical College in 1866. Orthopaedic surgeon and one of the original staff surgeons at the Presbyterian Hospital, Philadelphia. Introduced his tissue forceps in 1883.
Babcock tissue forceps	William Wayne Babcock, 1872–1963 Surgeon at the Samaritan and American Stomach Hospital, Philadelphia. Described a new operative technique, the Babcock operation, for thoracic aneurysm in 1926, and designed a surgical method for abdominal aneurysm repair in 1929.
Brown–Adson dissecting forceps	Thomas Brown of Dublin Founded the Brown Institute of the University of London that was destroyed in an air raid in 1944.
Chitwood–DeBakey forceps	Randolph Chitwood Jr Professor and chairperson, Department of Surgery, Center for Minimally Invasive and Robotic Surgery, Brody School of Medicine, East Carolina University, USA.
Crile forceps	George Crile, 1864–1943 Chief surgeon, Cleveland Clinic, Ohio. He carried on his father's famous thyroid clinic. One of the founders of the American College of Surgeons in 1912. Elected honorary Fellow of the Royal College of Surgeons of England in 1913.
DeBakey forceps, vascular needle holder, vascular clamps	Michael Ellis DeBakey, 1908– Of Lebanese extraction, born Michel Dabaghi, he graduated from Tulane University in New Orleans. While a medical student at Tulane he invented the roller pump used for heart–lung bypass. During military service in World War II, developed the concept of the Mobile Army Surgical Hospitals (MASH) for which he was awarded the Legion of Honour in 1945. From 1948 he was chairperson of the Department of Surgery at Baylor University, Houston, Texas.

He developed Dacron vascular grafts, devised several procedures for aortic aneurysm repair, performed the first carotid endarterectomy in 1953 and the first successful aorto-coronary artery bypass with autogenous vein graft in 1964. In 1968 he led a team in a historic multiple transplantation of heart, lung and kidneys from one donor to four recipients. At the age of 97 he suffered an aortic dissection and became the oldest person to undergo the operation for which he was responsible. He survived and was still alive in his hundredth year at the time this book went to print.

Durham retractor	Arthur Edward Durham, 1834–1895 Pioneering neurosurgeon and Professor of Clinical Surgery and Dean of the School of Medicine at the University of Pennsylvania. In 1919, he succeeded in cutting the sensory root of the trigeminal nerve for the relief of pain in tic douloureux.
Gillies forceps, skin hook	Sir Harold Delf Gillies, 1882–1960 New Zealand-born pioneer in plastic surgery, renowned for reconstructive and burns surgery during the two world wars. Later a consultant surgeon at St Bartholomew's Hospital, London.
Gwillim clamp	Calvert Merton Gwillim, 1899–1972 Born in Ceylon, schooled in South Wales, graduated in medicine in 1922 at St Bartholomew's Hospital, London. Devised a method for vaginal repair and hysterectomy.
Halsted mosquito forceps	William S Halsted, 1852–1922 General surgeon at Johns Hopkins, Baltimore. Popularised the radical 'Halsted' mastectomy, and pioneered work on the use of cocaine in local anaesthesia.
Hartmann forceps	Arthur Hartmann, 1849–1931 Otorhinolaryngologist from Berlin. Devised a number of instruments and invented the audiometer.
Jarit needle forceps	Jarit is a private American instrument company manufacturing instruments in Tuttlingen, Germany.

STERILE INSTRUMENTS

CHAPTER 5

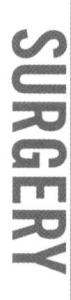

Table 5.1 Names behind the instruments *(cont.)*

Kocher clamps	Emil Theodor Kocher, 1841–1917
	General surgeon, Professor of Surgery at University of Bern Surgical Clinic, Switzerland. Devised 'Kocker's incisions' for thyroidectomy and cholecystectomy, a technique for duodenal mobilisation, and a manoeuvre for reduction of a dislocated shoulder. First to perform thyroidectomy for thyrotoxicosis. Awarded Nobel Prize in 1909 for his work on the physiology, pathology and surgery of the thyroid gland.
Langenbeck retractor	Bernhard von Langenbeck, 1810–1887
	Professor of Surgery and leading surgeon in Berlin, pupil of Theodor Billroth.
Mayo–Hegar needle holder	William Worral Mayo.
	General surgeon and father of surgeon brothers William and Charles, with whom he opened St Mary's Hospital, Rochester, Minnesota in 1889. This 13-bed hospital went on to become the Mayo Clinic.
McIndoe scissors	Sir Archibald Hector McIndoe, 1900–1960
	New Zealand-born plastic surgeon, cousin of Sir Harold Gillies with whom he worked in London. Postgraduate studies at Mayo Clinic. Built up famous plastic surgical unit at Queen Victoria Hospital, East Grinstead, treating burned RAF airmen. Described techniques for hypospadias repair and vaginoplasty.
Moynihan gall-bladder forceps	Lord Berkeley A Moynihan, 1865–1936
	General Surgeon, Leeds Royal Infirmary.
Pott scissors	Percival Pott, 1714–1788
	Obtained Grand Diploma of the Barber Surgeon's Company (now RCS) in 1749, and became surgeon at St Bartholomew's Hospital. Pioneered the lecture–demonstration style of teaching. Described 'Pott's' ankle fracture– dislocation.
Sims speculum	James Marion Sims, 1813–1883
	Surgeon, Alabama, was working in the UK when he devised his speculum and described the 'Sim's position' for vaginal examination and surgery. Established the State Hospital for Women in New York in 1853.

FURTHER READING

Friedin J, Marshall V. Illustrated Guide to Surgical Practice. Melbourne: Churchill Livingstone, 1984. Chap. 4, The Operation.

McGregor A, McGregor I. Fundamental Techniques of Plastic Surgery. 9th ed. Edinburgh: Churchill Livingstone, 1995. Chap. 3, Free Skin Grafts.

Thompson RVS. Primary Repair of Soft Tissue Injuries, Melbourne: Melbourne University Press, 1969. Chap. 3, Basic Instruments for Outpatient Reparative Surgery.

CHAPTER SIX

A GUIDE TO SUTURE MATERIALS AND SURGICAL NEEDLES

The three Fates were Clotho (who held the distaff), Lachesis (who spun the thread of life), and Atropos (who cut it off when life was ended).

E. Cobham Brewer, *Dictionary of Phrase and Fable: Fates* (1894)

INTRODUCTION

Common to all surgical specialties is the use of threads for suturing (sewing) and ligating (tying and securing). Over the centuries, many materials have been used for these purposes, including such unusual items as giant ant heads (the bodies having been ripped off after the bite had closed the wound), vegetable fibres wound figure-of-eight around giant thorns passed through both wound edges, and sterilised barbed wire in Japanese prisoner-of-war camps.

Modern sutures consist of a range of highly refined materials, some designed specifically for suturing. Most are presented in sterile packaging for single-patient use. Constant demand on the suture industry for improved performance, using better and cheaper materials, has led to huge advances in suture and needle technology. Organic materials such as catgut, linen and silk have been supplanted by synthetic materials that are more consistent and reliable, and cause much less tissue reaction.

SURGICAL NEEDLES

Needles are an integral part of suture technology, and an understanding of the basic concepts of their design will facilitate appropriate use. Most needles are made from corrosion-resistant stainless steel wire. The size, shape and curve, tip, and cross-sectional profile are selected according to the requisite function. Needles should be as thin as possible to minimise tissue trauma and drag, while being rigid enough to penetrate the tissue without bending, and ductile enough to deform without breaking. The point must be sharp enough to reliably penetrate tissues and large enough to carry the suture with minimal tissue trauma. The needle must have a three-dimensional shape that permits secure handling within the needle holder, without the risk of slippage and subsequent tissue trauma (Table 6.1).

Table 6.1	Desirable properties of a surgical needle
1.	Corrosion-resistant material, e.g. stainless steel
2.	Rigid enough to penetrate tissue without bending
3.	Ductile enough to deform without breaking
4.	Slim enough to cause minimal damage to tissues
5.	Wide enough to draw the thread though tissue without undue abrasion
6.	Sharp enough to penetrate tissues easily
7.	A method of thread attachment, e.g. eye or swage
8.	Stable when grasped or used in an instrument

Source: Compilation assisted by information from the *Wound Closure Manual*, Ethicon Inc, 1994.

Anatomy of a surgical needle

A standard set of terms is used to describe the common features of a surgical needle. *Needle point* is self-explanatory. Suture thread is attached to the needle by a *swage*, a pre-drilled hole at the base of the needle into which the thread is bonded. *Chord length* is the straight-line distance from the point to the swage. *Needle length* is the distance from point to swage when measured around the needle's outer surface. *Radius* is the distance from the centre of a circle, described by the arc of the needle, to the needle itself. *Needle diameter* is the thickness of a needle at any part of the needle body (Fig. 6.1).

Surgical needle characteristics

The most important characteristics of surgical needles are:
- shape and curvature
- needle length and diameter
- tip and cross-sectional shape
- attachment to the suture material.

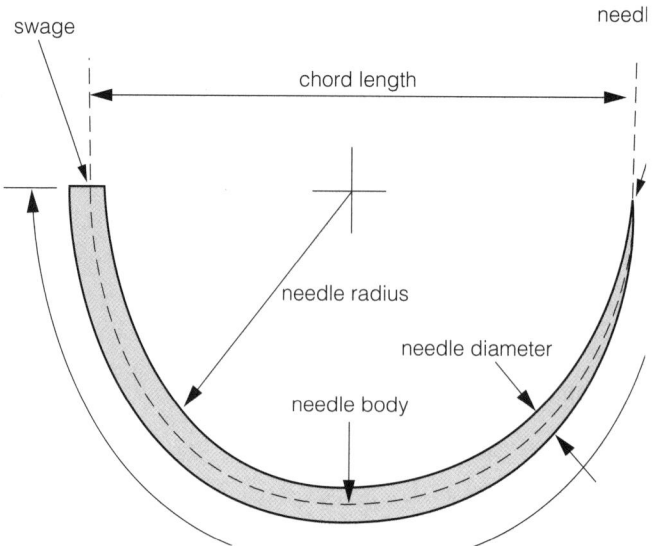

Fig. 6.1 Characteristics of a surgical needle

Shape and curvature

The shape and curvature of a needle will often dictate its function. Certain specialised needles are used for specific circumstances, for example J-shaped (Fig. 6.2).
- 1/4 circle: Ophthalmic and microsurgery
- 3/8 circle: General use in all tissues
- 1/2 circle: General use in all tissues
- 5/8 circle: CVS and 'cavities' (oral, nasal, pelvis, umbilicus, etc.)
- Straight: General use (but discouraged as hand-held)
- J-shaped: Similar to 5/8 (femoral hernia).

Needle length and diameter

The rigidity, ductility and strength of the wire used to make a needle of a particular length dictate the diameter required. The length of a needle depends on the thickness of tissue through which it will be driven. The diameter of a needle should match its functional requirements, its length and the suture it must carry. In general, long needles made from heavier gauges of wire are used for fascia and skin closure, while shorter and finer needles are used in visceral, vessel or fine-structure surgery. It is important to select a needle-holding forceps of appropriate weight for the diameter of the needle.

Tip and cross-section

The point of a needle is that part from the extreme tip to the maximum cross-sectional diameter. Beyond the point, the body may retain the same shape or change. The main point types are cutting, reverse cutting, taperpoint, tapercut and blunt.

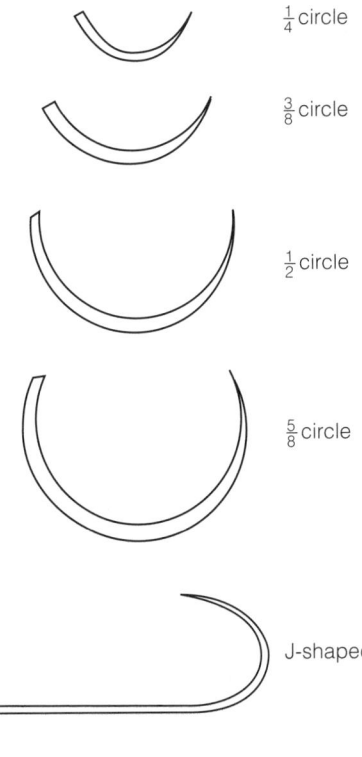

$\frac{1}{4}$ circle

$\frac{3}{8}$ circle

- 3/8 and 1/2 circle are by far the commonest patterns used.
- J-shaped needles have special applications in deep cavities.
- Straight (hand-held) needles have not been shown as their use is now generally discouraged.

$\frac{1}{2}$ circle

$\frac{5}{8}$ circle

J-shaped

Fig. 6.2 Common needle shapes and curves

Conventional cutting and *reverse cutting* needles are sharp-pointed needles with cutting edges on a triangular cross-section. They cut through tissue and so are used mainly on skin, periosteum, tendons and sclera. The upwards-facing cutting edge on the conventional cutting needle gives it a tendency to incise upwards into tissue when using a standard suturing technique; this may result in sutures cutting through the tissue being repaired. The reverse-cutting needle, which has the cutting edge on the outer curve, presents a flat edge upwards, and so is less likely to cut out. The latter is the more commonly used of these two (Fig. 6.3). There are several other variations of the cutting point tip, such as spatula, diamond and lancet points. These all have specialised functions and will not be dealt with here.

Taperpoint needles have a round body that tapers to a sharp point. They initially penetrate with this sharp tip, but then push (or split) the tissues apart with the round body. This works well with viscera and most fascia; however, tough, densely fibrous tissues such as skin, tendon and scar are less amenable to this type of needle. Although taperpoint needles will penetrate these tissues, the extra force required, and the resultant tearing of tissues, make them a vastly inferior choice.

Tapercut needles are a variation on the tapered needle, with a cutting trocar point and tapering round body. Tapercut needles penetrate denser fascia more easily than

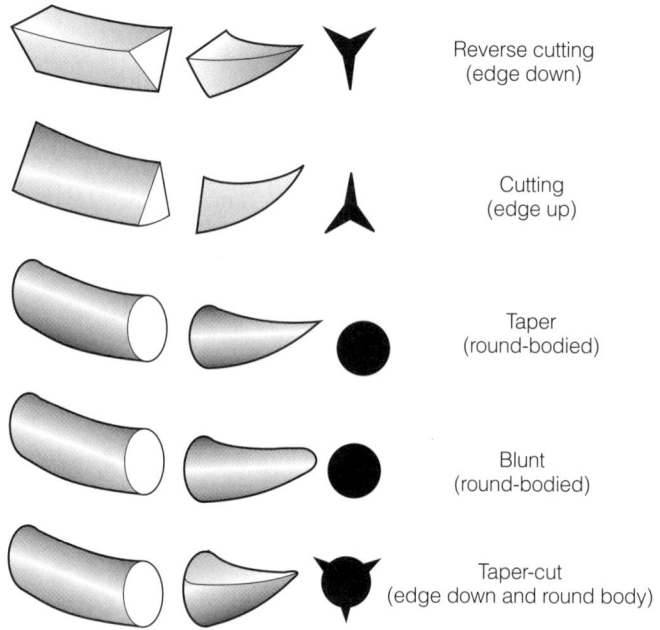

Fig. 6.3 Shapes of needle points and body shapes

taperpoint needles, but because they do not have cutting edges, they do not cut out as easily as cutting needles.

Blunt needles are a variation of the taperpoint needle; they were developed to reduce the chance of needlestick injury. They have a standard tapering circular body cross-section with a point that is gently rounded at the tip. As this is quite fine it will still penetrate fascia easily but is *far less likely to penetrate glove material or skin*. The round-needle body then passes as a normal taperpoint needle by splitting tissues. Blunt needles are particularly useful in liver repair and vascular regions where they will slide past (not penetrate) vessels, and in safer fascial closure with respect to the potential for needlestick injuries.

Needle bodies may retain the same cross-section for their entire length, or may flatten out on the inner and outer curves to facilitate grasping by a needle holder. Some needles have roughening or grooves on them to further improve this grip, or may be coated with silicone or other materials for smoother penetration.

Attachment to suture materials

Needles usually come with threads attached. This was not always so, as the technology to allow this has only been developed in the last few decades. Traditionally all needles were eyed, and the threads were inserted by the scrub nurse prior to use. Eyed needles are still manufactured but are rarely used.

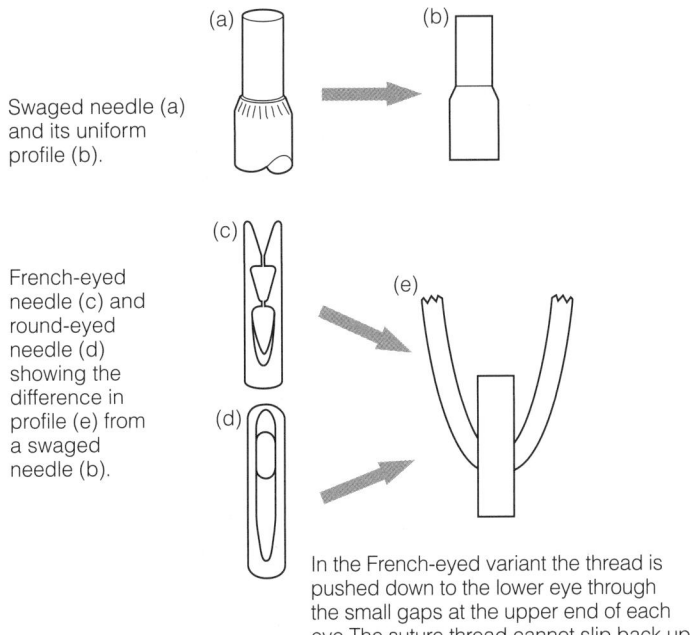

Swaged needle (a) and its uniform profile (b).

French-eyed needle (c) and round-eyed needle (d) showing the difference in profile (e) from a swaged needle (b).

In the French-eyed variant the thread is pushed down to the lower eye through the small gaps at the upper end of each eye. The suture thread cannot slip back up

Fig. 6.4 Swages and eyes

Swaging may be accomplished in two ways (Fig 6.4). In the first, a hole is drilled in the end of the needle, the suture is inserted into this and the end is pressed in (crimped) on four sides to secure it. In the second method, a split is made down the centre of the needle and the suture is inserted. The two sides are then crimped together to hold the suture in place.

There are several advantages to swaging. It reduces tissue trauma, because the thread is virtually the same size as the needle (rather than having a double thickness of thread through an eyed needle). This reduces the chance of leakage at anastomotic sites, particularly in vascular surgery, as the thread fills the entire needle hole. Swaged needles are more convenient and safer because there is no need for the scrub nurse to thread the needle.

SUTURE SIZES

The sizing of sutures initially followed a pattern set by the United States Pharmacopeia (USP standard) (Table 6.2), a standards organisation. This classification is based on the minimum and maximum diameters of the material in inches, and the minimum knot pull strength. Different standards were developed for organic absorbable sutures and other (non-absorbable and synthetic absorbable) sutures. An alternative European Pharmacopoeia (EP) system—also known as the metric system —is based on millimetre thicknesses and different knot pull tests (Fig 6.5).

The most commonly used suture sizes are in the range of 5/0 to I. Tissues that are thicker, or more collagen rich, require larger sutures and heavier needles (Table 6.2). Finer sutures, under 6/0 in size (about the diameter of a human hair), often require magnification with loupes or a microscope to be used accurately. They are used mostly for microvascular work or plastic microsurgery.

Table 6.2 | Suture selection

Size	Comparison	Uses
12/0 (to 7/0)	Quarter the size of a human hair	Exclusively microsurgical
6/0	Human hair size. Generally the smallest suture used with naked vision	Face, blood vessels
5/0		Face, neck, blood vessels
4/0		Mucosa, neck, hands, limbs, tendons, blood vessels
3/0		Limbs, trunk, gut, blood vessels
2/0		Trunk, fascia, stomach, viscera, blood vessels
0–1	Small pencil lead	Abdominal wall closure and other heavy fascial uses

SUTURE MATERIALS

The main properties of each suture material can be classified within three broad categories:
- the fabrication material
- the construction of the thread, and
- the pattern of breakdown in tissues.

Suture materials may be a natural substance (silk, linen or catgut), metal (stainless steel) or synthetic polymer. The first synthetic polymer was nylon, but there is now a wide range of polymers with different properties used for the manufacture of sutures. Sutures are constructed either as a single, solid monofilament or as a twisted or braided multifilament strand. The breakdown characteristics of a suture material are broadly absorbable or non-absorbable, although there is some overlap, with some substances (such as silk) eventually undergoing degradation in tissues.

Braided sutures have more drag through tissues, and are more likely catch or to cut out. Some manufacturers apply a lubricant coating to reduce this problem. Monofilament sutures slide more easily through tissues, and excite far less tissue reaction than multifilament sutures. Infection and scarring are much reduced with the

Percentage volumetric reduction with decreased size of suture

USP	EP	mm	% reduction
3	6	0.60–0.69	
2	5	0.50–0.59	28
1	4	0.40–0.49	33
0	3.5	0.30–0.39	31
2/0	3	0.25–0.29	27
3/0	2	0.20–0.24	51
4/0	1.5	0.15–0.19	40
5/0	1	0.10–0.14	49
6/0	0.7	0.07–0.099	54
7/0	0.5	0.05–0.069	50
8/0	0.4	0.04–0.049	44
9/0	0.3	0.03–0.039	40
10/0	0.2	0.02–0.029	50

Fig. 6.5 Relative suture sizes and reductions

use of monofilament sutures because they do not harbour the micro-organisms that collect in the interstices of a multifilament suture (Fig 6.6). Some braided absorbable sutures are impregnated with antibiotics to reduce the infection risk.

Other attributes of sutures that may influence selection include the initial tensile strength, the rate of strength degradation, stretch, handling qualities, knotting characteristics, and the tissue reaction to the material. When used for apposition rather than tension, the required suture strength is often overestimated. Sutures are more likely to break at knots than elsewhere, and correct knot technique is at least as important as the tensile strength of the suture itself. A certain amount of stretch in

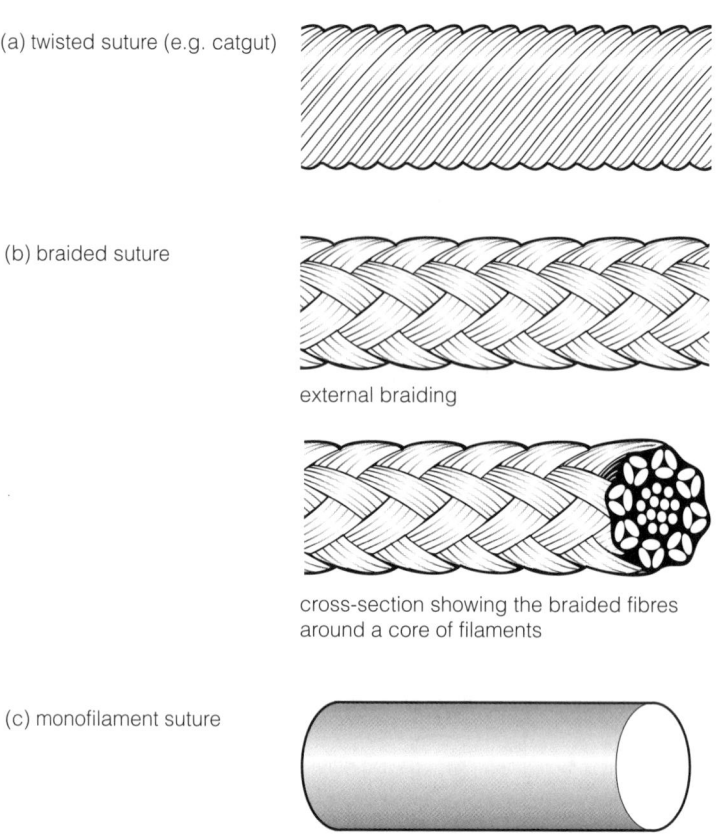

(a) twisted suture (e.g. catgut)

(b) braided suture

external braiding

cross-section showing the braided fibres
around a core of filaments

(c) monofilament suture

Fig. 6.6 Suture materials

the suture material is often an advantage, as it allows for tissue oedema and subsequent resolution of swelling. Some threads, particularly monofilaments, exhibit significant 'memory' properties that can make their handling more difficult.

In general, absorbable sutures leave no residue. Such sutures are used on tissues where healing will take place quickly, and continued tissue strength will not depend on the strength of the suture material e.g. subcutaneous tissue, ties on vessels etc. Material that absorbs slowly is required for tissues that are slow to heal, while in situations where long-term suture strength is required, a non-absorbable material is appropriate. The need for non-absorbable sutures was overemphasised in the past. Their knots have a propensity to erode adjacent tissue and may cause suture sinuses if close to the skin. Cumulative experience with slowly absorbable material such as polydioxanone has demonstrated that non-absorbable sutures are not usually necessary for fascial closure (such as in the abdominal fascia). Where reduced tissue reaction or avoiding infection is desirable, such as in skin or deep fascial closure, a monofilament should be used.

PROPERTIES OF COMMON SUTURE MATERIALS

Polyamides (nylon)

Synthetic, multi/monofilament, non-absorbable

Nylon is usually a monofilament but may be braided. It has poor handling and knotting qualities and therefore requires multiple throws and knot burying. It has a strong 'memory' and some loss of strength over time, but minimal absorption or breakdown. When used for abdominal fascial closure or hernia surgery, there is a small risk of suture sinuses developing due to erosion of knot tails through the skin. Nylon is available in many sizes (10/0 to 2) and virtually all needle types.

Common uses

- Fascial closure
- Skin closure
- Hernia repair
- Vascular surgery
- Neurosurgery.

Polypropylene

Synthetic, monofilament, non-absorbable

Another non-reactive polymer, with minimal tissue reaction, polypropylene and related formulations, polyvinylidine and hexafluoropropylene–VDF have high tensile strength like nylon, with smoother handling, less weakening and far less memory. These properties make general use and knotting easier. They also have good knot security and lose virtually no strength over time. Available in 10/0 to 2 on all needle types, polypropylene is a popular suture choice.

Common uses
- Fascial closure
- Vascular anastomosis
- Subcuticular (skin) closure
- Tendon repairs
- Ophthalmology
- Neurosurgery.

Polybutester, polyether

Synthetic, monofilament, non-absorbable

These polymers are very supple with good handling and tying characteristics. They excite minimal reaction in tissues. They have low tissue drag, good knot rundown and first-throw security. They have high tensile strength and permanent tissue retention. They have marked elasticity and recoil to original size without permanent distortion or damage. Products are available in 10/0 to 2 on a full range of needles. Some have a lubricant coating to further reduce tissue drag.

Common uses
- Skin closure (plastics)
- Ophthalmology
- Fascial closure (general).

Polyester

Synthetic, multi/monofilament, non-absorbable

Yet another polymer, it has high and permanent tensile strength and excites minimal tissue reaction. Most companies have a variety. It has excellent handling and tying characteristics with good knot security after 5–6 throws. In monofilament form there is some gauged elastic recoil. To improve tissue run, some presentations of the braided form are coated with silicone or teflon. The fibre is also woven into vascular grafts. Comes in sizes 6/0 to 1 in all needle types.

Common uses
- Cardiac valve surgery
- Tendon suture
- Orthopaedics
- Ophthalmology.

Polyglycolic acid (PGA)

Synthetic, multifilament, absorbable

A polymer of glycolic acid, the monofilament form is too brittle for use, so the extruded filaments are stretched and braided to attain high tensile strength. PGA is stronger, loses less strength in knotting and excites less inflammatory reaction than catgut. It is absorbed by hydrolysis in 10–90 days in a predictable and uniform way. Suture strength is lost over 3–4 weeks.

Tissue drag and abrasion due to braiding are alleviated by coating the suture with a dry lubricant but this reduces knot security. As there is no slip in knotting, the first throw of each knot must be placed with precise tension and accuracy. It is produced in sizes 5/0 to 2 and is available on a wide range of needles. It replaces catgut in many situations, but retains strength longer and so has several other applications.

Common uses

- GI anastomosis
- Muscle and fascial closures
- Subcuticular skin closure (undyed suture).

Polyglactin 910

Synthetic, multifilament, absorbable

A relative of PGA, polyglactin 910 is a copolymer of glycolide and lactide. The braided filaments may be impregnated with the antibacterial agent triclosan, and are coated with a mix of polymer and calcium stearate to reduce drag. Absorption, by hydrolysis, commences at around 20–40 days and is complete by 60–90 days. Strength is lost over a 3–4 week period. Strength and knotting are similar to PGA and the material evokes a similar, minor, inflammatory reaction. An alternative formulation allows much more rapid hydrolysis, with strength retention for 7–10 days and complete absorption in 40–60 days. It comes in a wide range of sizes (8/0 to 2) and needles.

Common uses

- GI anastomosis
- Muscle and fascial closure
- Subcuticular skin closure.

Trimethylene/glycolic acid

Synthetic, monofilament, absorbable

This monofilament polymer is synthetic, non-antigenic and non-pyrogenic with a high tensile strength. There is minimal tissue reaction or patient discomfort. Non-enzymatic hydrolysis is uniform in all patients and is generally completed in 180–210 days. Strength reduces by 50% over 5–6 weeks in a predictable pattern, giving it good long-term wound support characteristics. It is available as 7/0 to 2 in a full range of needles.

Common uses

- GI anastomosis
- Fascial closure
- Caesarean section.

Polydioxanone

Synthetic, monofilament, absorbable

This is a polyester polymer heat-extruded into monofilaments. Impregnation with triclosan antibacterial is an option. Although absorbable, strength at implantation is very high. There is little pyrogenicity or antigenicity and tissue reaction is minimal. Absorption by hydrolysis starts at 90 days and is completed by 6 months. It exhibits good handling, and usually requires four throws to knot securely. It is useful in slow-healing areas, but local infection markedly accelerates loss of strength. It can also be made into clips and staples that are absorbed and therefore do not affect magnetic resonance imaging. The suture is available in 6/0 to 2 on a full needle range.

Common uses
- GI anastomosis
- Fascial closure
- Subcuticular (skin) closure.

Poligecaprone 25

Synthetic, monofilament, absorbable

This absorbable synthetic is a copolymer of glycolide and caprolactone. Antibacterial coating may be added. It has good tissue run characteristics, being a monofilament, and handles and ties well. The polymer is non-antigenic and pyrogenic with little tissue reaction. Its absorption profile is predictable (fully absorbed in 90–120 days) and all tensile strength is lost by 21 days. It is available in sizes 5/0 to 1 in a range of needles.

Common uses
- Subcuticular (skin) suture
- Ligation
- Subcutaneous suture.

Stainless steel

Natural, multi/monofilament, non-absorbable

A rarely used suture, it retains great strength and excites minimal response. Tissue passage is good but 'knot tying' is extremely difficult (and in fact, stainless steel is most commonly twisted together and bent over). This is the strongest of all suture materials, and comes in sizes 4/0 to 7 on a limited range of needles.

Common uses
- Sternal closure
- Hernia (Shouldice repair)
- Contaminated wounds
- Orthopaedics.

Catgut

Natural, multifilament, absorbable

Catgut is effectively obsolete in modern surgical practice. It is produced from sheep or cow intestinal submucosa, which is split, twisted, dried and polished to a monofilament profile. It may be chrome tanned ('chromic') to delay absorption. Catgut is digested by proteolytic enzymes from phagocytic cells in 80–120 days but there is little tensile strength left by 10 days. This loss may be even quicker (24 hours) when used in stomach or ileum. Chromic gut takes about twice as long to lose strength. Tissue reaction to catgut is prominent. While a wide range of sizes and needles are available, most must be stored in a fluid medium or the suture dries out and becomes rigid. Marked memory, a tendency to fray, and difficulty in tying when dry all contribute to the decline in use given the newer, better alternatives.

Common uses

- All but abandoned.

Silk, cotton, linen

Natural, multifilament, non-absorbable

Less commonly used now, due to the available alternatives. They are easy to handle but silk loses strength by enzymatic digestion as it, unlike cotton and linen, is a protein. All three excite marked inflammatory reactions.

Common uses

- All but abandoned.

CHAPTER SEVEN
ENERGY SOURCES IN SURGERY

I have witnessed the tremendous energy of the masses. On this foundation it is possible to accomplish any task whatsoever.

Mao Zedong (1893–1976), September 1958

INTRODUCTION

A vast array of surgical instruments has been designed to exploit the unique tissue effects of various energy sources. An understanding of the principles underlying the physics and mechanism of tissue effects is important if such surgical devices are to be used safely and effectively.

ELECTROSURGICAL DIATHERMY

Introduction

By far the most common and important energy source in surgery is electrosurgical diathermy. This is most frequently used in operations to achieve haemostasis by coagulating small blood vessels. It can also be used to cut tissue, or to perform a combination of both of these effects.

History

The first surgical diathermy machine capable of both cutting and coagulation was designed by William Bovie, a Harvard physicist, and Harvey Cushing, a neurosurgeon. This machine was first used at Peter Bent Brigham Hospital in 1926 by Harvey Cushing. Ironically, Bovie sold the patent to his machine for one dollar and reputedly died a poor man. His important contribution to the development of electrosurgical diathermy in surgery is reflected in the fact that even modern electrosurgical machines are sometimes still referred to as 'Bovies', particularly in the United States.

Principles

An electrosurgical generator provides the source of the electron flow and voltage. An electrical circuit is created whereby current flows from the generator, through an active electrode into the patient's tissues, and back to the generator through a return electrode (also known as the 'passive' or 'indifferent' electrode, and sometimes incorrectly referred to as the 'ground plate'). In *monopolar diathermy* the return electrode is located away from the site of surgery (Fig. 7.1). The patient's body actually forms part of the circuit. It is impedance to the passage of current through the tissues that causes heating. The area of contact between the return electrode and the patient is very large, resulting in low impedance, low current density and negligible heating at this site. At the active electrode (e.g. pencil diathermy), a high current passes through a small area. This high current density causes intense heating that coagulates or cuts tissue (Fig. 7.2).

If the patient is actually part of this circuit then why is he or she not electrocuted? Late in the nineteenth century, French physiologist Jacques-Arsène d'Arsonval showed that neuromuscular stimulation and risk of electrocution mainly occurs when alternating current below 100 kHz is passed through the body. Electrosurgical generators convert 50 Hz alternating current into safer high frequencies (300–3800 kHz) to achieve cutting and diathermy with minimal neuromuscular stimulation. Such

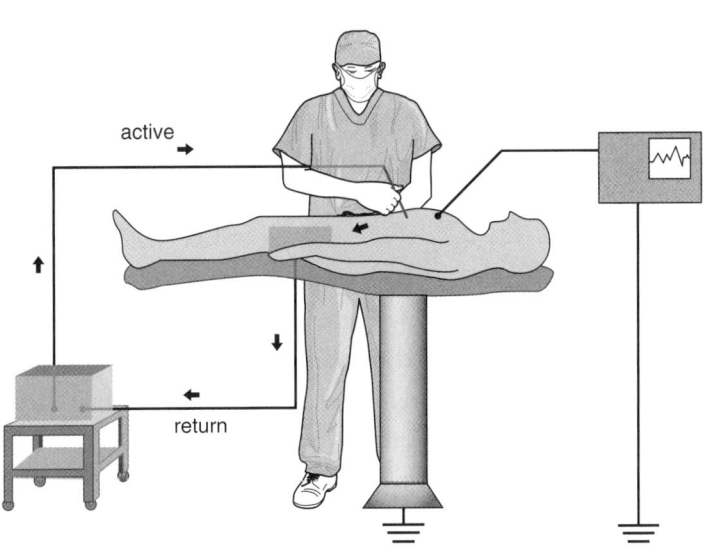

Fig. 7.1 Monopolar electrosurgical diathermy

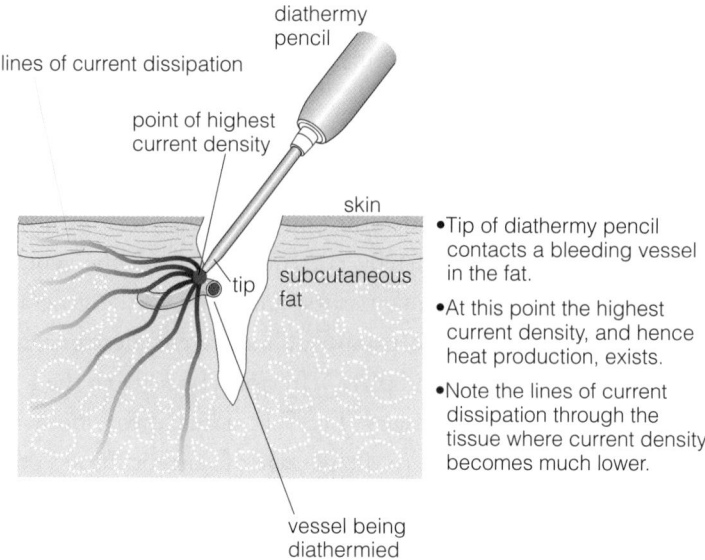

- Tip of diathermy pencil contacts a bleeding vessel in the fat.
- At this point the highest current density, and hence heat production, exists.
- Note the lines of current dissipation through the tissue where current density becomes much lower.

Fig 7.2a Dissipation of diathermy current

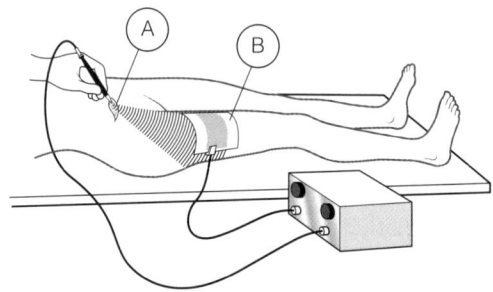

Current flows from the diathermy electrode at A to the plate at B and back through the machine. In this way the patient is an active part of the circuit.

Fig 7.2b High current density at A causes intense heating, whereas the same current returning through a large surface area return electrode at B results in a low current density and minimal heating

frequencies lie in the radiofrequency (RF) electromagnetic spectrum and therefore electrosurgical generators are sometimes referred to as 'radiofrequency devices'. The waveform of this current is altered to achieve varying tissue effects of cutting and coagulation (Fig. 7.3). These waveforms are adjustable on the electrosurgical machine, and the surgeon can activate 'cut' or 'coagulation' modes by depressing the appropriate finger- or foot-operated switch. The 'cut' current is typically a continuous waveform, whereas the 'coagulation' current uses higher voltages delivered in short bursts. By adjusting power output and peak voltage it is possible to combine cut and coagulation waveform characteristics into 'blended' current.

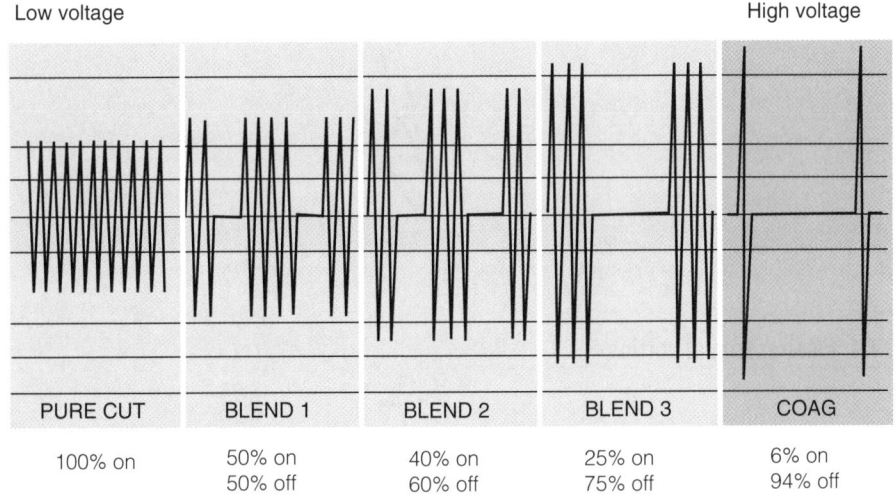

Low voltage   High voltage

| PURE CUT | BLEND 1 | BLEND 2 | BLEND 3 | COAG |
| 100% on | 50% on 50% off | 40% on 60% off | 25% on 75% off | 6% on 94% off |

Fig. 7.3 Electrosurgical waveforms

It should be noted that the different waveforms only change the rate at which heat is produced at the site of the active electrode. If heat is produced rapidly, then tissue vaporisation and consequent cutting will result; whereas if heat is produced more slowly, coagulation will occur (Table 7.1).

Table 7.1   Thermal effects on tissue

Approximate tissue temperature °C	Biological effect
37–60	Warming and protein denaturation
> 60	Coagulation and blanching
~100	Boiling and vaporisation of cellular water
300–400	Tissue carbonisation and ablation
> 500	Burning and evaporation of non-water tissue components

Clinical application

To achieve efficient cutting the active electrode should be held slightly away from the tissue to create a spark, which maximises the current density. This continuous arc from electrode to tissue results in rapid heating, intracellular boiling, and consequent cellular vaporisation (Fig. 7.4).

Electrosurgical diathermy is most commonly used to achieve haemostasis of small blood vessels. Such coagulation can be achieved by *desiccation* or *fulguration*. *Desiccation* ('drying') occurs when the electrode is held against the tissue directly and coagulation or cutting current is allowed to flow (Fig. 7.5). Less heat is

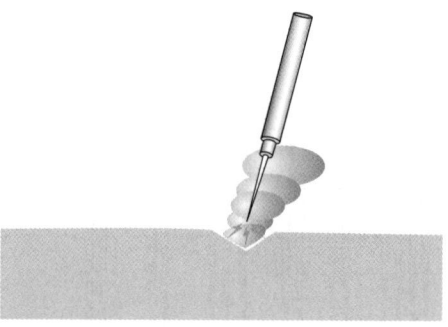

Fig. 7.4 Electrosurgical cutting

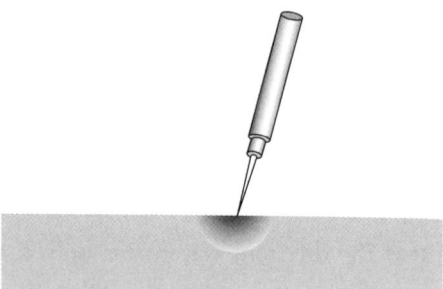

Fig. 7.5 Desiccation

produced and this results in spasm of vessel walls with denaturation of proteins, desiccation of tissue and thrombus formation. The current density is lower than if a spark is allowed to bridge the gap between the active electrode and tissue to cause cellular vaporisation and cutting. In common practice, the active electrode is touched against a conductive haemostat or forceps that grasps the bleeding end of the vessel. In this way the instrument itself becomes part of the circuit. Heating of the tissue at the tip of the forceps is caused by high current density and the impedance of the tissue, in just the same way as if the active electrode itself been applied directly to the tissue.

Fulguration refers to using a coagulation waveform and short bursts of high voltage to overcome the high impedance of air in order to spark across a broad front from the active electrode to the tissue. This results in coagulation and charring over a wide area, with deeper tissue destruction (Fig. 7.6).

Many surgeons routinely 'cut' using a coagulation waveform by adjusting the power settings and active electrode configuration. Likewise, cutting current can be used to coagulate if the electrode is held against the tissue. This reduces current density and slows the rate at which heating occurs, causing coagulation rather than vaporisation. Remember, however, that coagulation current uses higher voltages than cutting current and this has implications for safety in minimally invasive surgery (discussed below).

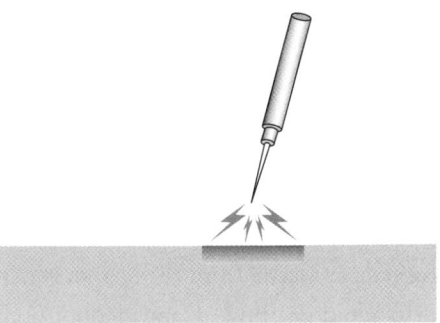

Fig. 7.6 Fulguration

Apart from the waveform, a number of other variables influence the effect of electrosurgical diathermy on tissues. The *size of the electrode* directly influences current density. Small electrodes (e.g. needle point electrodes) generate higher current density and can be used at lower power settings for the same tissue effect. Prolonging the *time of application* results in production of more heat, with thermal spread to adjacent tissue. *Manipulation of the electrode* to change the area of tissue contact changes the tissue effect. Direct tissue contact tends to produce coagulation, whereas sparking across the electrode/air gap results in more efficient cutting. The *type of tissue* is another important determinant of tissue effect since tissues vary widely in electrical resistance. For instance, fat tends to have a high resistance and cuts poorly. In the cut mode, some diathermy units have the ability to sense variation of tissue resistance and adjust voltage and current output automatically to maintain constant cutting performance. This minimises power output and thus reduces collateral thermal damage, neuromuscular stimulation, electromagnetic interference with other operating room electronic devices, and capacitive coupling (discussed below). *Eschar* on the tissue or on the electrode tip itself increases resistance and impairs performance. Where a stainless steel electrode tip is used, a 'scratch pad' is employed to clean the tip. Modern electrode tips coated with Teflon® (PTFE: polytetrafluoroethylene) or elastomeric silicone reduce eschar build up and can be wiped clean on a gauze swab.

Hazards

Although modern electrosurgical diathermy is very safe, there are potential dangers that can result in inadvertent injury to the patient or surgeon.

Particular caution should be taken when applying monopolar diathermy to structures with a narrow pedicle. High current density may be generated in the base of the pedicle, potentially resulting in enough heating to cause vessel thrombosis and sometimes catastrophic ischemia. Such a *channelling effect* must be avoided in structures such as the penis or testis (Fig. 7.7). Similarly, during a cholecystectomy care should

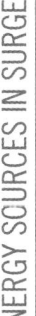

ENERGY SOURCES IN SURGERY | CHAPTER 7

be taken when applying monopolar diathermy energy to the gall bladder when it is only attached by the cystic duct to the common bile duct. Protection against the channelling effect can be achieved by laying the organ against the body to increase the return area and thus decrease current density. Reducing power settings will also help. Alternatively, by using bipolar diathermy (discussed below) risks from the channelling effect are completely eliminated.

Ignition of flammable material can occur from the sparks generated by electrosurgical diathermy. It is essential to avoid pooling of any alcohol used to prepare skin prior to surgery. Particular attention should be paid to any pooling in the umbilicus or from runoff between the patient and the bed. Ignition of alcohol by diathermy in this setting can result in disastrous patient burns. Electrosurgical diathermy should be avoided in the presence of flammable anaesthetic gases, and it is recommended that diathermy is not used to open the bowel in cases of gastrointestinal obstruction, following poor bowel preparation, or following the use of mannitol for bowel preparation where potentially flammable bowel gases may ignite.

Return plate burns may result from poor contact between the patient and the return electrode. Note that the so-called 'passive' electrode only differs from the 'active' electrode in having a much greater surface area and high conductivity, thus greatly reducing current density and heating. Anything at this electrode that concentrates the current into a smaller area risks increasing current density and causing a return electrode burn (Figs 7.8 and 7.9).

Table 7.2 summarises the important considerations in preventing return plate burns.

Most modern electrosurgical generators incorporate circuitry to check the integrity of the connection between the return plate and the patient. This highly desirable safety device continuously monitors the impedance at the return electrode by using an interrogation circuit through a split pad. If impedance at the return electrode is dangerously high, the machine deactivates to prevent a return plate burn (Fig. 7.10).

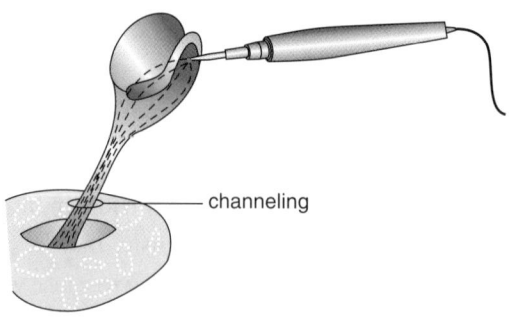

channeling

Fig. 7.7 Channelling of current through a pedicle creates heating and potential vessel thrombosis

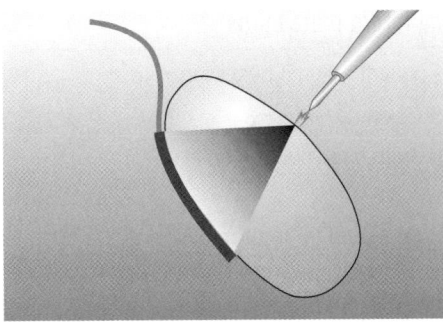

Fig 7.8 Proper return electrode contact minimises current density at the exit site

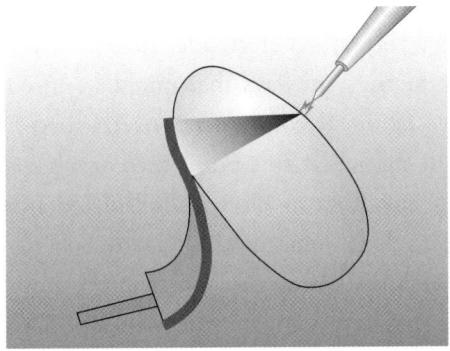

Fig. 7.9 Incomplete contact of the return plate electrode increases current density and the risk of a return electrode burn

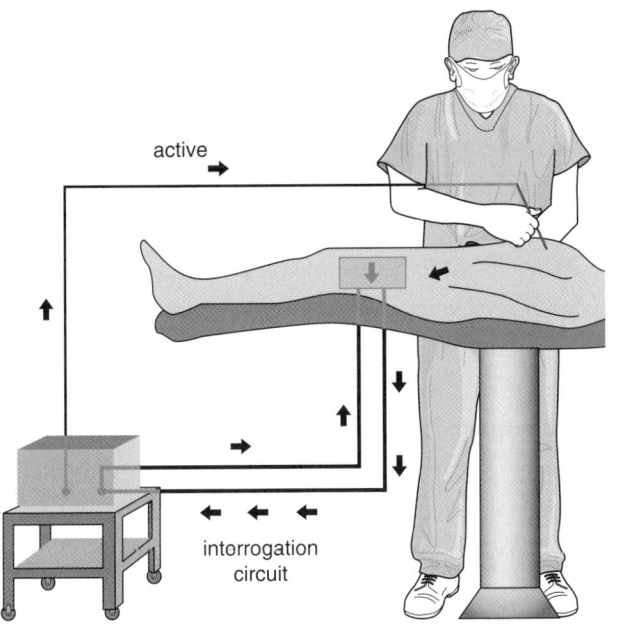

active

interrogation
circuit

Fig 7.10 Return electrode montioring

Table 7.2	Minimising return plate burns
	Shave the patient's skin if necessary
	Apply to dry skin
	Use a plate with large surface area
	Don't fold
	Position close to and on the same side as the operative site
	Choose a well-vascularised muscle mass
	Avoid bony prominences or scar tissue
	Don't apply over prostheses

Older electrosurgical generators were electrically grounded. This meant that rather than returning via the return electrode, current could potentially return to earth via alternate conductive pathways that might be in contact with the patient such as ECG electrodes or metal components of the bed ('current diversion'). If current density was high enough at this point then an *alternate site burn* could occur. Modern electrosurgical generators are electrically isolated and do not return current to ground, thereby effectively eliminating this hazard.

Inadvertent activation of a diathermy device may cause unintentional burns to the patient. For this reason it is very important to store the active electrode in a clean, dry, non-conductive quiver when not in use. As a safety measure, electrosurgical generators generate an audible sound to alert the surgeon when the active electrode has been activated. The tone is different for coagulation and cutting.

Although electrosurgical diathermy uses high-frequency current because this does not stimulate nerve or muscle, *neuromuscular stimulation* may occur as a result of demodulated low-frequency alternating currents ($< 100\,\text{kHz}$). Filter circuitry in the electrosurgical generator is designed to remove these demodulated currents from the current delivered to the patient. However, demodulated currents can be produced locally, particularly following open circuit activation of a diathermy device (i.e. activation of the active electrode before any tissue contact). This results in generation of a high voltage with consequent arcing as the activated active electrode is brought into contact with the haemostat grasping the tissue. Activation of diathermy close to a nerve or large mass of skeletal muscle may cause strong and sudden muscular contractions. This can be particularly problematic during transurethral resection of bladder tumours lying on the lateral bladder wall, close to the obturator nerve.

If the electrosurgical machine is not working properly, avoid merely turning up the power settings as a first response. Check all connections, the patient/plate contact and the generator settings.

Surgical diathermy may affect *permanent pacemaker (PPM) function*. Generally, electrosurgical diathermy may cause temporary inhibition of pacemaker function, though sometimes it may result in PPM reprogramming. This can be overcome by the application of a magnet. Rarely, PPM damage may result from application of high electrosurgical currents near the device. Therefore, avoid the use of monopolar electrosurgery in the presence of a PPM if possible, and use bipolar diathermy or electrocautery (see below) instead. If monopolar diathermy must be used, ensure that the return electrode is positioned well away from the pacemaker unit, and use short, intermittent applications of current. Ensure that a magnet, defibrillation and external pacing equipment are available. *Internal cardiac defibrillators* should be deactivated prior to surgery.

The return plate should not be placed over *prostheses*. Uneven patterns of electrical resistance through and around such devices may result in localised areas of high current density causing thermal injury.

As current follows the path of minimum impedance from the surgical site to the patient return electrode, it may preferentially travel via any *metal jewellery*. For this reason, all metal jewellery should be removed from the patient preoperatively to help prevent burns. The distance between the surgical site and the return electrode should also be minimised to make this current diversion less likely.

There are particular hazards of electrosurgical diathermy when applied to minimally invasive (particularly laparoscopic) surgery. *Direct coupling* occurs when the active electrode is allowed to accidentally activate another conducting instrument which in turn produces an unintentional diathermy burn. This may occur if the two instruments are touching at the time of activation or are even just in close proximity (Fig. 7.11). Arcing from one instrument to another is most likely when the electrode is activated while not in contact with the target tissue ('open circuit activation'). The particular danger during laparoscopic surgery is that direct coupling may occur outside the field of view and cause hidden injury. Direct coupling can be reduced by using only insulated instruments and taking care not to activate the electrode close to conductive objects such as the laparoscope, staples, or other metal instruments.

Insulation failure may provide an alternative exit path for current. If the current density at this point is high enough, then an unintended burn will result. This is especially the case when using the high voltages associated with coagulation diathermy. Such voltages can potentially breach areas of thin but otherwise intact insulation (Fig. 7.12). Current leakage is more likely with open circuit activation. Some electrosurgical generators help protect against insulation failure during minimally invasive surgery by monitoring current in the active electrode.

Capacitive coupling may occur when a diathermy electrode is activated within a laparoscopic cannula. A capacitor consists of two conductors separated by a non-

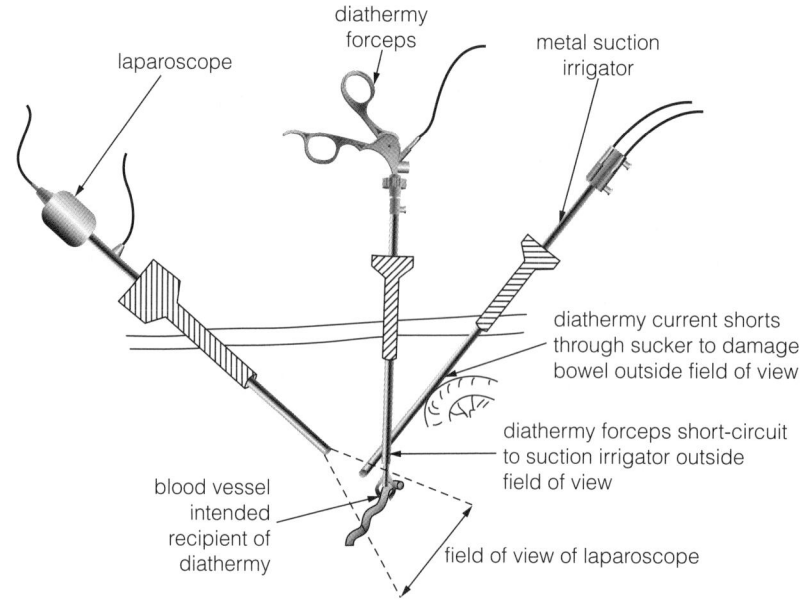

Fig. 7.11 Direct coupling

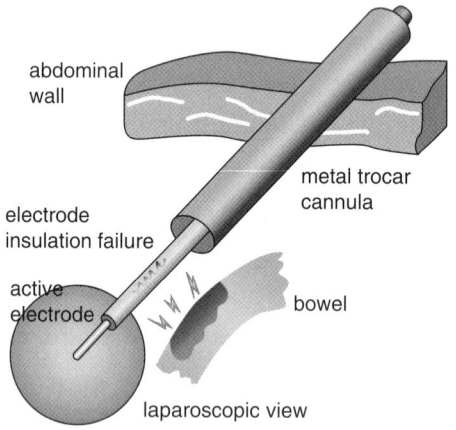

Fig. 7.12 Insulation failure

conductor. An electrostatic field is generated between the two conductors, and as a result an alternating current in the active conductor can induce an alternating current in the second conductor. Such an arrangement is inadvertently formed when a diathermy device (comprising a central conductor surrounded by an insulating sheath) is placed within a conducting metal cannula. Current can be transferred to the metal cannula, even though the insulation remains completely intact (Fig. 7.13). This occurs to a much greater degree across a 5 mm port than a 10 mm port, and has potential to cause an inadvertent burn. Capacitive coupling is more likely to occur with open circuit activation and when using high-voltage diathermy (coagulation and fulguration modes).

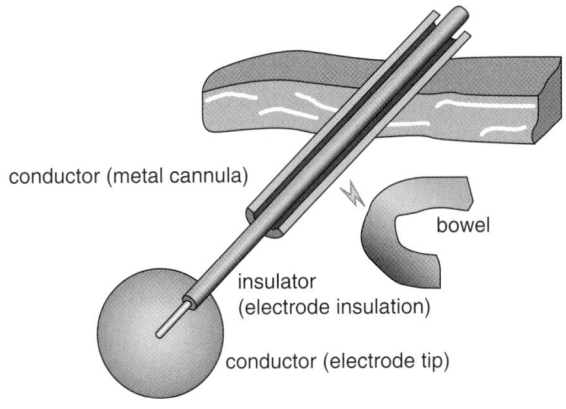

conductor (metal cannula)

bowel

insulator
(electrode insulation)

conductor (electrode tip)

Fig. 7.13 Capacitive coupling

Use of a non-conductive plastic cannula will minimise the chance of capacitive coupling, but it will not completely eliminate it because the patient's conductive tissue surrounding the sheath completes the definition of a capacitor. Capacitive coupling is most dangerous when a hybrid cannula system is used. Such a system comprises a non-conductive plastic sheath surrounding the metal cannula where it traverses the abdominal wall. This effectively stops current from dissipating through the abdominal wall but coupled current can still exit from the metal cannula within the abdominal cavity, potentially causing occult visceral damage (Fig. 7.14).

Following prolonged diathermy activation, the tip of the electrode may remain quite hot for some time after the current is switched off. This *retained heat* may be sufficient to cause tissue damage.

Electrosurgical diathermy presents certain possible risks not only to the patient but also to the operating surgeon and theatre staff. Vaporisation of tissue by electrosurgical

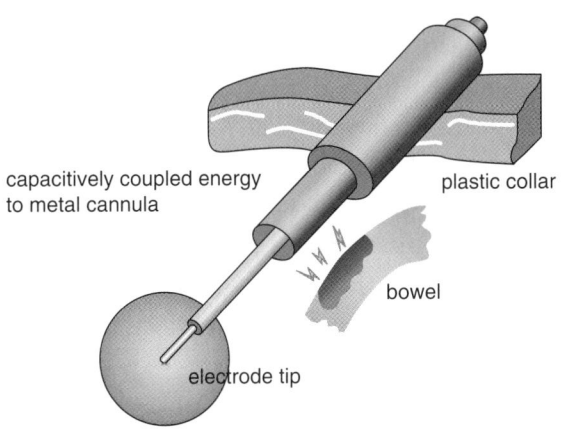

capacitively coupled energy
to metal cannula

plastic collar

bowel

electrode tip

Fig. 7.14 Capacitive coupling in a hybrid cannula system

diathermy generates *surgical smoke*. This smoke may contain a variety of noxious agents including viral DNA, carcinogens, mutagens and various chemical irritants. To minimise the inhalation risks to staff it is therefore recommended that a dedicated smoke evacuation device is employed. This may be an integrated suction device that attaches to the diathermy pencil. *Burns* can occasionally occur through the surgeon's or assistant's glove. These are commonly attributed to pre-existing holes but more commonly result from electrical breakdown of the glove. It has been postulated that this occurs through three different mechanisms. *Direct current conduction* occurs if impedance of the glove reduces sufficiently to allow current to pass. This occurs more readily as the glove hydrates. *Radiofrequency capacitive coupling* may occur across the insulating glove with induction of current in the surgeon's hand. Lastly, *high-voltage dielectric breakdown* results when the glove cannot withstand the high energy generated by the electrosurgical machine. This is more likely when high voltages (coagulation) and power settings are used and where a small area of contact is made between the haemostat being touched by the active electrode and the hand holding it. Glove burns are also more likely when open circuit activation occurs prior to touching the active electrode to the haemostat. Burns to the surgeon's hand are much less likely to occur if the surgeon is not in any other direct or indirect contact with the patient at the time of electrode activation. This prevents an alternative current pathway being formed through the surgeon.

Beware of *needlestick injuries* from the use of needle point diathermy electrodes. Use of these electrodes should be avoided if possible.

BIPOLAR DIATHERMY

Principles

In bipolar diathermy, the active and return plates are combined at the site of surgery in one instrument. Only the tissue grasped is included in the electrical circuit, therefore no patient plate is required (Fig. 7.15). This makes bipolar diathermy very much safer to use on pedicled structures such as the digits or penis. Cutting is virtually impossible (except when using a dedicated bipolar cutting instrument) and there is minimal surrounding tissue damage. As a consequence, bipolar diathermy is used extensively in neurosurgery (Fig. 7.16) and ophthalmology. Other advantages of bipolar over monopolar electrosurgery are detailed in Table 7.3.

Most modern electrosurgical generators have provision for providing current for bipolar diathermy devices. When using bipolar electrosurgical instruments, remember that the tines of the forceps need to be held slightly apart and not touching to achieve a tissue effect.

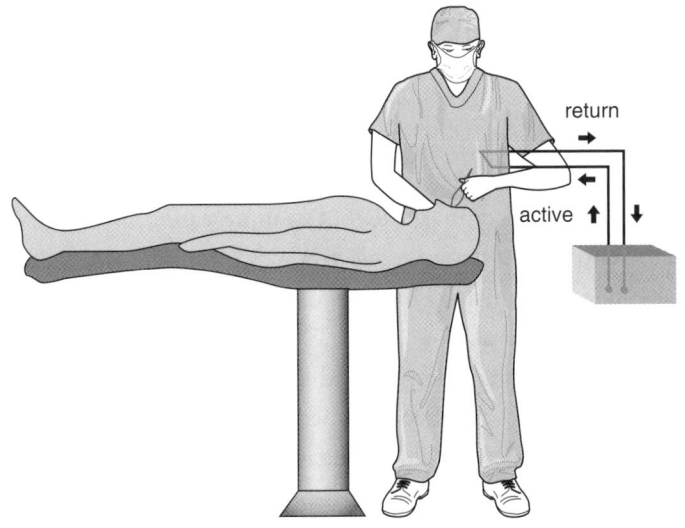

Fig. 7.15 Bipolar diathermy

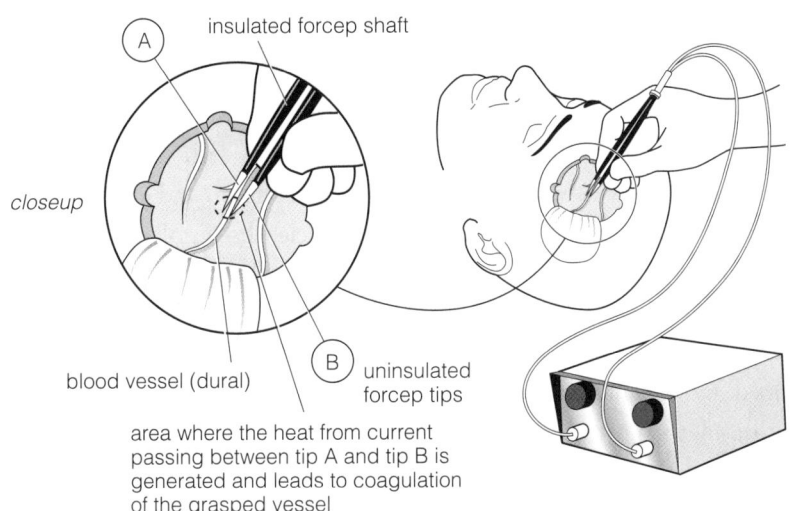

A — insulated forcep shaft

closeup

blood vessel (dural)

B — uninsulated forcep tips

area where the heat from current passing between tip A and tip B is generated and leads to coagulation of the grasped vessel

Fig. 7.16 Bipolar diathermy in neurosurgery

Table 7.3	Advantages of bipolar electrosurgery
	Safe to use on pedicled structures
	Minimal tissue damage
	No possibility of return electrode burns
	No possibility of alternate site burns
	Minimal risk of capacitive coupling
	Minimal risk from insulation failure
	Minimal risk of direct coupling

OTHER DIATHERMY DEVICES

Argon beam diathermy

Principles

Argon gas is inert and non-combustible, but is more easily ionised than air. When argon is sprayed alongside the activated electrode, it is ionised, and creates a pathway which is more conductive than air. This spreads current over a wide surface, resulting in rapid fulguration and coagulation of tissue. Argon beam diathermy results in less smoke and odour with less drag and tissue adhesion than conventional diathermy. In coagulation mode there is no direct contact between the electrode and the tissue, and the argon gas tends to blow away blood and fluids from the area being coagulated (Fig. 7.17). A thinner, more flexible eschar is produced.

Argon beam coagulation is difficult to manage in laparoscopic surgery because the high flow of argon gas into the abdominal cavity increases intra-abdominal pressure.

Electrosurgical vessel sealing

Several specialised electrosurgical generators and instrumentation are available for reliable vessel sealing as alternative to using ligatures or clips. Systems use a combination of feedback-controlled bipolar diathermy with instrumentation that apply pressure to the vessel wall to achieve fusion of collagen and elastin and creation of a permanent seal. During the energy delivery cycle, the bipolar generator delivers pulsed energy that is feedback-controlled and constantly modified according to the tissue response. The generator delivers a high-current (4 A), low-voltage (200 V) output. When the seal is complete the output to the instrument is automatically discontinued and a generator tone sounds. Vessels up to 7 mm in diameter can be sealed with a mechanical strength that is comparable to ligatures or clips. The seal withstands up to three times systolic blood pressure. Importantly, pedicles can be sealed without the need for dissection or vessel isolation which itself may sometimes result in bleeding. Both open and laparoscopic instrumentation are available.

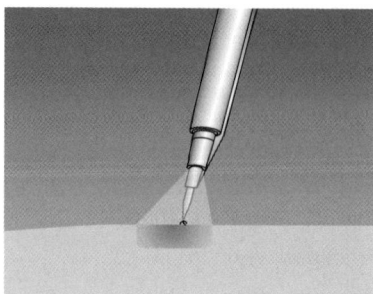

Fig. 7.17 Argon beam coagulator

Electrovaporisation

By engineering ridges or spikes on an electrosurgical 'rollerball' and using high power settings, very high current densities can be generated. This results in tissue vaporisation and ablation. Such rollerballs can be used to ablate benign prostatic enlargement (transurethral vaporisation of the prostate—TUVP) or can be used to achieve endometrial vaporisation.

Electrocautery

Electrocautery refers to the use of direct current to heat a wire, which in turn is used to coagulate vessels by dissipating the heat that it has stored. Unlike electrosurgery, the patient is not part of the circuit. Such devices are often built into a disposable pen and are often used in ophthalmic or minor skin surgery.

LASER

Principles

External energy applied to certain materials can be used to excite electrons into higher metastable states. If a photon arrives that has an energy exactly equal to the difference between the metastable state and the vacant lower energy level, the photon will cause the electron to fall to the lower energy level. The original photon continues on its way and a new photon is released with exactly the same direction and phase as the original photon. This process is known as *stimulated emission*. By reflecting the photons back and forth along the same axis they create yet more photons of the same energy and coherence (*light amplification*) (Fig. 7.18). The laser (*Light Amplification by Stimulated Emission of Radiation*) light so produced has a single monochromatic wavelength that is determined by the composition of the lasing medium. Lasers are therefore named according to the type of lasing medium used which may be solid, liquid or gas. Laser

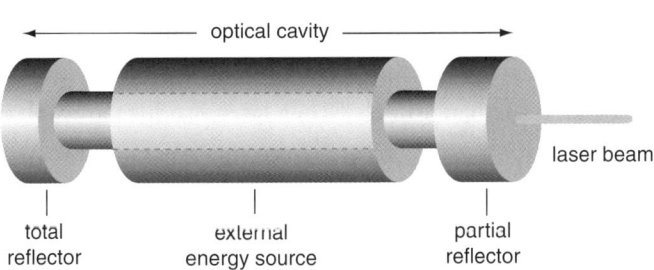

Fig. 7.18 Diagrammatic representation of a laser

light is highly collimated (i.e. the photons travel parallel to each other with minimal divergence) and it may be pulsed or continuous.

Tissue effects

Interaction of laser radiation with tissue may cause thermal, photochemical and photomechanical effects. Absorption and scatter are the most important mechanisms responsible for the *thermal effects* of laser radiation. The resultant tissue effects vary according to the temperature generated (see Table 7.1). When very high power density is delivered in very short pulses, ionisation and plasma sparks are generated, producing acoustic shock waves that cause mechanical damage to the absorbing medium. This *photomechanical effect* may be used to fragment urinary tract stones. *Photochemical effects* occur when short-wavelength ultraviolet light is absorbed causing excitation of electron bonds and breakage of organic bonds. In *photodynamic therapy* a photosensitive drug is administered that is taken up by malignant cells. This is activated by low-power laser light resulting in destruction of the malignant tissue. *Tissue welding* may also be achieved using laser energy.

Generators and uses

Laser energy is used across a wide range of medical and surgical specialties. The *carbon dioxide* laser produces far-infrared energy that is rapidly absorbed by water, causing tissue vaporisation with minimal thermal spread. Applications include ablation of endometriosis deposits in gynaecological surgery or destruction of genital condylomata acuminata. The *neodymium:yttrium–aluminium–garnet (Nd:YAG)* laser produces a spectrum of light that penetrates around 5 mm into tissue and is mainly absorbed by haemoglobin. This results in a wide zone of thermal damage. Uses include palliative ablation of obstructing gastrointestinal tumours or treatment of bladder and external genital lesions. *Laser lithotripsy* uses high-energy pulses from a *holmium:YAG* laser to produce photomechanical destruction of renal or ureteric calculi. The energy is delivered via a fine flexible quartz fiberoptic fibre that is passed up the working channel of the endoscope to contact the calculus. The holmium: YAG laser can also be used to cut tissue. *Erbium:YAG* laser offer precise ablation and are used for cosmetic skin resurfacing. Hair removal can be achieved using high-powered *diode* laser that produce a wavelength of light selectively absorbed by melanin present in the hair follicle. *Argon* laser produce a visible wavelength of light that is selectively absorbed by melanin and haemoglobin. These lasers are used in ophthalmology to treat retinal diseases, and in cosmetic medicine to treat cutaneous hemangiomata. Ophthalmologists also use *UV excimer* laser to reshape the cornea to correct refractive errors. This laser has also been used for coronary angioplasty. The wavelength of *dye* laser can be 'tuned' for maximum absorption and consequent ablation of pigmented skin lesions.

Precautions and safety

The eye is the organ most susceptible to laser damage and most laser injuries to this organ occur by reflection. The pattern of damage to the eye depends upon the wavelength, intensity and the angle of incidence of laser radiation. Corneal burns occur with wavelengths of > 1400 nm whereas retinal damage occurs with wavelengths of around 400 to 1400 nm. Everyone within the 'nominal ocular hazard area' must therefore use appropriate eye protection (including the patient). The nominal ocular hazard area is defined as the area within which exposure to direct or scattered laser light may exceed the maximal permissible exposure. It is essential that the protective eyewear worn is specifically suited to the particular wavelength of laser light being used.

Skin must be protected from inadvertent laser exposure to prevent burns. During ablative laser procedures, a plume of *smoke* with similar properties to that produced by electrosurgery can be produced and this must be efficiently evacuated to prevent occupational exposure. Heat generated by laser energy can potentially cause *ignition of flammable material*. When using a laser fibre down an endoscope it is imperative that the fibre tip be kept in view at all times whilst lasing. If the laser is fired within the working channel then significant *endoscope damage* will result.

Specific working rules are required for each particular type of laser. Medium- and high-powered (classes 3B and 4) lasers must only be operated in controlled areas with visual warning notices interlocked to the laser operation.

ULTRASOUND

Introduction

Ultrasound is used extensively throughout medical and surgical practice. Low energies are typically used for imaging, whereas high energies can be used to produce thermal and cavitation effects on tissue. Ultrasound cutting and coagulation devices generate high-frequency longitudinal sound (pressure) waves that are propagated through a medium to an active blade element.

Ultrasonic scalpel

Principles

The ultrasonic scalpel utilises ultrasonic energy to cause tissue cavitation, coagulation or cutting. Electrical energy is converted into mechanical energy by a piezoelectric crystal in the handpiece of the instrument (an *electrostrictive* transducer). Mechanical vibrations are amplified and transmitted to the tip of the instrument, which vibrates at a frequency of 50 000 Hz. Adjusting the power setting of the generator varies the longitudinal extension of the instrument tip between 60 μm and 100 μm.

Generators and instrumentation

The ultrasonic scalpel system comprises a generator, footswitch, handpiece and attachable instruments. There is a wide range of blades, shears and coagulating instruments designed for both open and laparoscopic surgery that can be connected to the handpiece (Fig. 7.19).

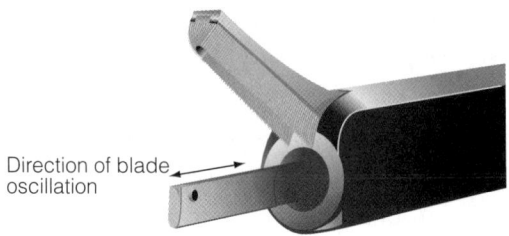

Direction of blade oscillation

Fig. 7.19 Ultrasonic coagulating shears

Tissue effects

The ultrasonic scalpel can be used to achieve three main tissue effects. *Cavitation* is caused by transmission of high-frequency vibrations to the tissue resulting in rapid volume changes and formation of vapour bubbles. This results in cellular vaporisation in parenchyma or dissection of tissue planes in connective tissue. *Coaptation / coagulation* occurs when ultrasound energy and pressure are applied together. Proteins are disrupted leading to the adherence of collagen molecules at low temperatures (coaptation). When the ultrasound energy is applied for longer periods, higher temperatures cause protein denaturation (coagulation). *Cutting* occurs when the tissue is rapidly stretched by the vibrating instrument tip beyond its elastic limit.

The balance between these tissue effects is determined by the combination of power setting, blade sharpness, tissue tension and grip force (pressure) applied. Higher power settings and sharper blades, along with greater tissue tension or higher grip pressures, result in faster cutting and less haemostasis. The water content and type of tissue along with the time of energy application also influence the result.

The ultrasonic scalpel avoids the disadvantages of transmitting electrical energy through the patient, particularly when used in minimally invasive (laparoscopic) surgery. It results in less charring, smoke and desiccation than electrosurgery and causes less lateral thermal spread and depth of tissue penetration, allowing for safer dissection near vulnerable structures.

Cavitational ultrasonic aspiration

Principles

The cavitational ultrasonic aspirator has two tissue effects. First, it causes rapid vibration of tissue in contact with the tip, resulting in tissue fragmentation. Second, it produces cavitation effects by producing localised pressure waves with the development and collapse of vapour pockets. Rather than use a piezoelectric transducer, the ultrasonic aspiration system utilises the phenomenon of *magnetostriction* to convert electrical energy into ultrasonic waves of 23–36 kHz. A nickel alloy is placed in a magnetic field created by electrical current to cause it to expand and contract by up to 35 µm. The handpiece and instrument tip amplify this motion up to tenfold and the amplitude can be adjusted on the machine. The system incorporates coaxial fluid delivery to the vibrating tip to keep it cool and to suspend fragmented tumour tissue, and an integrated suction apparatus to aspirate this away.

Use

Ultrasonic aspiration systems are used to perform tumour and tissue ablation with minimal trauma to surrounding healthy tissue. Such systems offer a degree of tissue selectivity since low water content or collagen-rich structures such as blood vessels and nerves require considerably higher energies to fragment than high water content structures such as the liver. These devices are particularly well suited to neurosurgical treatment of intracranial and intraspinal tumours and are also promoted for use in liver resection.

Others

Ultrasound energy is used in a variety of other surgical devices. *High-intensity focused ultrasound* (HIFU) causes thermal and cavitational effects, and has been used to ablate tissues such as benign prostatic enlargement or prostatic adenocarcinoma. *Ultrasonic contact lithotripsy* uses the jackhammer effect of vibrations at the tip of a probe to fragment urinary tract calculi. *Extracorporeal shock-wave lithotripsy* (ESWL) focuses ultrasonic shock waves from outside the body onto urinary or biliary calculi to cause fragmentation, and can also be used to treat certain musculoskeletal disorders.

OTHER ENERGY SOURCES

Tissue ablation through heating can be achieved by using several other modalities. *Radiofrequency ablation* (e.g. transurethral needle ablation of the prostate) utilises low-level radiofrequency energy to cause thermal tissue damage. *Microwave energy* can be directed into tissue using a microwave antenna. This has been used to treat benign prostatic enlargement.

Cryotherapy refers to the use of cold to destroy tissue by freezing cells. Liquid nitrogen is often used in general and dermatological practice to destroy skin cancers. Under ultrasound control, a cryoprobe tip can be placed into primary or secondary tumours of the liver, kidney, prostate or other organs. Several freeze/thaw cycles are then used to destroy the tumour.

Urinary stone fragmentation can be achieved using several other energy sources. *Electrohydraulic lithotripsy* (EHL) utilises a high-voltage discharge between two underwater electrodes to create a shock wave very close to a stone. Another shockwave lithtripsy system uses compressed air is used to propel a metal projectile to strike against the base of a probe. This ballistic energy is transmitted along the shaft of the probe to its tip to produce a mechanical jackhammer effect.

Water jet devices utilise a fine high-pressure laminar flow jet of water to achieve tissue selective dissection and precision cutting. Advantages include minimal trauma to surrounding tissues with no thermal damage.

CONCLUSIONS AND THE FUTURE

The role of energy sources in surgery along with their related technologies and instrumentation is ever expanding. This chapter provides an overview of the most important modalities, their tissue effects and common applications. However, it must be remembered that the devices themselves are no substitute for sound surgical judgement and technical competence. It is incumbent upon the surgeon to understand the indications, limitations and proper use of all the energy modalities in the surgical armamentarium and to apply them judiciously.

FURTHER READING

General

Valleylab website: http://www.valleylab.com

Jallo GI. CUSA EXcel Ultrasonic Aspiration System. Neurosurgery 2001;48:695–6.

LigaSure tissue fusion system website: http://www.valleylab.com/ligasure-usa/index.htm

MacLellan DG, Quail AW. The operation/operating theatre safety and hazards module. Surgical Trainees Educational Module. Melbourne: RACS, 2000.

UltraCision—The Harmonic Scalpel and The Harmonic Scalpel—System Components. In: Feil W, Lippert H, Lozac'h P, Palazzini G, Amaral J, eds. Atlas of Surgical Stapling. Heidelberg: Johann Ambrosius Barth, 2000; 47–65.

Lasers

Waynant RW, ed. Lasers in Medicine. 1st edn. CRC Press Inc., 2001.

Electrosurgery

Valleylab Electrosurgery Products website: http://www.valleylab.com/product/es

2003 Standards, Recommended practices, and Guidelines with official AORN statements. AORN Inc., 2003.

Zinder DJ. Common myths about electrosurgery. Otolaryngol Head Neck Surg 2000; 120: 450–5.

Harmonic® devices website: http://www.harmonic.com

CHAPTER EIGHT
ERGONOMICS IN SURGERY

Strength of heart
And might of limb, but mainly use and skill,
Are winners in this pastime.

Alfred Lord Tennyson (1809–1892),
Idylls of the King: The Last Tournament, line 197

INTRODUCTION

Ergonomics is the scientific study of the relationship between people and their working environment. In surgery as in industry, the aims of ergonomics include better productivity and quality of work, and also better outcomes for individual patients and the benefit of society at large. It considers equipment design, workplace layout, environmental factors such as lighting, and other matters such as skill, productivity and safety. The best surgeons, like other good craftspeople, engineers and managers, are good intuitive ergonomists. Today, as technology becomes more complicated, a more calculated approach is needed than formerly.

Hippocrates, more than 2000 years ago, wrote that surgeons should work in a good light, be seated comfortably, have the relevant part of the patient presented in a convenient way and have assistants who help promptly and in silence. For modern surgery he would consider a complex team, instruments for special tasks such as microsurgery, minimally invasive surgery and robotics and other technology, management of budgets and the wider society. Such modern surgery dates from the first general anaesthetic in 1846. Post-modern surgery began in the 1960s when technologies such as the operating microscope, and laparoscopic and robotic systems began to intervene between operators, their instruments and the patient.

The subject of ergonomics for surgeons would need a thick textbook (yet to be written) to cover topics and details adequately, and this chapter can only sketch out the subject, relying on references (at the end of the chapter) to complete descriptions and explanations adequately. A model of the surgeon at work (Fig. 8.1) provides a convenient framework to introduce the discussion.

There are three elements in this model—operator, instrument and tissue—and two interfaces: the ergonomic interface between surgeon and equipment, and the bioengineering interface between instruments and tissue.

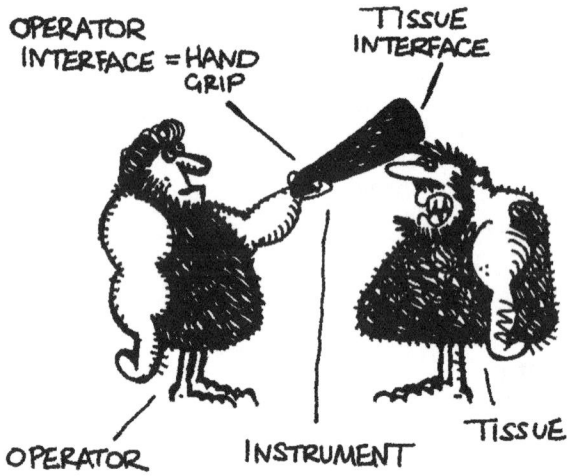

Fig. 8.1 Ergonomic model of the surgeon at work (Cartoonist: Stephen Stanley)

The bio-engineering (instrument–tissue) interface must take into account the tissue property of viscoelasticity. This is what differentiates soft tissue management from carpentry or engineering (or handling hard tissue such as bone). The Romans first used teeth in surgical instruments to better control tissue: the teeth generate high enough pressures to overwhelm the creep and stress relaxation that constitute the viscoelasticity of living tissue. Postmodern instruments have been designed with respect for viscoelasticity and incorporate chamfers, bevels and compliant inserts to control tissue by working with its biomechanical properties.[1, 2, 3]

The ergonomic interface starts at the surgeon's hands, extends outward to the immediate environment and operating room design, considers specific types of work like microsurgery and laparoscopic surgery, and then considers issues like skill, fatigue, safety and health at work, organisational culture and information design. Further interfaces can be added, for example between instruments and equipment, and how well the jaws of a needle holder grip the needle.[4]

HAND GRIPS

Surgeons use five main types of hand grip:[5]

1. *Power grip*, for large instruments like a hand-held abdominal retractor (Fig 8.2a).
2. *External precision grip*, the classical type of pen hold for writing, when the instrument is at about 45° to the working surface (Fig 8.2b).
3. *Internal precision grip*, the common scalpel grip in general surgery; the instrument is practically parallel to the work surface. A variant is used for scissors and ring-handled tools, when a common mistake is to put the fingers too far into the rings. This results in clumsiness due to the loss of fine finger tip touch and the loss of proprioceptive feedback from the 'missing' joints, and makes it difficult to let go of the instrument (Fig 8.2c).
4. *Pinch grip* (not shown).
5. *Double grips* are used to maintain traction on a suture or to stretch tissue with one hand. *Storage grips* are used to tuck instruments into the palm of the hand with the ring and little fingers.

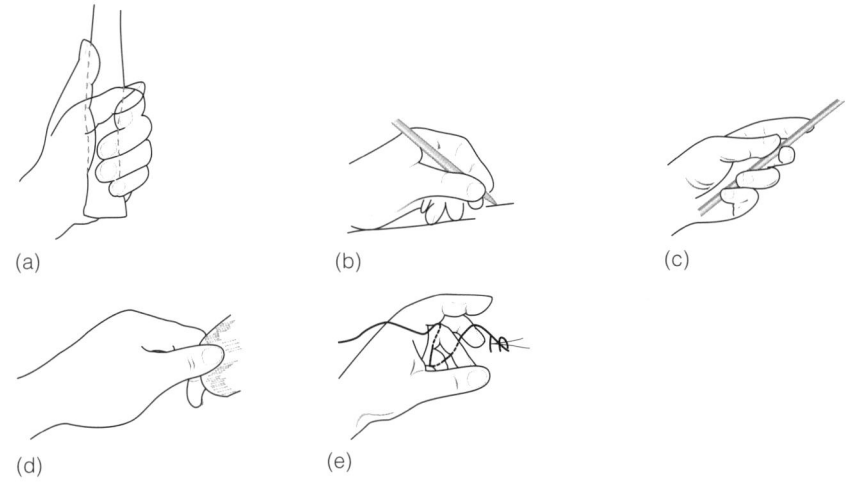

(a) (b) (c)

(d) (e)

Fig. 8.2 Grips

Handles can be designed logically for better use. For use in the power grip the length should be greater than the normal palm width of about 12 cm, the diameter should be 2–3 cm to maximise skin contact area, the handle should be slightly flattened to control rotation without friction, and should have flattened areas for the thumb and index finger for more sensitive tilt control. Sharp projections should be avoided as they inhibit voluntary grip strength. A small pommel and hilt should be provided to prevent slip when muscles acting on the hand relax a little, and often a bend, perhaps 30° where the handle joins the shaft, is helpful to avoid ulnar deviation of the user's wrist for long periods of time. A detailed checklist contains more than 60 items.[6] Similar considerations apply to pedals and other controls.

For the finest work, a microsurgical needle holder should be just over 12 cm long, cylindrical in shape and about 1 cm in diameter at the fingertip pulp when the jaws are closed, and should have a low stiffness of about 50–70 g weight (about 0.5–0.7 Newton) to avoid aggravating normal hand tremor. Concavo–convex jaws give more secure needle grip, and offsetting them by about 30° affords more accurate control of suturing.[7]

WORKPLACE ARRANGEMENT

As equipment in operating rooms (ORs) has multiplied, the older standard dimensions for them have become inadequate, and storage areas for disposables and large mobile items such as image intensifiers have also had to increase. Unfortunately, bureaucrats start their architectural planning with a fixed plot size into which to squeeze professional activities. In contrast, an ergonomic approach should start by describing the work to be done and only then defining the area required, while also allowing for future expansion. The problem of communicating with architects can be improved using simple 1:10 plans with movable components.[8]

There are simple lessons from office and factory ergonomics that apply in the operating room. Equipment should be placed within the natural areas of reach for the hand, forearm and shoulders. Video monitors should be positioned in line with the hands so that the operator does not have to extend or twist his or her neck The top of the monitor should be several centimetres below eye level, allowing the viewer to gaze comfortably below the horizontal (Fig 8.3b). Optimal viewing distance is usually five to seven screen heights from the operator, closer for high definition. Additional monitors may be required for assistants. Too frequently, the monitor is placed on the top shelf of a 'tower', demanding an (unconsciously) uncomfortable position (Fig. 8.3a). No clerical union would tolerate this for its members. Poor monitor placement becomes one of the cumulative challenges threatening the success of longer, more complex videoscopic procedures.

Operating tables should be selected so they can be made low enough for the surgeon to avoid having to abduct their arms in a 'chicken-wing' posture, which causes both fatigue and less accurate manipulation (Fig. 8.4). There are implications, with which Hippocrates would have sympathised, for positioning of the patient, and placement of incisions and endoscopic ports.

The current generation of 'operating rooms of the future' is designed with information and cabling systems that keep the floor clear of obstructions and improve workflow, in line with current ideas on management, but older sites can

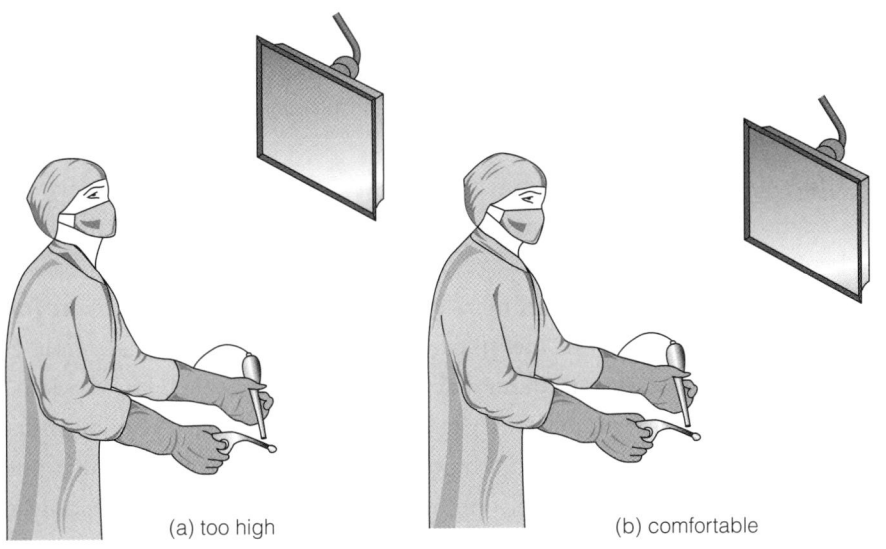

Fig. 8.3 Monitor placement

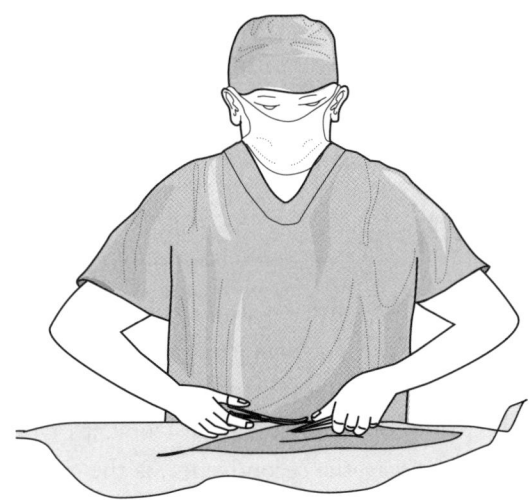

Fig. 8.4 Inappropriate table height

also be improved with such concepts in mind. Much can be learned by simply asking surgeons what they would like changed in ORs.[9, 10]

ENVIRONMENTAL CONDITIONS

Productivity is highest when working in a ambient temperature of about 18 °C (which should be controllable in the OR without having to send for a technician), with measurable humidity, and little noise.

Lighting is one of the main determinants of visual acuity and perception. As far as surgeons are concerned, acuity depends on several factors.[11]

1. *Illumination intensity:* within broad limits, visual acuity is proportional to the logarithm of the lighting intensity.[12]

2. *Glare* near the line of sight.[13] Shiny instruments produce more glare; matt or satin finish of instruments is an advantage, but a matt black finish is even better.

3. *Colour contrast:* Colour discrimination is a key element of edge recognition, and is very important in identification of anatomy during dissection. Some theatre lights give better colour discrimination than others. Early video chips compromised colour resolution, particularly in the red range, making structures more difficult to delineate in a bloody endoscopic field. There are a number of ways to improve colour discrimination. Use of a tourniquet and dyes like methylene blue are practical examples of techniques to improve colour contrast. Imaging such as sentinel node scanning could be considered a visual aid.

4. *Other factors:* binocularity, visual health, trained perception, magnification, directional lighting, colour rendering from light sources, filters and reflectors, flicker, and unwanted effects such as heating. Lighting levels should increase in proportion to magnification. A total approach would consider the ergonomics of light positioning and controls.

SKILLS ACQUISITION

Surgical skills can be studied in the same way as skills in sport, industry or music.[11] The process of skill acquisition can be considered in three stages. *Coding,* the first stage, is learning to relate a particular movement to a particular end result, such as pressing middle C on the piano, or squeezing an instrument or tissue with a given amount of force. *Temporal organisation,* the second stage, is the arrangement of coded movements into a sequence, such as the notes of a melody or the movements of tying a surgical knot. *Hierarchical organisation,* the final stage, is a mental 'programme' or 'sub-routine' ready to be called on by the operator, modified according to other sensory input, but which cannot be interrupted halfway through. This is a smooth rhythmic performance, saving time because it does not have to be repeated. It is a feature of the skills of the best workers, artists and athletes.

Many elements of surgical skill can be described as 'heuristics' (Greek 'eureka', discovery). Heuristics are rules of thumb derived from experience. Experts are often unaware of the heuristics they use automatically, and therefore cannot teach them.[14] For example non-rigid tissue is best cut at right angles to lines of tension. A double hand grip by the operator allows one hand to stretch tissue to facilitate cutting it with the other (Fig. 8.2). Tensing a structure over the index fingertip provides very accurate information about the thickness of the layer being created, and the presence of intervening structures (Fig. 8.5). It allows more accurate and easier dissection of a hollow adherent structure such as some hernial sacs, a difficult duodenal stump, or a gall bladder.

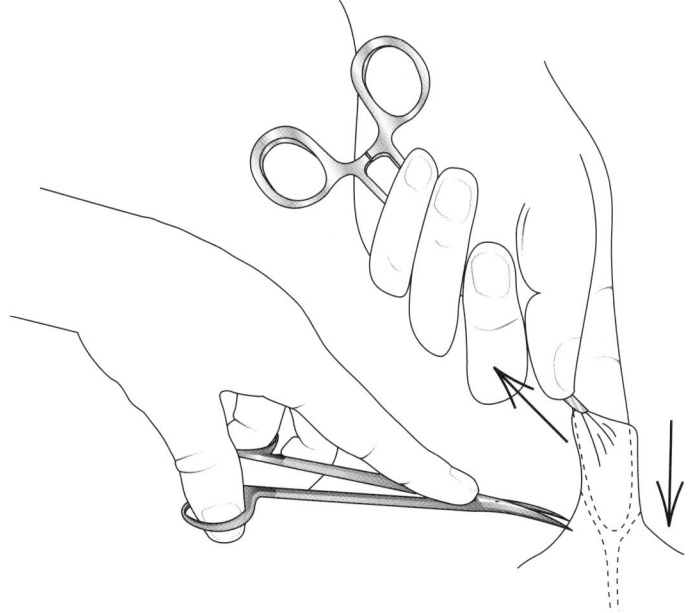

Fig 8.5 A double hand grip for dissecting a difficult hollow structure

The three heuristics just described are not for the fledgling surgeon, who should concentrate more on tensing tissue that is usually attached at one end to the weight of the body. If tissue is limp, it will not separate when pushed against even by a blade, but will simply indent, an ineffective movement. The more skilful surgeon may not move more quickly than the beginner (perhaps even more slowly, to absorb more information before and during movements) but will perform many fewer ineffective movements. Expert surgeons perform fewer 'ineffective movements' and more 'effective movements' in a task such as mobilising the oesophagus during a Nissen fundoplasty.[15] Analysis of skill in surgery should eventually give many more examples of explicit knowledge which replaces implicit or subconscious knowledge.

A further component of skill in operative and clinical surgery as well as other physical activities is the ability to judge the magnitude and timing of forces applied to instruments and tissues. Sir Hugh Devine, an outstanding abdominal surgeon of his time, wrote:[16]

After prolonged use of these scissors — always of exactly the same weight — I have been able to develop with them a sense of touch that enables me to recognise, with the tips of the scissors, the slightest difference of tissue density and therefore to identify blood vessels and other structures by the feel of them.

He was probably speaking of a difference in feedback of touch of less than 50 g of force (0.5 Newton) transmitted to his fingers through the handles of the scissors. This is not all that difficult to perceive through scissors whose blades are not held tightly by the screw joint, if the user thinks consciously of his or her fingers, not being distracted by the stress of other problems at the time of surgery, and practises this mental skill. Recent conferences on surgical simulation[17] have yielded a growing number of measurements of force exerted, for example during laparoscopic suturing, pelvic examination and estimation of abdominal tenderness.

Work management

One important way of improving surgery is by the same team carrying out a procedure frequently, with properties of the learning curve applied to the group rather than just to the individual and the gradual evolution of improvements, like musicians practicing and playing together. The same operating team carrying out many hip replacements, liver resections or cleft palate repairs will achieve a rhythm of work impossible with changing staff and infrequent procedures. Surgeons who are not naturally good leaders should take an interest in this subject and work to improve their skills in it.

Techniques should be standardised and simplified, complicated new procedures rehearsed, and lists of instruments and sutures and special requirements updated for each procedure.

Ergonomics and microsurgery

Some aspects of this have already been mentioned.[11] The push to apply ergonomics here came because the natural ability of many surgeons was not sufficient to overcome the deficiencies of poor work systems. One problem was that some instruments required a kilogram weight of force to close, about 15 times too much.

Overall, the important considerations are comfortable adjustable seated posture at the microscope with support for the forearms and hands, good quality binocular image, instruments designed to fit the external precision grip of the hand, and attention to factors that affect hand tremor. These questions were resolved by the end of the 1970s. The only later enhancement has been the ability to control fine movement by means of robotics and enhanced visual and haptic feedback.

Ergonomics and laparoscopic surgery

Unlike microsurgery, the ergonomic problems of laparoscopic surgery are far from solved.[18] One is the optimal design of handles to allow accurate manipulation of the working ends, together with trigger functions to work and lock the jaws. The underlying problem is a fulcrum halfway along the shaft. This is aggravated if the operator's arms are abducted because the table is not low enough and no platform is there to stand on. (Problems escalate: the platform needs a lip to stop foot controls sliding off.) Some simple compensations are possible, for example steadying the hand with the outstretched ring finger on the port if a diathermy handpiece is used without a trigger type control (Fig. 8.6).

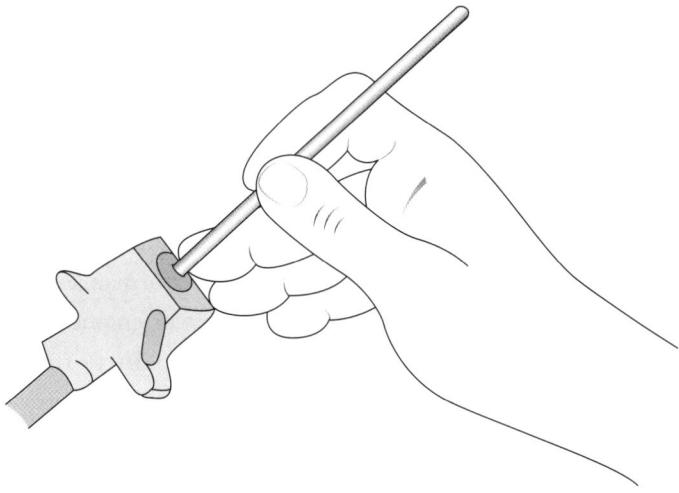

Fig. 8.6 Improving control of a diathermy handpiece

Monitors are often placed too high (see Fig. 8.3a) and too far away. Working from a flat screen means that of the 18 cues which convey depth perception, seven important ones are lost.[18]

Some of these problems are solved by the Da Vinci surgical robot, which has excellent seating, binocular vision and finger controls giving each arm six degrees of freedom. However this is at a heavy financial cost which makes it impractical for most institutions, and the robot has a long set-up time. Both these barriers should diminish.

Fatigue and fitness

Pilots recognise three patterns of fatigue, each with different qualities and requirements for recovery. Fatigue associated with a single trip is analogous perhaps to a hard day at work; some exercise, nutrition and a sound sleep are required for optimal performance the next day. Fatigue associated with a tour of duty calls for a proper holiday; experience suggests that two weeks is a minimum. The surgical lifestyle, priorities and pattern of practice can make it difficult to achieve regular recuperative breaks and the result can be chronic fatigue. Chronic fatigue is related to burnout and depression and can be recognised as a state where one no longer cares, creating important implications for safety, teamwork and the quality of one's work. Life balance, general fitness and nutrition are too easily neglected, yet they are vital to day-to-day morale and motivation, and play an important role in surgery.

Cognitive error and information design

Modern surgery developed in an unforgiving culture based on a myth of infallibility and perfect human performance. If there were failures (and there were) it had to be because one 'didn't know enough, didn't do enough or didn't care enough'. This flawed perspective continues to cause misery for thousands of surgeons and trainees and the emotional cost has been compounded by bewilderment and inability of traditional organisations to learn from mistakes made under such assumptions.

Modern industries such as aviation and power generation as well as traditional industries such as mining, transport and the military would be floundering if they had not addressed the very real limitations of human performance demonstrated by recent advances in cognitive psychology and human factors engineering. Surgery has been slow to adopt these lessons but has been catching up. Error theory, root cause analysis, debriefing and disclosure are encouraging developments in contemporary surgery. Cognitive psychologists have demonstrated the extent to which patterns of error are 'hard wired' and predictable. It is essential to understand how the mind works and errs under normal and abnormal conditions in order to understand how errors occur and how they might be avoided or mitigated. A full explanation of this engrossing field is beyond the scope of this chapter and readers are directed to the review by Lucian Leape.[20]

Implications and future developments[21]

By their temperament and training, surgeons are well equipped to make practical use of the rich existing fund of ergonomic knowledge, aided by new habits of observation, concentrating on the operator and their hands and eyes instead of on the patient, and by the use of video recording technology now readily available. Many problems are still managed by flair, intuition and heroic compensation instead of scientific analysis, despite a wealth of practical guidelines in the ergonomic literature. With concepts already available, their application awaits only the interest and energy of some young surgeons. It is easier for a surgeon to learn ergonomics than for an ergonomist to learn enough surgery to bridge the gap between the two disciplines. Only the stimulus for such work has been missing up till now. The application of ergonomics, in the correct context of surgical pathology, should result in better handiwork during operations, more satisfaction and less worry for the operator, and a better result for the patient.

REFERENCES

Much of the material referred to in this chapter can be accessed at Michael Patkin's archives website at http://www.mpatkin.org.

1. Cartmill JA, Shakeshaft AJ, Walsh WR, Martin CJ. High pressures are generated at the tip of laparoscopic graspers. ANZ J Surg 1999;69:127–30.

2. Marucci D, Cartmill J, Walsh W , Martin C. Patterns of Failure at the Instrument–Tissue Interface. J Surg Res 2000;93:16–20.

3. Cartmill JA, Shakeshaft AJ, Walsh WR, Martin CJ. Curved edge moderates high pressure generated by laparoscopic graspers. Surg Endosc 2001;15:1232–4.

4. Patkin M. The hand has two grips: an aspect of surgical dexterity, Lancet 1965;1,1384–5.

5. Patkin M. Selection and care of microsurgical instruments. Advances in Ophthalmology 1978,37,53–63.

6. Patkin M. Surgical instruments and effort, referring especially to ratchets and needle sharpness. Med J Aust 1967,1:225–6.

7. Patkin M. A checklist for handle design [cited 2007 Nov 6]. Available from: http://mpatkin. org/ergonomics/handle_checklist.htm.

8. Vickers DW. A new microsurgical needleholder. Aust N Z J Surg. 1977 Jun;47(3):381–4.

9. Patkin M. Operating room design for minimally invasive surgery. Minim Invasive Ther Allied Technol. 2001 May,10(3):129–31.

10. Patkin M. What surgeons want in operating rooms. Minim Invasive Ther Allied Technol 2003;12(6):256–62.

11. Matern U, Koneczny S. Safety, hazards and ergonomics in the operating room, Surg Endosc. 2007 Nov;21(11):1965–9.

12. atkin M. Ergonomics and the operating microscope. Advances in Ophthalmology 1978,37:23–33.

13. Lythgoe, RJ. The measurement of visual acuity. M.R.I. Special Report Series No. 173. London: H.M.S.O., 1932.

14. Luckiesh M, Moss, FK. The new science of seeing. In: Interpreting the science of seeing into lighting practice, 1, 1927–1932. Cleveland: General Electric Co.

15. Patkin M. Surgical Heuristics. ANZ J Surg (in press June 2008).

16. Leeder PC, Patkin M, Stoddard J, Watson DI. Dissection efficiency during laparoscopic oesophageal dissection. Minim Invasive Ther Allied Technol. 2005;14(1):8–12.

17. Devine H. Surgery of the Alimentary Tract. Bristol: John Wright & Sons Ltd, 1941.

18. Westwood JD et al. eds. Medicine Meets Virtual Reality 14—Accelerating Change in Healthcare: Next Medical Toolkit. Volume 119 Studies in Health Technology and Informatics. USA: IOS Press, 2005.

19. Patkin M, Isabel L. Ergonomics, engineering and surgery of endosurgical dissection. JRCSED 2000;40:120–32.

20. Leape L. Error in Medicine. JAMA 1994; 272:1851–7.

21. Patkin M. History of Ergonomy in Surgery. In: Bruch H-P, Kockerling F, Bouchard R, Schug-Pass C, eds. New Aspects of High Technology in Medicine. Proceedings of the World Congress of High Tech Medicine, Hanover, Germany, 15–18 October 2000. Bologna: Monduzzi Editore.

FURTHER READING

Ergonomics in general

Dul J, Weerdmeester BA. Ergonomics for Beginners: a Quick Reference Guide. 2nd ed. New York: John Wiley, 2001.

Kroemer KHE et al. Ergonomics: How to Design for Ease and Efficiency. 2nd ed. Englewood Cliffs: Prentice Hall, 2000.

Ergonomics applied to surgery

Patkin M. Ergonomic aspects of surgical dexterity, Med. J. Aust. 1967;2:755.

Patkin M. (a) Ergonomics for surgeons; (b) Selection and care of surgical instruments. In: Burnett W, editor. Clinical science for surgeons. London: Butterworth, 1981.

CHAPTER NINE
BASIC OPERATIVE SKILLS

A journey of 1000 miles must begin with one step.

Lao-zi, *Dao de jing*, 6th century BCE

INTRODUCTION

There are hundreds of documented methods for the surgical repair of tissues and many variations in technique for most operations. Within this diversity, however, lies a common thread: those techniques and operations that are successful are built upon the foundation of basic skills. It is competence in the basic skills that underpins mastery of complex procedures.

This chapter introduces the basic surgical skills necessary to embark upon the course of becoming a master surgeon: the operative environment, suturing, knot tying, debridement and haemostasis.

THE OPERATIVE ENVIRONMENT

The entire theatre team, including surgeon(s), anaesthetist(s), technicians, assistants, scrub nurses and circulating nurses all have a direct responsibility for maintenance of an optimal operative environment. As a work environment, the operating theatre is governed by sets of conventions and rules. These have developed over time to increase the effectiveness of the operating team and the safety of patients. For example, the Royal Australasian College of Surgeons endorses the practice of taking 'time out' to check correct patient, correct procedure and correct site immediately prior to commencing a procedure. In addition, less obvious environmental factors may be important in some situations. This means that distractions such as conversation and music should be kept to a minimum unless specifically requested, and the surgeon's concentration should not be broken by unnecessary interruptions. This also applies to the anaesthetist who may require silence for concentration on a difficult situation before, during or after the operation.

Maintenance of the operative field

The site of operation and its surrounds are generally referred to as the 'operative field'. The operative field, as defined by the visible area within the drapes, must be large enough to allow easy and comfortable access for all steps of the operation. Surfaces within the draped sterile field should also be kept tidy to maximise technical efficiency and safety. Bright, concentrated light should illuminate all parts of the operative field but be directed primarily onto the area where tissue is being manipulated. The assistant should alter the lighting when necessary, often many times during a procedure. Additional illumination may be needed from a headlight or lighted retractor for working in deep cavities.

The conventions followed for establishing and maintaining the operative field are underpinned by the need to ensure sterility and tidiness. These two principles, in practice, relate to prepping and draping the patient and instrument management.

Prepping and draping the operative site

This refers to the preparation of the operative field by the application of antimicrobial solutions to the site of operation (prepping) and the exclusion of other areas with sterile towels or sheets (draping). Preparation of the surgical site is discussed more fully in Chapter 4.

Instrument management

Most of the instruments required for an operation are laid out on trolleys and managed by the scrub nurse. Safety and sterility are optimised when all instruments and sharps are 'owned' by the scrub nurse. This means that the surgeon is merely 'borrowing' them and that they must be returned personally to their 'owner', not just dropped in the operative field. This approach ensures that all instruments are accounted for and that no sharps are left in an unexpected position.

The only instruments that belong on the operative field are the diathermy, sucker, instrument scabbard and any clamps or self-retaining retractors while *in situ*. Unfortunately, the last two may catch other instruments, hands or threads, resulting in damage to tissues or tangling. To minimise this, exposed instruments may be covered with a drape.

Positioning the patient

Preoperative positioning of the patient on the operating table is the responsibility of both the surgeon and anaesthetist, with assistance from other members of the operating theatre team including nurses and technicians. Positioning for specific operations is outside the scope of this book; however it is an integral part of learning for any surgeon. The overriding concern in positioning the patient must be safety and the prevention of complications. All staff should be attentive to simple details such as avoiding contact between skin and metal, padding of bony prominences and avoiding pressure on peripheral nerves (the ulnar nerve is particularly vulnerable at the elbow), ensuring joints are not overextended and checking the patient is secure on the table.

Exposure

Good vision of the operative site is a prerequisite for safe surgery, and the ability to achieve this is a key surgical skill. Preparation of the operative field and positioning the patient are preliminary steps. Planning of anaesthesia is also important as for many procedures adequate anaesthesia is vital to keep the patient relaxed to facilitate access to deep structures. If during the procedure exposure becomes suboptimal then the maxim 'check lights, check anaesthesia, enlarge incision, get more assistance' is a time tested strategy.

The operative team

The complexity of modern surgery requires a multidisciplinary team, each member having special skills and roles. At different stages of a procedure primary responsibility for patient care may rest with different medical members of the team—anaesthetists or surgeons. Effective teams have a clear understanding of members' roles and responsibilities, respect for the skills of all members, an open attitude to learning together and good communication. For a full discussion of surgical conduct, see Chapter 1.

Assistance during the procedure

Skilled assistance is invaluable. Anatomy will be best displayed, tensions maintained and other conditions optimised by operating with an assistant who understands the procedure being performed. Experience derived while assisting an experienced surgeon is also an ideal way to learn and appreciate operative surgery. Assisting skills are elaborated at the end of this chapter.

Surgical ergonomics

To increase efficiency of operating and avoid muscle strain due to poor posture, a basic understanding of the ergonomics of surgery is essential. Surgeons should plan every manoeuvre and be constantly mindful of things that will make a task easier to perform. Consider body position or posture (including significant adjustments such as sitting or moving to the other side of the patient), placement of assistant or retractors, table height, repositioning lights, moving monitors, and so on. In times of doubt or stress the basic principles should be strictly adhered to.

All people have a resting tremor and this is exacerbated by the anxiety of operating. To minimise the effect of this tremor both instruments and hands can be steadied against a firm base. This may be as simple as resting an elbow on the table to steady the forearm complex or bracing the operating hand against the patient or the other hand. Instruments such as scissors can be balanced against fingers of the opposite hand to ensure stability while cutting.

See Chapter 8 for a full discussion of surgical ergonomics.

SURGICAL KNOT TYING

The ability to tie secure knots rapidly in any situation or body cavity is an essential part of surgical practice. The life of the patient may depend on the security of one ligature at a virtually inaccessible point. Slippage of such a tie may result in death from exsanguination or major morbidity from blood loss and its haemodynamic sequelae.

Principles of knot tying

The formation of a knot in a suture can be described as the 'intertwining of threads for the purpose of joining them' (Kirk 1995). What we call a knot, however, is strictly a *bend* or *hitch* as the definition of knot is 'a knob or node' in the arboreal sense. The security of any tied suture is improved by the use of certain patterns of knot and the friction between the threads. Friction is affected by the size of the contact area between threads, the tightness of tying, and the suture material that is used. Unfortunately, kinking of the thread or inadequate tightening can reduce knot security by either slippage or breakage.

A *reef knot* is the basic pattern from which all surgical knots derive (Fig. 9.1a). This may have two turns of the thread, as opposed to the standard single turn, and is then called a *surgeon's knot* (Fig. 9.1b). The main advantage of this pattern is the greater friction between threads, leading to improved security of the first throw.

The basic element of the reef knot is a *half-hitch*. This refers to the single intertwining throw of one thread around the other. To complete a secure *reef* knot a mirror image of the first half-hitch is performed. If the reverse throw is performed a less secure *granny knot* is formed (Fig. 9.1a), which is more prone to thread breaking.

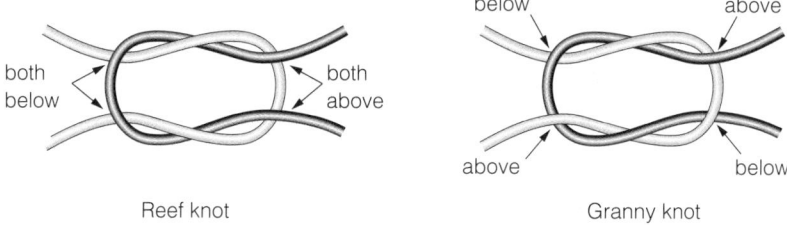

When tying a reef knot, note how the two free ends of one suture emerge from either above or below the loop created by the other suture. In a granny knot the free ends emerge one above and one below each loop.

Fig. 9.1a Reef versus granny knot

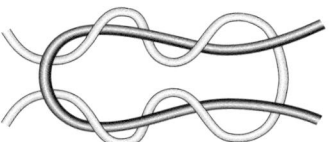

The surgeon's knot follows the same pattern as the reef knot except there are two throws on each side of the knot instead of one.

Fig. 9.1b Surgeon's knot

To ensure correct orientation and good security of the knot, the ends of the thread should be pulled at 180° to each other. This will 'lay down' the knot as flat as possible and prevent the thread pulling into a *sliding hitch* (Fig. 9.2). Depending on the suture material, up to four throws may be required to ensure security of a standard knot and as many as eight when tying slippery monofilament.

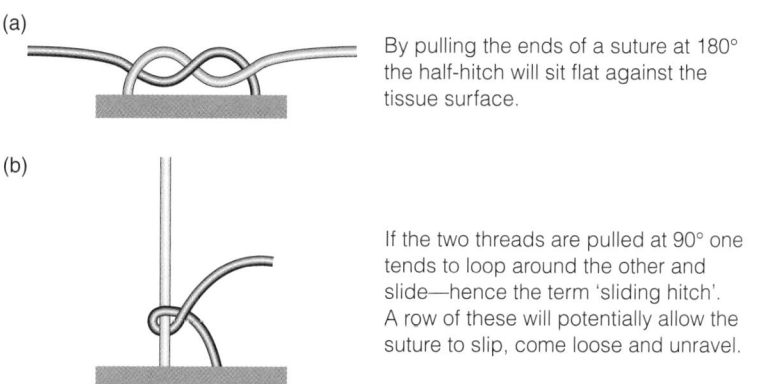

(a)

By pulling the ends of a suture at 180° the half-hitch will sit flat against the tissue surface.

(b)

If the two threads are pulled at 90° one tends to loop around the other and slide—hence the term 'sliding hitch'. A row of these will potentially allow the suture to slip, come loose and unravel.

Fig. 9.2 Flat 'laid-down' knot versus sliding half-hitch

The next two sections deal with two different ways of tying the same knot. The first and simplest to learn is the instrument-tied reef knot. The second is a one-handed technique for tying reef knots. A two-handed technique is the third common method of tying a reef knot. A surgeon should be able to tie one- and two-handed knots with either hand dominant. Hand ties are more often used for tying ligatures or heavier sutures. An instrument is most often employed to tie a suture when a needle holder has been used to insert the suture, or when one end of the thread is very short.

Instrument knot

Using a needle holder to tie a reef or surgeon's knot is probably the most frequently used method of tying sutures in the skin and subcutaneous tissues. It is more economical on thread than a hand tie.

Step 1

Insert the suture and pull it through so that there is a long end which still has the needle attached and a short end on the other side of the wound. Ergonomic technique will usually have the long end on the side of the wound closest to you (Fig. 9.3a).

Step 2

Hold the long end of the suture in the left hand and pull it vertically upwards to straighten (but not put tension on) the thread. Conceptualise the two ends of the thread emerging to form a 'U' shape (Fig. 9.3a). Proper instrument tying requires that the needle holder *always* start inside this 'U'. With needle holder held in the right hand, play a tennis forehand shot towards the straightened thread (Fig. 9.3b).

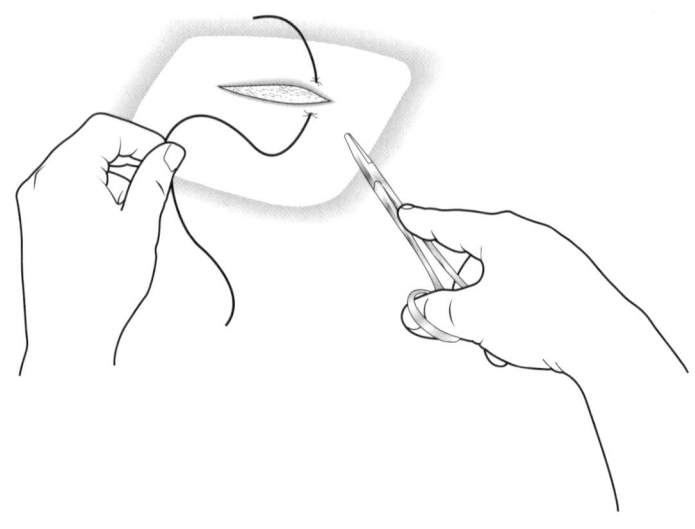

Fig. 9.3a Step 1

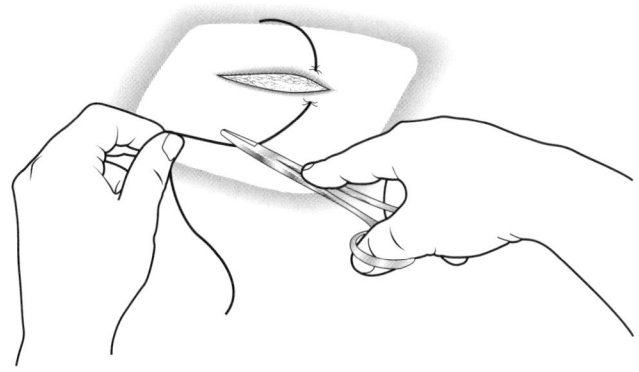

Fig. 9.3b Step 2

Step 3

When the needle holder makes contact, the long end of the thread is wound over and around the jaws of the needle holder, in a clockwise spiral, and back around to the vertical. This may be done twice to create the double loop of a surgeon's knot. Then grasp the tip of the short thread in the needle holder (Fig. 9.3c).

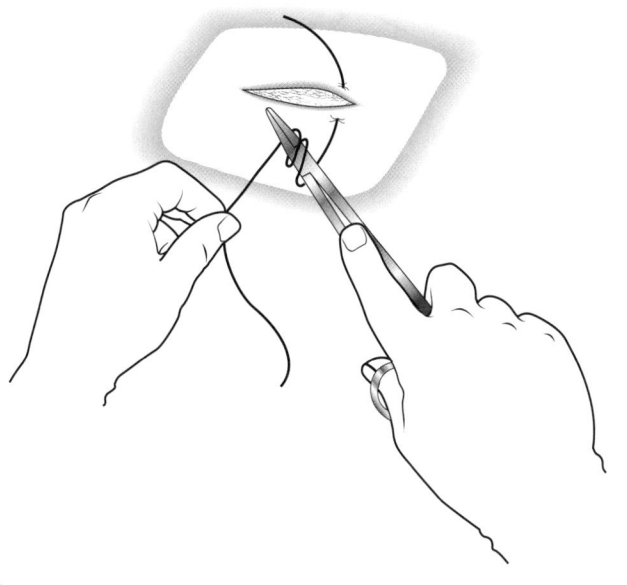

Fig. 9.3c Step 3

Step 4

The short end of the thread is drawn through the loops wound around the needle holder, and out across the wound, with the needle holder following through the tennis forehand shot (Fig. 9.3d).

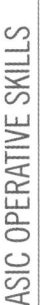

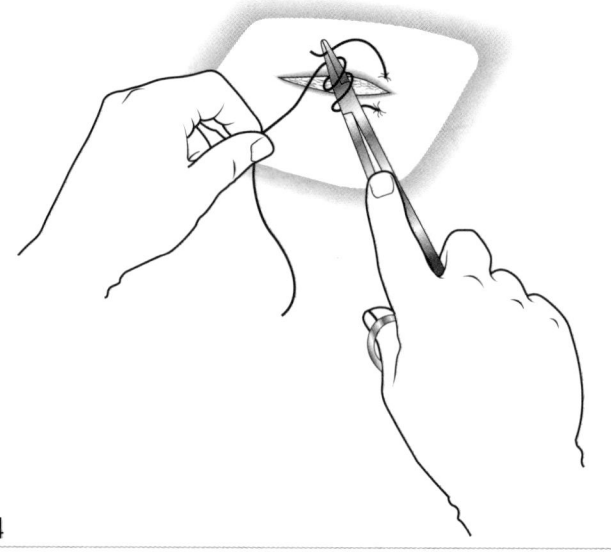

Fig. 9.3d Step 4

Step 5

The long thread end is tensioned in the opposite direction so that the throw is brought down flat in the line of the inserted suture (Fig. 9.3e).

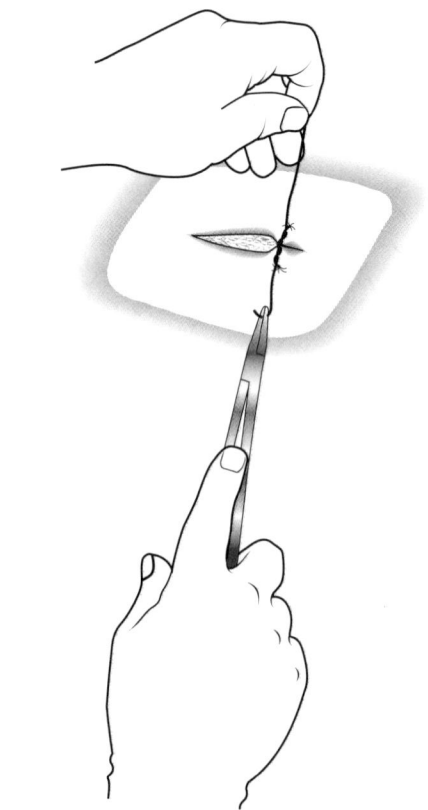

Fig. 9.3e Step 5

Step 6

To make the second, locking throw, once again draw the long end of the thread vertically with the left hand. Ensure that this is not done so hard as to loosen the tightened first throw or to convert it into a hitch. With the needle holder still held in the right hand, play a tennis backhand shot towards the straightened thread (Fig. 9.3f).

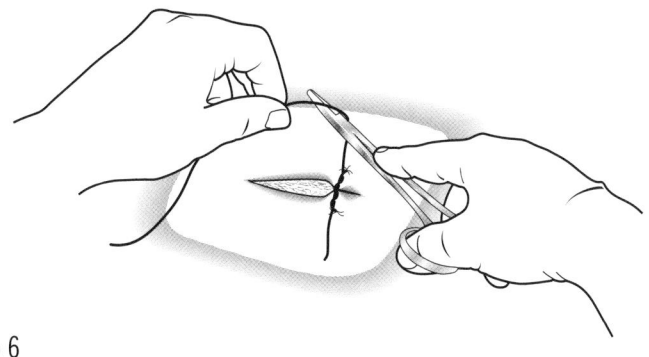

Fig. 9.3f Step 6

Step 7

When the needle holder contacts the thread, wind the thread over and around the jaws of the needle holder in an anti-clockwise spiral over the instrument and back around to the vertical. Once again, this may be done twice to create the double loop of a surgeon's knot (Fig. 9.3g).

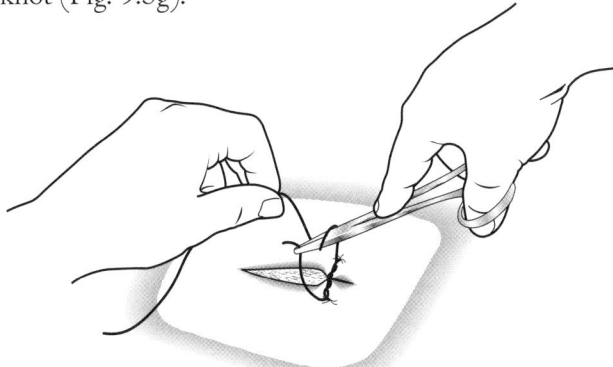

Fig. 9.3g Step 7

Step 8

Grasp the short end of the thread and draw it through the loops of thread around the needle holder and out in the opposite direction from the first throw. Tighten the knot by pulling the ends at 180° to each other. This completes the reef or surgeon's knot (Fig. 9.3h).

Note that the hands change sides every time that a new throw is laid down; this is essential to form a proper reef knot. It is critical that the threads are laid down at

180° to each other to avoid formation of a slip knot. Remember that the topology of a slip and a reef knot are exactly the same: the type of knot formed is entirely determined by how each throw is laid down.

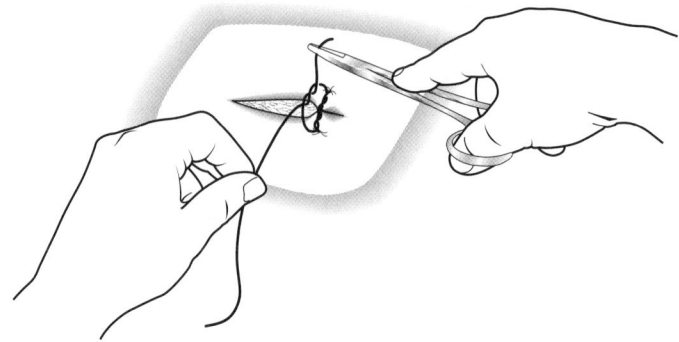

Fig. 9.3h Step 8

Step 9

Repeat steps 2 to 8 as required, producing the appropriate number of throws to secure the suture. Remember the principles of forming a secure reef knot outlined in Table 9.1.

Table 9.1	The important principles for forming a secure reef knot
1.	The needle holder always starts inside the 'U' formed by the emerging threads.
2.	The hands always change side as each throw is laid down.
3.	The threads must be laid down at 180° to each other.

One-handed knot

While called a one-handed knot, two hands are required to tie it. The name comes from the fact that the second hand is merely an anchor for one of the threads, all throws of the knot being made by the fingers of one hand only. Both hands are required to secure the knot down snugly.

This description is for right-handers, as the left hand is used for tying. This means that an instrument in the right hand (usually a needle holder with needle) does not have to be placed down on the patient while tying the knot. Instead it may be palmed while the right hand anchors the long end of the thread. This description also assumes that the short (tag) end of the thread is away from you and the long (needle) end is closer (Fig. 9.4a).

There are two distinct phases to tying this knot. Phase one generates the first throw of the knot and is shown in steps 1–9. The second throw is described in steps 10–13.

Step 1

Both ends of the thread are grasped in an 'underhand pinch' grip between the thumb and middle fingers of both hands. Both forearms should be in the mid-prone position (Fig. 9.4a).

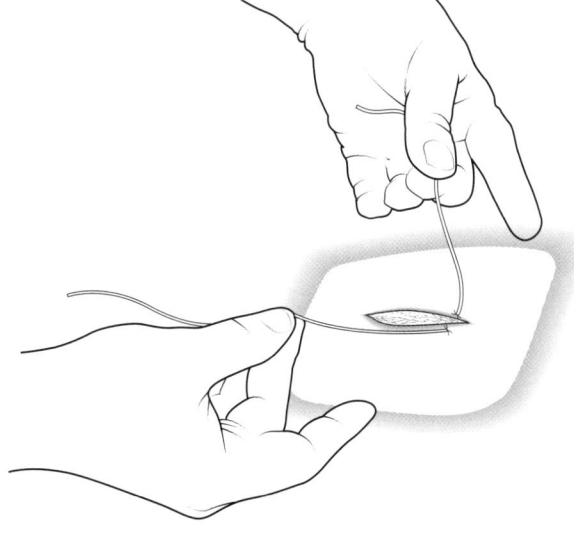

Fig. 9.4a Step 1

Step 2

The left index finger is placed *under* the thread held by the left hand and over the thread held by the right hand (Fig. 9.4b).

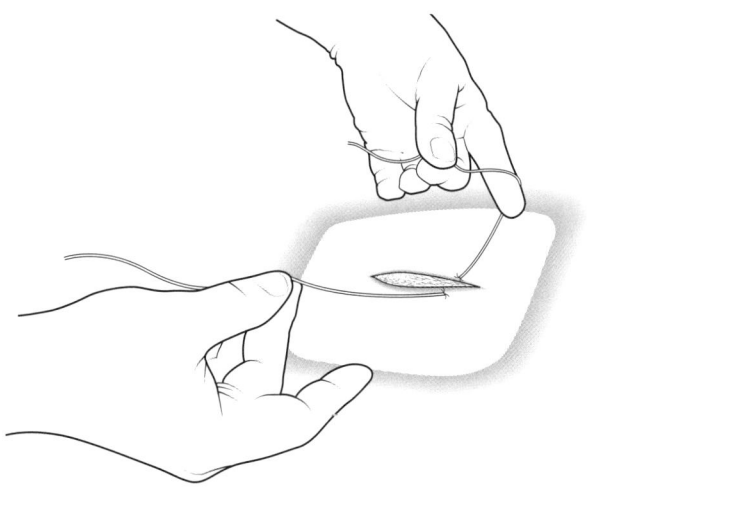

Fig. 9.4b Step2

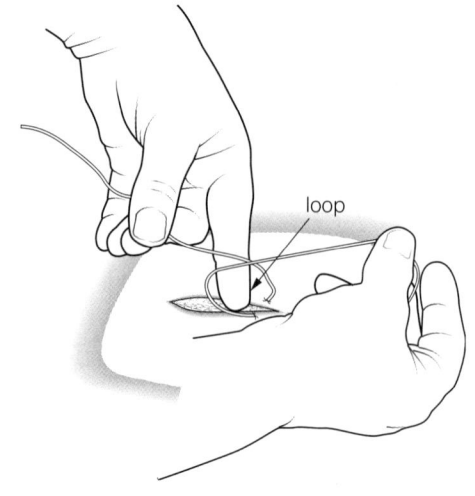

Fig. 9.4c Step 3

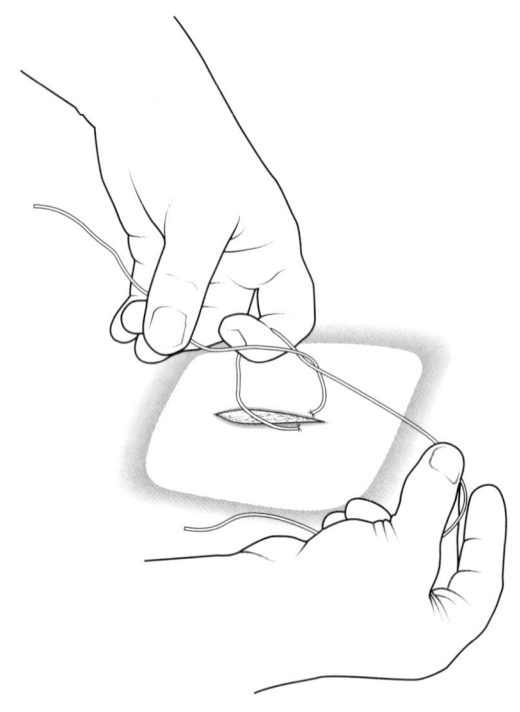

Fig. 9.4d Step 4

Step 3

The right hand is then pushed forward, drawing the thread over the index finger, and the two threads form a loop (Fig. 9.4c).

Step 4

The left index finger is flexed (curled up) so that it lies below the left hand's thread but at the same time traps the right hand's thread in the flexed distal interphalangeal joint (Fig. 9.4d).

Step 5

Extension of the interphalangeal joints of the left index finger, while the metacarpophalangeal joint is still flexed, will pick up the left hand's thread in preparation to use the back of the finger to sweep it through the loop mentioned in step 3.

Step 6

Full extension of the metacarpophalangeal joint of the left index finger is combined with extension of the wrist, and at the same time the left-hand thread is released. This manoeuvre will draw the left-hand thread through the loop (Fig. 9.4e).

Step 7

The left-hand thread is then re-grasped in an 'overhand pinch' grip between the thumb and index finger of the left hand with the left forearm fully pronated (Fig. 9.4f).

Step 8

The throw is then laid down by bringing the left hand towards the operator and pushing the right hand (still in its original orientation) directly away from the operator. This should be done with the threads at 180° and will result in the first half of the reef knot lying flat against the tissues (Fig. 9.4g).

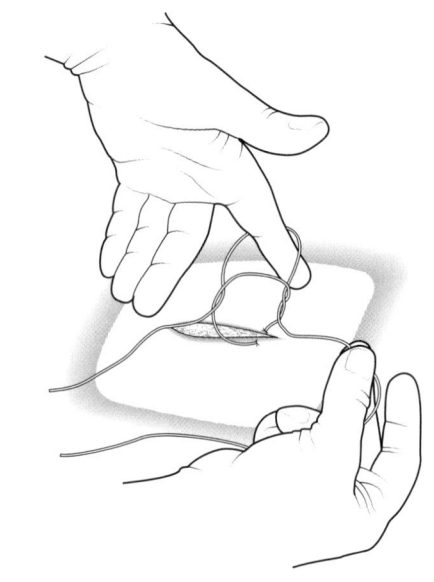

Fig. 9.4e Step 6

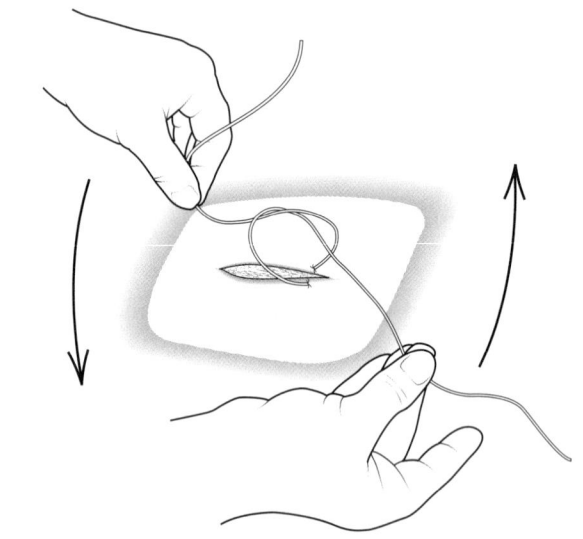

Fig. 9.4f Step 7

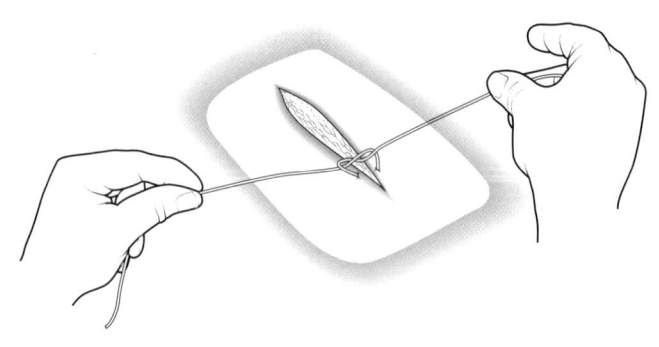

Fig. 9.4g Step 8

Step 9

Next, fully supinate the left forearm with the thread still held between the thumb and index finger but with these two fingers above the plane of the palm. The left-hand thread should now run down and towards the operator, around the little finger or ulnar side of the hand, and back to the wound, creating a *bridge* (Fig. 9.4h).

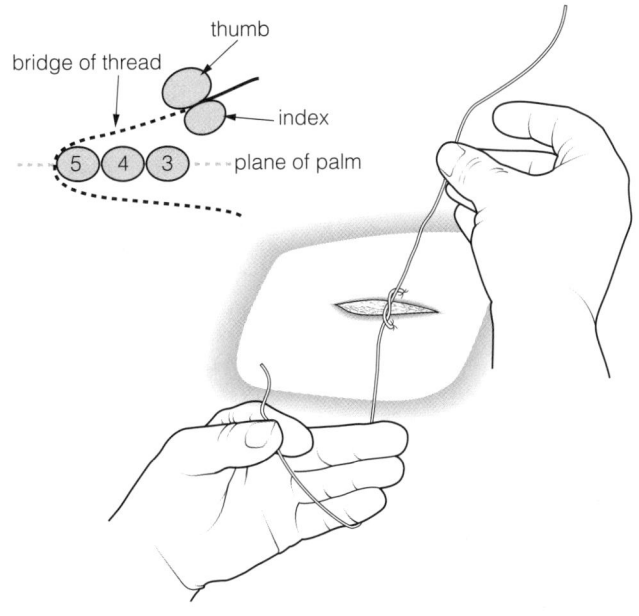

Fig. 9.4h Step 9

Step 10

The right-hand thread must now be brought back towards the operator and laid flat on the three outstretched fingers of the left hand at the level of the PIP joint. The right hand should now be closer to the operator than the left hand. This also creates a loop of thread behind the left hand (Fig. 9.4i).

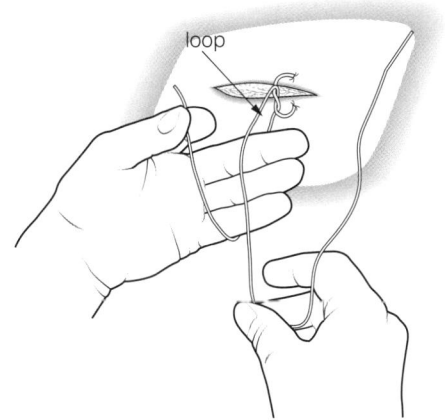

Fig. 9.4i Step 10

Step 11

The middle finger of the left hand is flexed over the thread lying flat on the palm and positioned underneath the *bridged* left-hand thread (Fig. 9.4j).

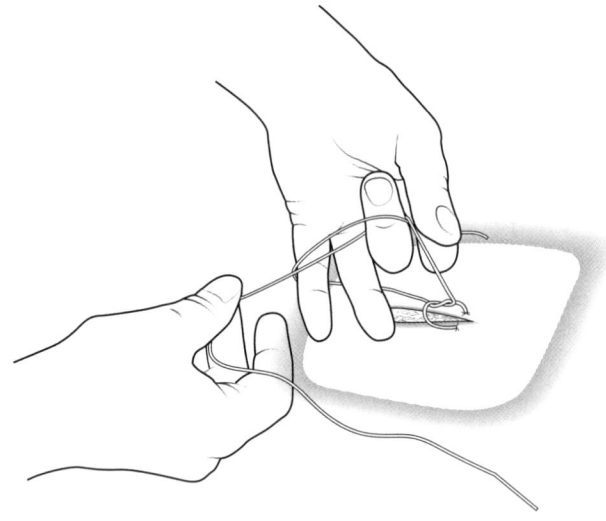

Fig. 9.4j Step 11

Step 12

Extension of the left middle finger will pick up the thread (Fig. 9.4k) and extension of the wrist will pull the thread through the loop described in step 10 (Fig. 9.4l).

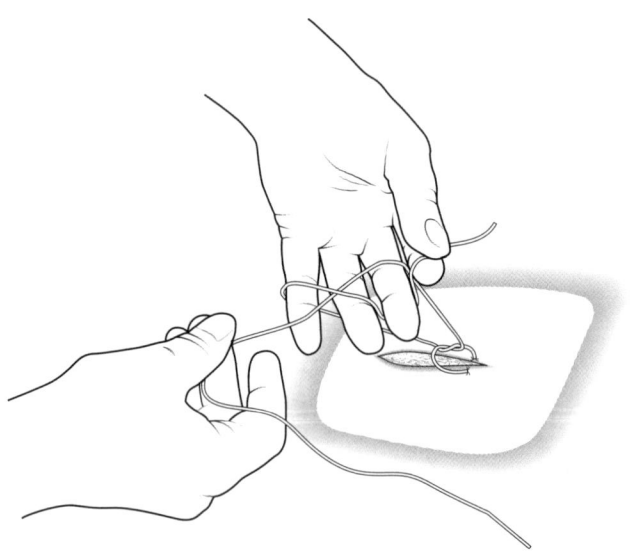

Fig. 9.4k Step 12

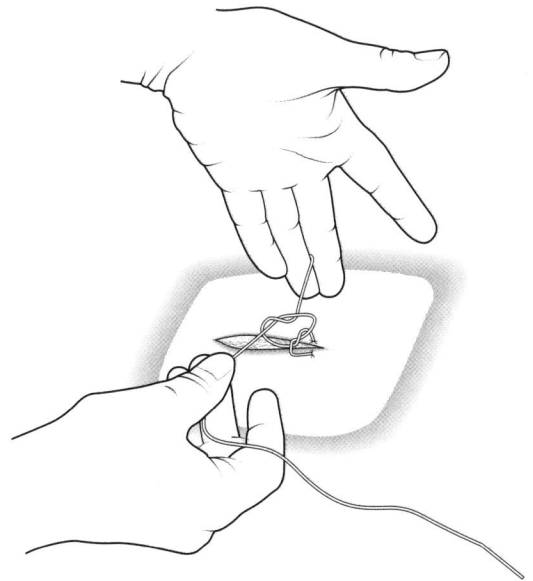

Fig. 9.4l Completing step 12

Step 13

The left-hand thread must now be firmly grasped between the thumb and middle finger of the left hand. This hand is pushed away from, and the right hand brought towards, the operator with the threads at 180°. This will lay the second throw of the reef knot flat against the tissues (Fig. 9.4m).

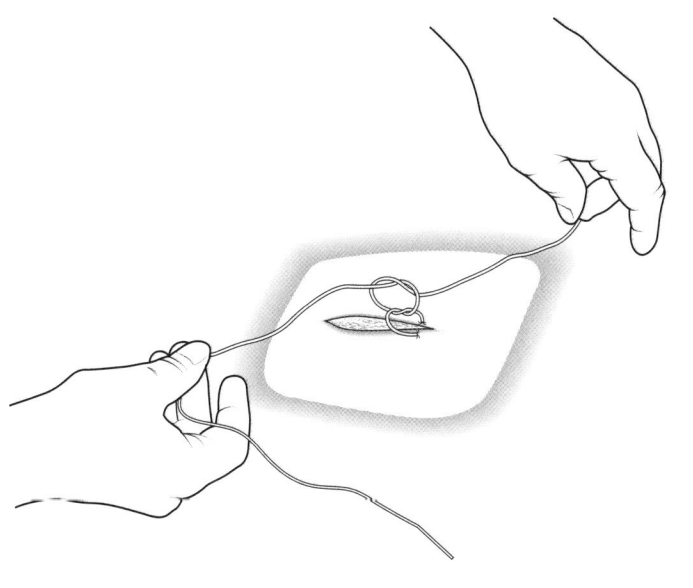

Fig. 9.4m Step 13

Step 14

Repeat steps 1 to 13 to create a double reef knot. As an added feature, two throws of the thread can be brought through the loops in steps 6 and 12 to create a surgeon's knot.

Two-handed knot

The two-handed method of tying a reef knot is most useful when it is desirable to maintain strict tension on both threads. This may apply when the structure is difficult to secure and must be kept compressed while tying. It is sometimes employed by surgeons when tying large vascular pedicles and is the technique of preference for some. It is also useful when tying very fine threads that are more difficult to control with the one-handed technique. It is important that all surgeons are competent in this technique. Like the one-handed knot, there are two distinct phases to the two-handed technique, outlined in steps 1–6 and 7–11 below.

Step 1

Start with the short end of the thread away from you and pick up that end between left thumb and index finger. Grasp the long end of the thread with the right hand in an overhand grip (Fig. 9.5a).

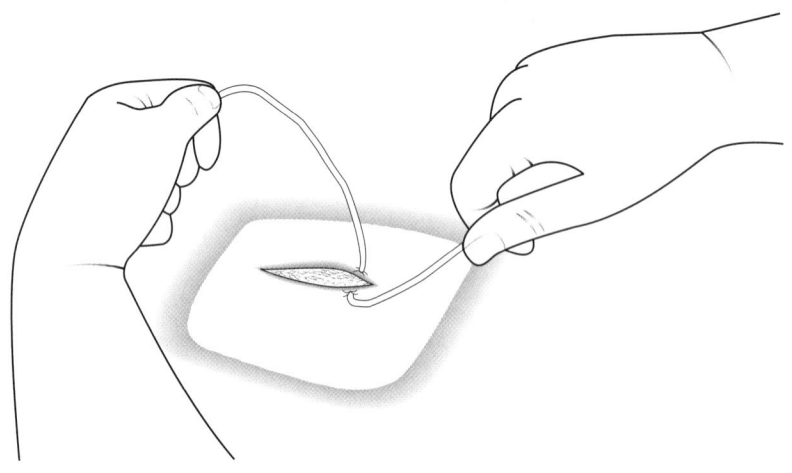

Fig. 9.5a Step 1

Step 2

Hook the right thumb underneath the long end and cross the threads over the thumb (Fig. 9.5b).

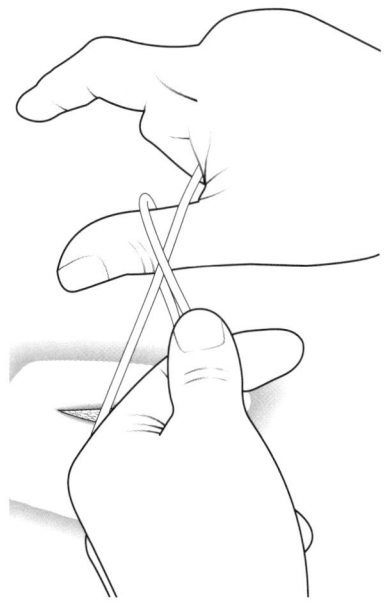

Fig. 9.5b Step 2

Step 3

Appose the right index finger and thumb (Fig. 9.5c), then supinate the right forearm to rotate the apposed digits beneath the crossed threads to the opposite side (Fig. 9.5d).

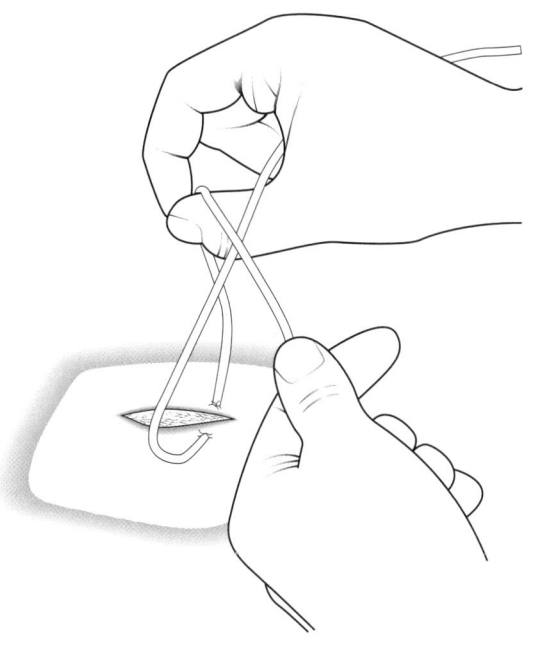

Fig. 9.5c Step 3

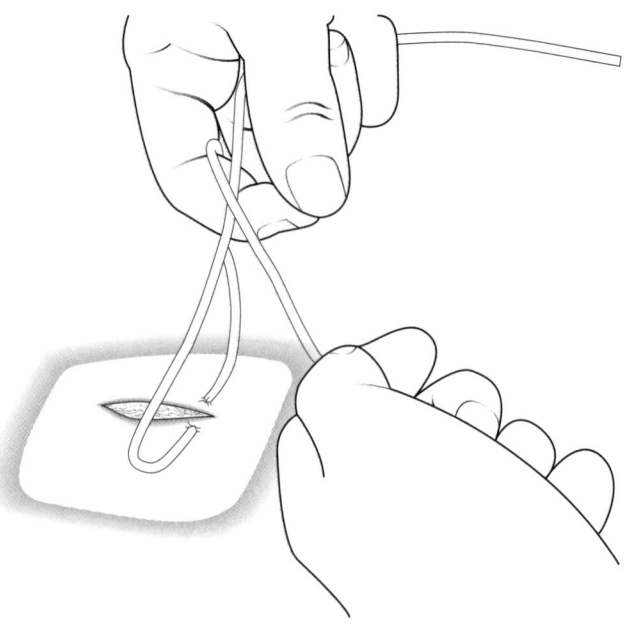

Fig 9.5d Completing step 3

Step 4

Transfer the short end of the thread from your left hand into the right hand finger–thumb grasp (Fig. 9.5e).

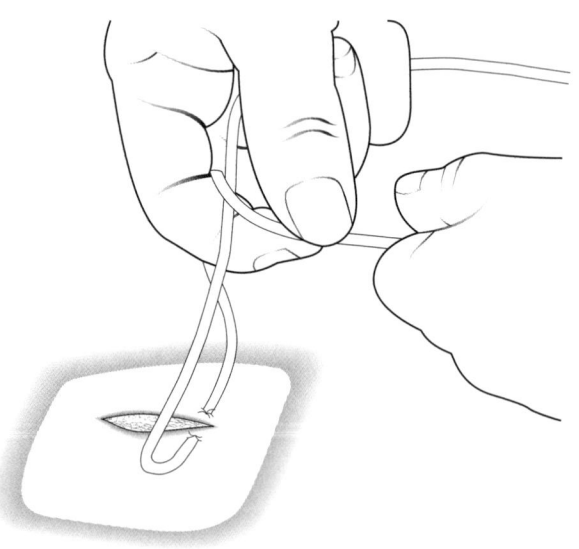

Fig. 9.5e Step 4

Step 5

Pronate the right forearm to bring the short end of the thread back beneath the crossed threads (Fig. 9.5f).

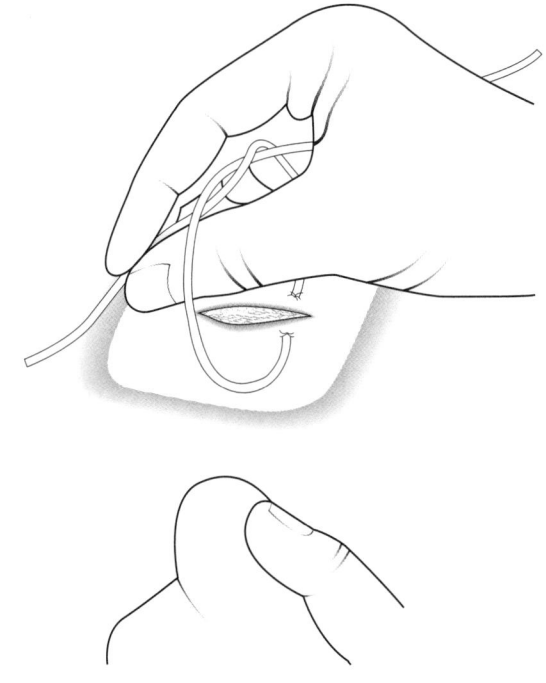

Fig. 9.5f Step 5

Step 6

Re-grasp the short end between the thumb and index finger of the left hand and lay the throw flat by drawing the right hand away from you and your left hand towards you, tensioning the threads at 180° to each other (Fig. 9.5g).

Step 7

Retain the long end in the right hand in an overhand grip, and then supinate the right forearm to hook the right index finger under this strand (Fig. 9.5h).

Step 8

Cross the threads over the right index finger (Fig. 9.5i).

Step 9

Oppose the right thumb and index finger again and pronate to rotate the opposed digits through the loop beneath the crossed threads (Fig. 9.5j, k).

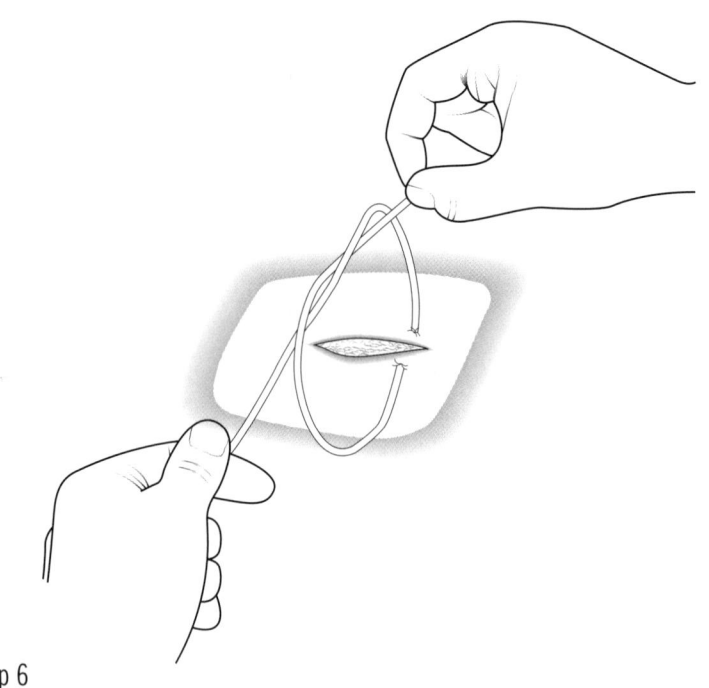

Fig. 9.5g Step 6

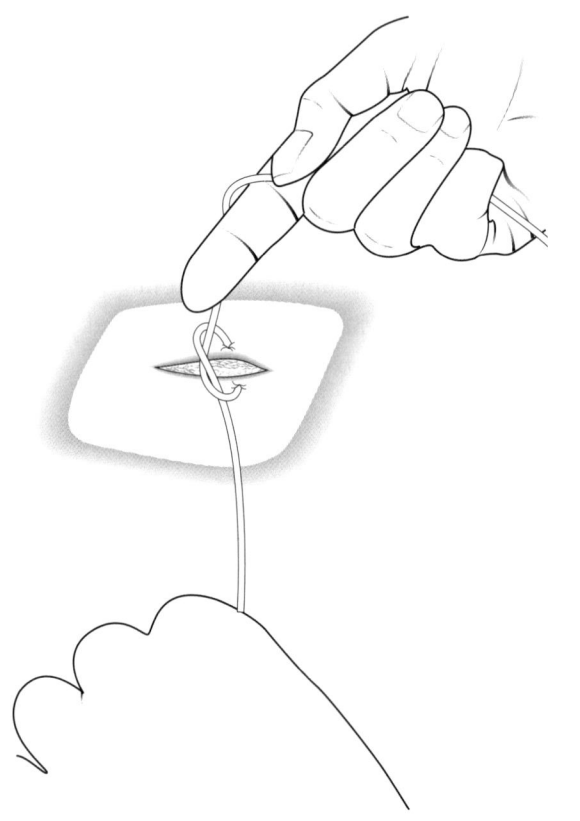

Fig. 9.5h Step 7

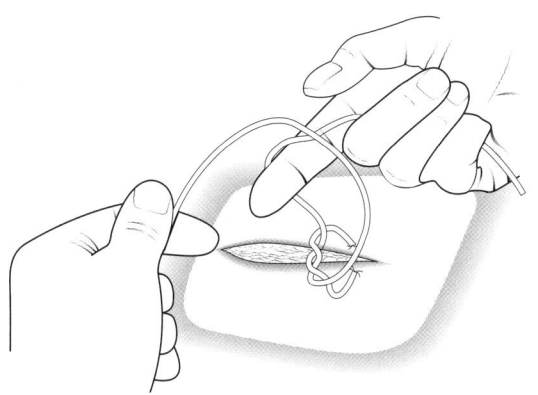

Fig. 9.5i Step 8

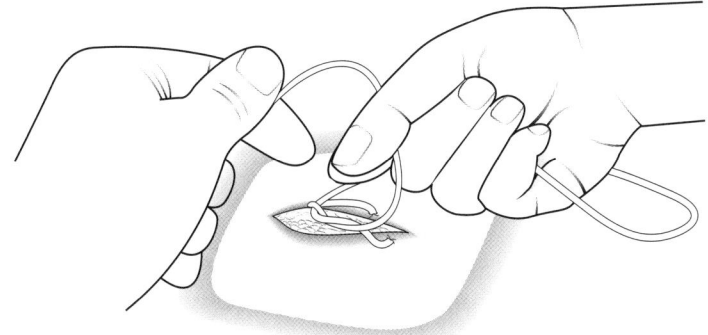

Fig. 9.5j Step 9

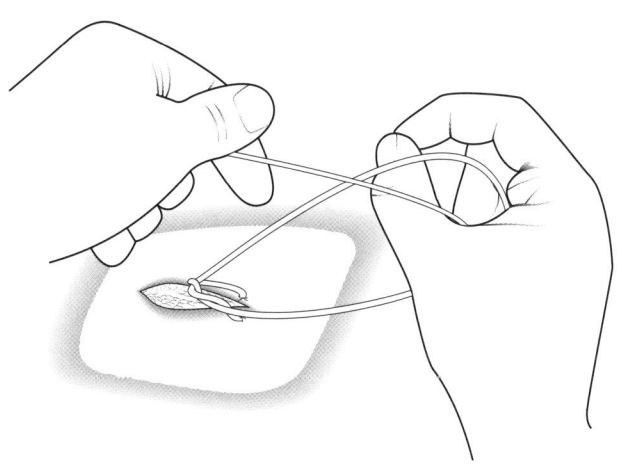

Fig. 9.5k Completing step 9

Step 10

Transfer the short end from the left hand to the opposed right index finger and thumb, and supinate to bring the thread back through the loop (Fig. 9.5l, m).

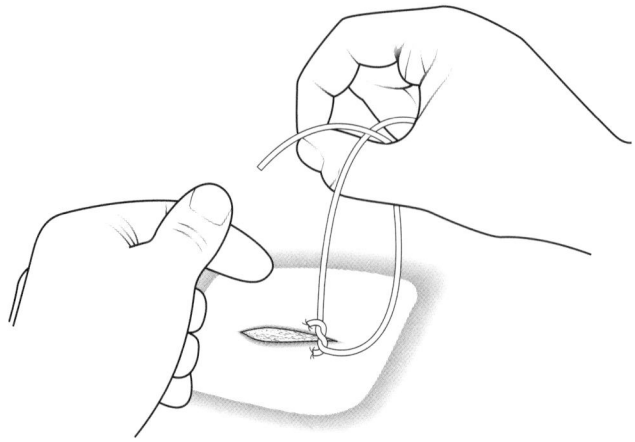

Fig. 9.5l Step 10

Step 11

Re-grasp the short end with the left hand and lay the throw down squarely upon the first throw by drawing your left hand away from you and your right hand towards you.

Notice how your hands change sides to tension alternate throws. Again lay the throw flat by drawing the threads at 180° to each other (Fig. 9.5n, o). Steps 1 to 11 are repeated as required.

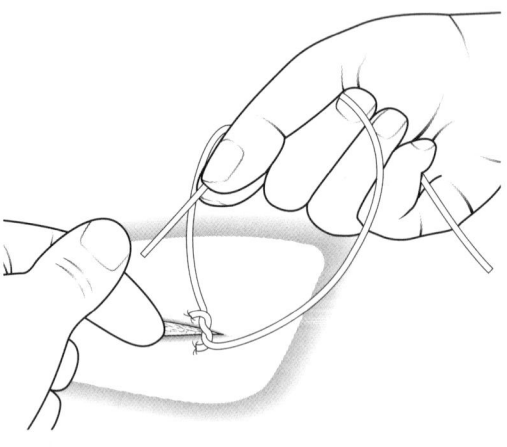

Fig. 9.5m Step 11

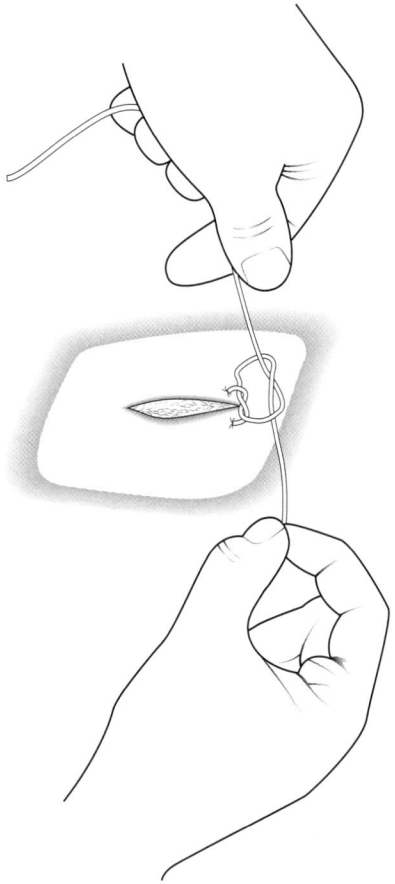

Fig. 9.5n Completing step 11

Slip knots

Sometimes, when tying at depth or bringing together edges under tension, it is helpful to tie an intentional slip knot and push this down. This is done by throwing two half hitches, pushing these down with the index finger and tightening, then securing with a reef knot according to the following steps. The slip knot is constructed using exactly the same steps as for a reef knot. The only difference is how the throws are laid down on each other: in a reef knot the threads are laid down at 180°; in a slip knot they are laid down at 90°.

Step 1
Make an initial one-handed throw, laying down the threads down at 90° to each other (Fig. 9.6a).

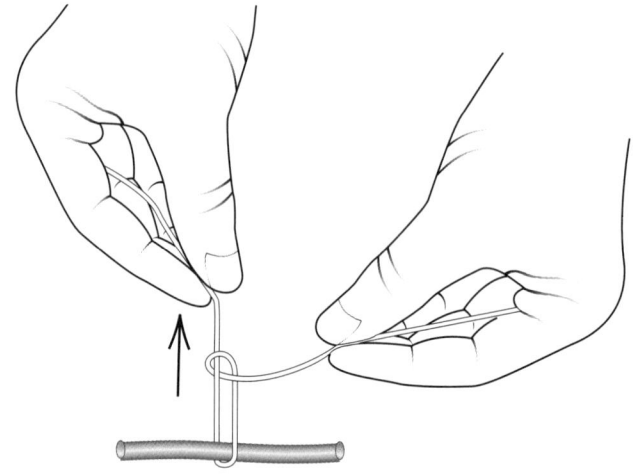

Fig. 9.6a Step 1

Step 2
Make a second one-handed throw, again laying down the threads down at 90° to each other (Fig. 9.6b).

Step 3
Push the slip knot to depth by holding the thread carrying the half hitches straight with the right hand and pushing the knot down with the left index finger (Fig. 9.6c).

Step 4
Complete the knot with two further throws to make a reef knot on top of the slip knot.

Endoscopic knot tying
Various endoscopic knot techniques utilise pre-tied slip knots pushed down into position with a knot pusher (Fig. 9.7). Alternatively, knots can be tied intracorporeally with the same technique as instrument tied knots described above, using laparoscopic instruments.

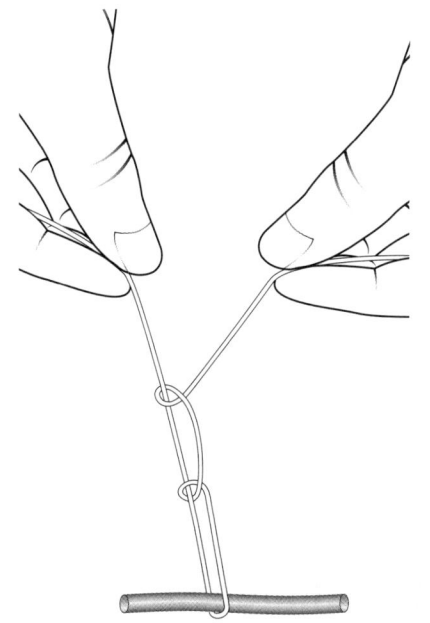

Fig. 9.6b Step 2

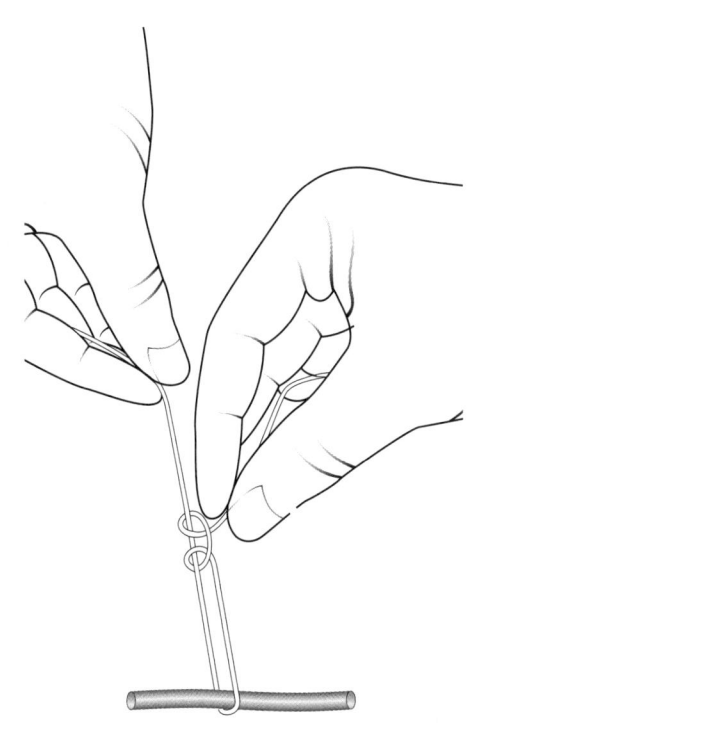

Fig. 9.6c Step 3

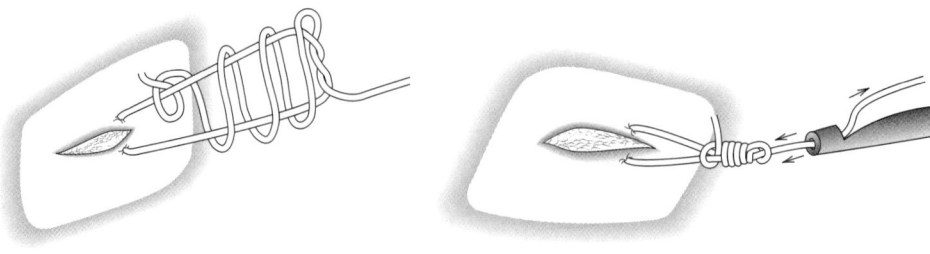

The Roeder knot is secured by
a knot pusher

Topology of the Roeder knot

Fig. 9.7 Extracorporeal slip knots—the Roeder knot

BASIC SUTURING TECHNIQUES

This section deals with basic suturing techniques used in the repair of skin and fascia. The combination of dexterity, instrument handling, tissue handling and the exposure to tissue tension make suturing and knot tying the perfect introduction to surgical skills.

Introduction to suturing tissues

Some simple conventions apply to the suturing of all tissues. *Round-bodied* or *taper* needles are used for fat and fascia and *reverse cutting* needles for skin. See Chapter 6 for a detailed discussion of needle types. The needle should be grasped in needle-holding forceps (see Chapter 5) of appropriate size. Tissues such as the skin edge should be handled lightly with a fine- to medium-toothed forceps (e.g. Adson or Gillies) or a skin hook to avoid crush damage. This same principle, with appropriate tools, applies to all types of tissues for suturing.

The objective is to achieve approximation of the wound edges, loosely and accurately, and to minimise dead space. The width and distance between sutures depends on the tissue, the suture material and the site of the wound. In general terms the suture should run as deeply as the distance from the skin edge to the suture entry point. The sutures should be balanced evenly, with equal bites taken on either side of the wound, and spaced as widely as the distance from entry hole to exit hole, thereby forming squares (Fig. 9.8a).

The knot is tied 'square', and laid to the side of best sit (Fig. 9.8b). The stitch itself should not indent the skin. Interrupted (individual) sutures should be equally spaced and the ends cut so as not to touch the next suture (Fig. 9.8a).

(a)

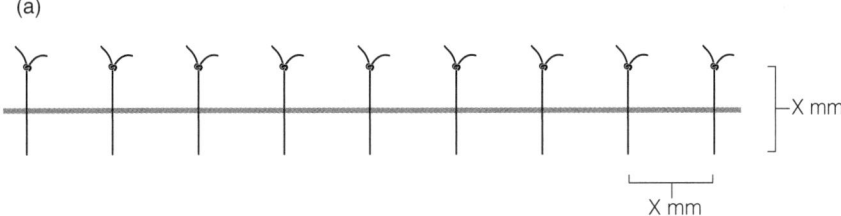

—X mm

X mm

Sutures along a wound are spaced at approximately equal intervals (X mm).
This corresponds with the width of the stitch and allows the sutures to form
a square (box) pattern.

(b)

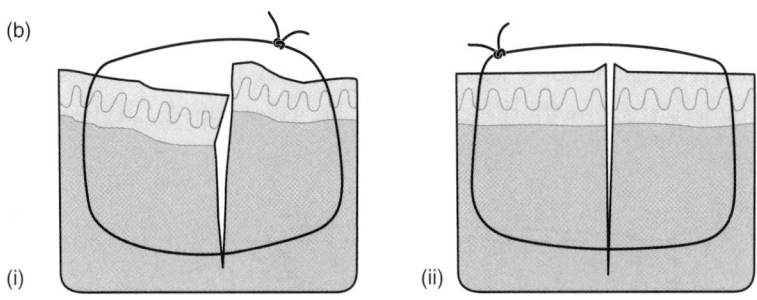

(i) (ii)

Demonstration of placing the knot on the side of the wound that allows the
skin to sit most evenly. When on the right (i) the skin is uneven but if the knot
is moved to the left (ii) this evens out.

Fig. 9.8 Placement of sutures

If sutures are too tight they will be painful, and postoperative swelling
may cause the suture to cut into epidermis leaving scarred 'train-tracks'. More
seriously, excessive pressure may cause ischaemia leading to wound-edge necrosis
and possible infection. These principles apply equally to deep tissues. Excessive
dead space allows haematoma formation, but tight sutures may strangulate and
necrose fat, muscle and fascia, causing pain and providing a nidus for infection and
subsequent wound weakness.

The most commonly used suture materials for interrupted and exposed skin
sutures are non-absorbable, synthetic monofilament fibres, which usually need to be
removed between the 5th and 10th postoperative days, depending on the site. Sutures
that are buried, or run in the skin (subcuticular sutures) are usually made from an
absorbable material. There are exceptions to these basic rules, but these basic options
will safely cover most common situations. See Chapter 6 for more detail about suture
types and selection.

Simple suture

As the name suggests, the simple suture (Fig. 9.9) is the basic pattern of suture and the one on which all others are based. It is useful in many situations and must be mastered as part of basic skill development.

The curved needle should be gripped in the tips of the forceps, two-thirds of the way from the point to the swage, and enter the tissue (skin) at 90°. It should traverse a *virtually* semicircular course to exit skin again at 90°. This is often performed in two separate bites, each describing a 90° arc. Once the needle enters the bottom of the wound it should be removed, reinserted into the holder and the second arc begun from the depths of the wound. (Fig 9.11)

The knot is tied and adjusted to give the best 'vertical' apposition of skin edges. If more deep tissue than superficial is taken the skin edges will evert (Fig 9.10a). Similarly, if less is taken the edges will invert (Fig 9.10b). This pattern of suture may also be used in deep tissues with the knot either buried or superficial (Fig. 9.10c).

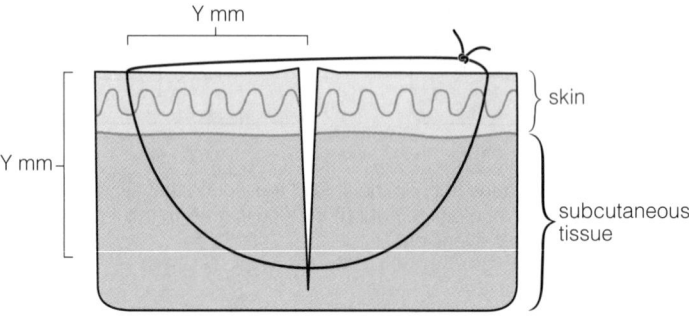

A schematic representation of the semi-circular simple suture. The depth of the bite and the distance from skin puncture site to the centre of the wound are both a 'radius' in distance (Y mm) and should be virtually equal.

Fig. 9.9 Simple suture

Vertical mattress suture

The vertical mattress suture (Fig. 9.12, pages 179–180) begins the same way as a simple suture, but after the needle has exited the skin, it is reversed in the needle holder and reinserted to pick up a small lip of each wound edge in the same line as the original stitch (Fig. 9.10a). This ensures eversion of the edges and better healing. The vertical mattress suture is best used in skin creases and areas of natural inversion (e.g. the back of a hand or other sites of loose skin).

The major potential problem with this suture is that it can cause excessive pressure on the tissues. If the sutures are so close and tight that they prevent dermal blood flow this may subsequently cause skin-edge ischaemia and necrosis. Attention to suture spacing will minimise this complication.

(a) everting simple suture

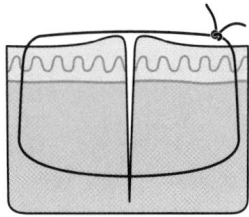

The everting simple suture picks up more subcutaneous tissue than the skin width and, when tied, this deeper tissue is squeezed superficially to evert the edges of the wound.

(b) inverting simple suture

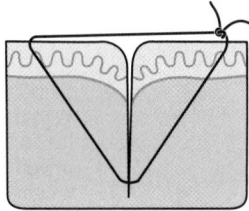

The inverting simple suture does the opposite of (i) and takes less deep tissue. This allows the more superficial tissues to roll in towards each other causing inversion. A suture like this should not be used in skin but is very useful for inverting bowel edges in anastomoses.

(c) buried simple suture

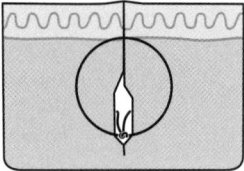

The buried simple suture is used to secure deep layers of tissue and approximates a circle rather than a semi-circle.

Fig. 9.10 10 variations on simple suture

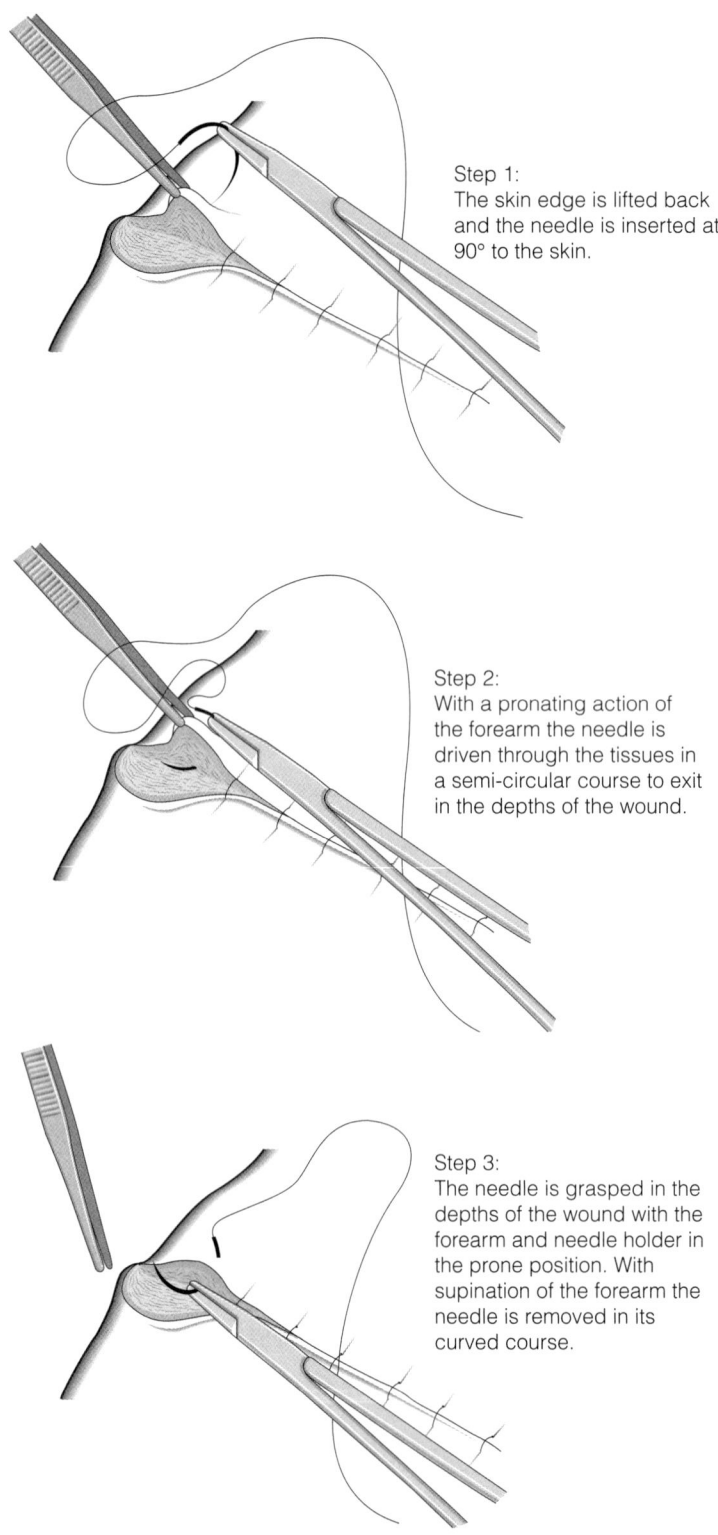

Step 1:
The skin edge is lifted back and the needle is inserted at 90° to the skin.

Step 2:
With a pronating action of the forearm the needle is driven through the tissues in a semi-circular course to exit in the depths of the wound.

Step 3:
The needle is grasped in the depths of the wound with the forearm and needle holder in the prone position. With supination of the forearm the needle is removed in its curved course.

Fig. 9.11 Inserting a simple suture

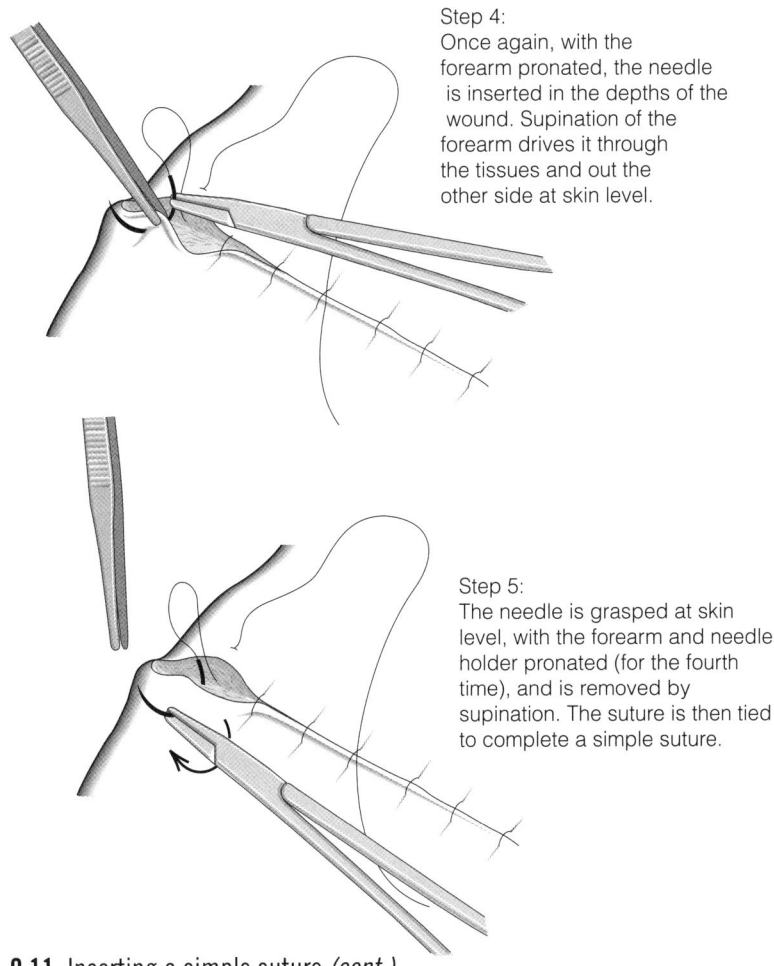

Step 4:
Once again, with the forearm pronated, the needle is inserted in the depths of the wound. Supination of the forearm drives it through the tissues and out the other side at skin level.

Step 5:
The needle is grasped at skin level, with the forearm and needle holder pronated (for the fourth time), and is removed by supination. The suture is then tied to complete a simple suture.

Fig. 9.11 Inserting a simple suture *(cont.)*

(a)

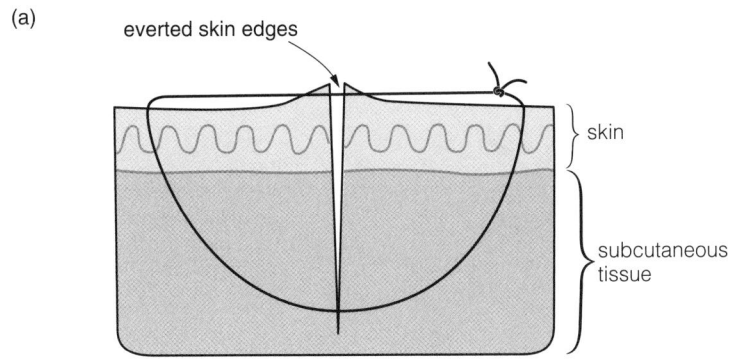

everted skin edges

skin

subcutaneous tissue

A schematic representation of the vertical mattress suture showing how the skin is picked up with a second 'mini-suture' in the same line as the main suture. This ensures eversion of the skin edges.

Fig. 9.12 Vertical mattress suture

(b) Inserting a vertical mattress suture

The first five steps correspond with Figures 9.11(a) to (e).

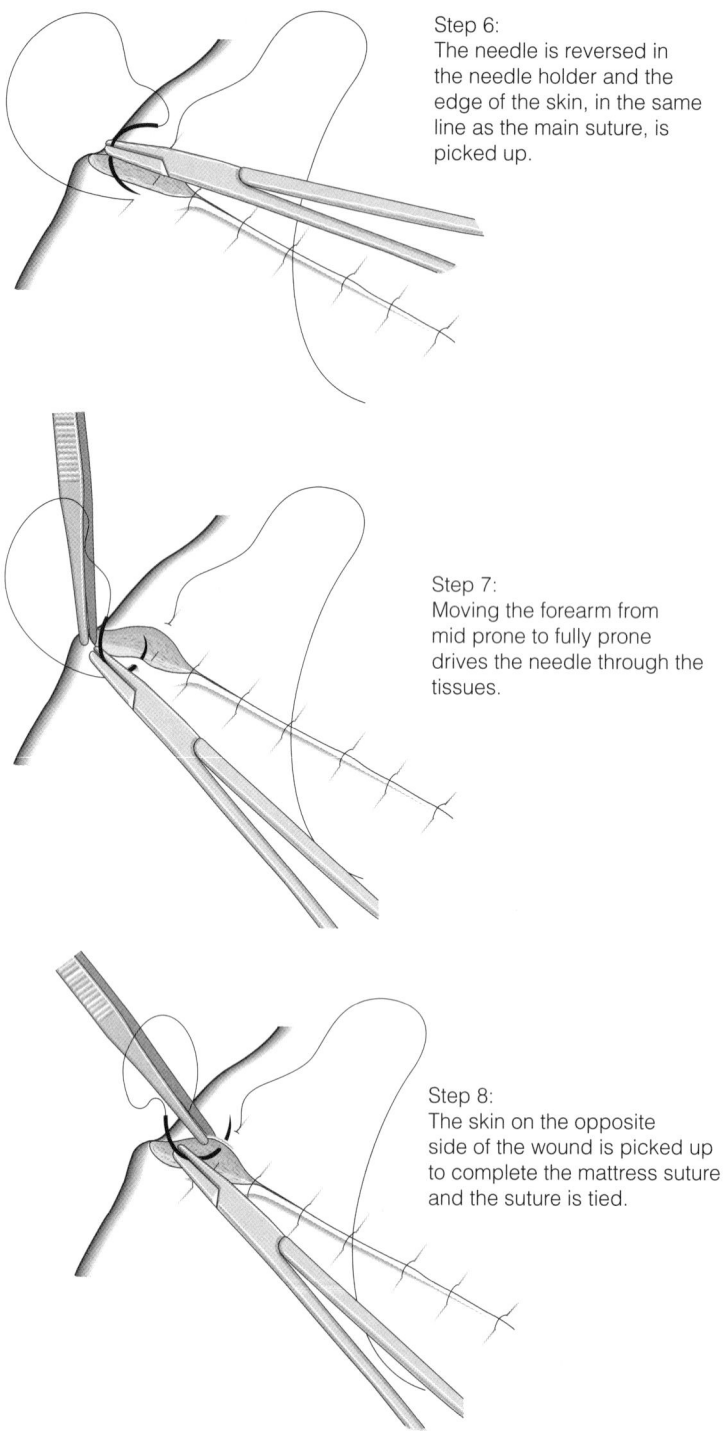

Step 6:
The needle is reversed in
the needle holder and the
edge of the skin, in the same
line as the main suture, is
picked up.

Step 7:
Moving the forearm from
mid prone to fully prone
drives the needle through the
tissues.

Step 8:
The skin on the opposite
side of the wound is picked up
to complete the mattress suture
and the suture is tied.

Fig. 9.12 Vertical mattress suture *(cont.)*

Horizontal mattress suture

The horizontal mattress suture (Fig. 9.13) is also useful for ensuring eversion of the skin. Like the vertical mattress suture, it begins with the first stitch of a simple suture. Then, instead of tying over the wound, the needle is reversed and moved a stitch length along the wound. A full-thickness bite is taken in the reverse direction, ending on the original side where the two ends are tied. In essence this creates two parallel simple sutures which have a bridge of suture joining them on one side of the wound and the two tied ends on the other. The mattress suture should appear to sit in a square configuration (Fig. 9.13a).

In tying this suture the tension must be just right. If tied too loosely the skin edges fall apart, and if too tightly the skin edges pout too far and do not appose correctly. With the correct amount of tension the dermis and epidermis evert but still meet for accurate healing (Fig. 9.13b). This type of suture is of particular use in flexures, on the backs of hands and any site with loose skin, as it gives an excellent everting result.

Continuous ('running') suture

The continuous suture runs the entire length of the wound and is formed from a single piece of thread (Fig. 9.14). The suture is tied at one end of the wound and then the pattern (simple, vertical mattress or horizontal mattress) is followed until the other end of the wound is reached and the suture is tied again. Apart from the previous variants, the simple suture may also be interlocked to improve the lie of the sutures. This can however increase the risk of tissue ischaemia.

Subcuticular suture

A subcuticular suture (Fig. 9.15) is an excellent way of closing skin without leaving unsightly cross-hatches in the scar. It is also far less ischaemic as the suture runs through the dermis (and therefore *in* the plane of the vessels) leading to reduced tissue pressure and ischaemia.

This suture is commenced either by burying a knot and bringing the suture up through the apex of the wound (using absorbable threads) or by entering from the outside to the apex of the wound and securing the completed suture outside (Fig. 9.15a(i)). Alternatively, the needle can enter from the outside to the apex of the wound then be secured using an Aberdeen knot. This technique can be mirrored at the distant end of the wound. The advantage of this technique is that the suture is soundly secured at either end of the wound with a knot that still has a long but completely buried tail (Fig. 9.15a(ii)). Bites are taken parallel to the skin surface but through the dermis. Unless these bites are at the same depth an uneven vertical overlap will occur (Fig. 9.15b).

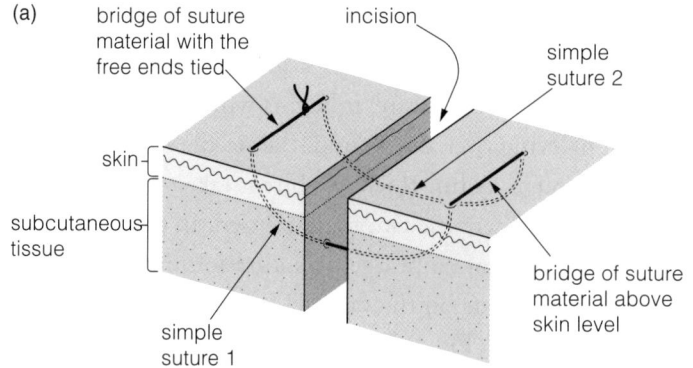

(a)

bridge of suture material with the free ends tied

incision

simple suture 2

skin

subcutaneous tissue

bridge of suture material above skin level

simple suture 1

The horizontal mattress suture comprises two simple sutures and two bridges of suture material above the skin. In rough terms, the positioning of suture bites and suture bridges should approximate a square.

(b)

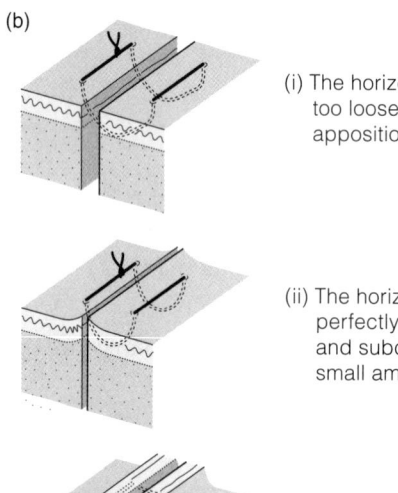

(i) The horizontal mattress suture tied too loosely, resulting in poor tissue apposition and gaping of the wound.

(ii) The horizontal mattress suture tied perfectly, with meeting of the skin and subcutaneous tissues and a small amount of eversion.

(iii) The horizontal mattress suture tied too tightly. The subcutaneous tissues meet but the eversion is so great that the skin sits apart preventing healing.

Fig. 9.13 Horizontal mattress suture

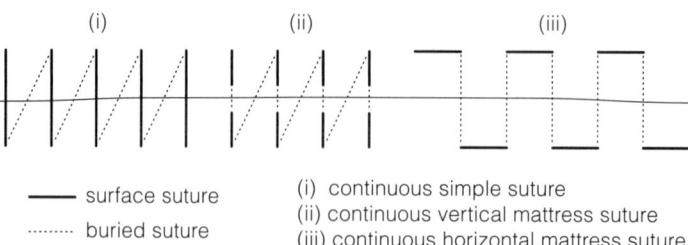

(i)   (ii)   (iii)

—— surface suture

········ buried suture

(i) continuous simple suture
(ii) continuous vertical mattress suture
(iii) continuous horizontal mattress suture

Fig. 9.14 Continuous suture – three versions

There are differing views about how much overlap should occur between suture bites, varying from none to almost 90%. The subcuticular suture technique usually employs an absorbable suture, which will not need to be removed. If a non-absorbable suture is used, it must be placed meticulously without kinks or knots that may impede later removal. If a non-absorbable suture has to be used for a long wound, a bridge stitch (loop of suture out onto the skin at intervals along the wound) may be placed to allow for easier removal (Fig. 9.13c).

If a non-absorbable suture is used it may be tied to itself at the ends of the wound, or tied over the wound to create a loop (Fig. 9.13d). Beads and crimped metal have also been used to retain the ends.

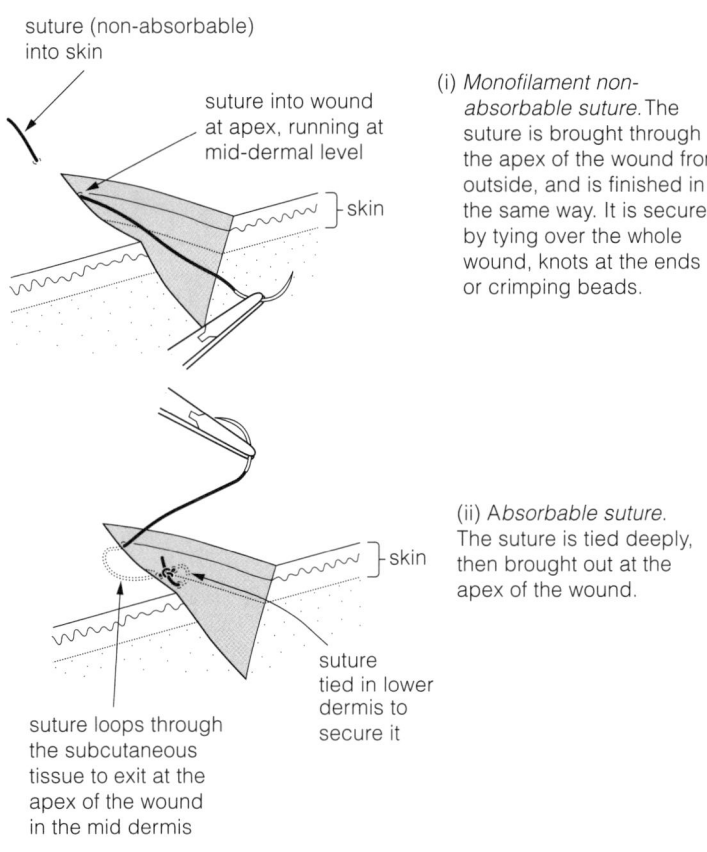

(a) Starting the subcuticular suture (2 methods)

suture (non-absorbable) into skin

suture into wound at apex, running at mid-dermal level

skin

(i) *Monofilament non-absorbable suture.* The suture is brought through the apex of the wound from outside, and is finished in the same way. It is secured by tying over the whole wound, knots at the ends or crimping beads.

skin

(ii) A*bsorbable suture.* The suture is tied deeply, then brought out at the apex of the wound.

suture tied in lower dermis to secure it

suture loops through the subcutaneous tissue to exit at the apex of the wound in the mid dermis

Fig. 9.15 Subcuticular suture

(b) Subcuticular suture placement

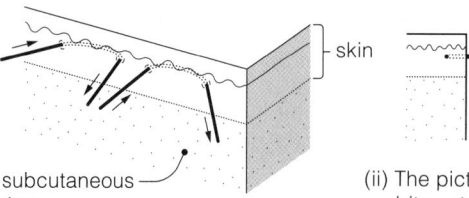

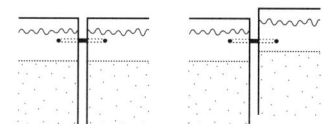
skin

subcutaneous
tissue

(i) The subcuticular suture should
enter and exit at approximately
the junction of the upper and
middle thirds of the dermis.

(ii) The picture on the left shows
bites at the same dermal level,
allowing even skin apposition.
The picture on the right shows
uneven bites at different dermal
levels, causing uneven apposition.

(c) Patterns of subcuticular stitch insertion

(i)

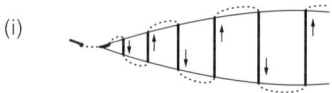

Suture is inserted straight across
from the exit point in the opposing
dermis.

(ii)

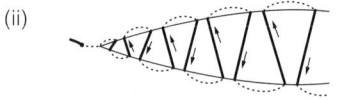

Suture is angled back towards the
exit point of the last suture on the
opposite side.

(iii)

subcuticular
suture   wound

bridge of suture
over the wound

bridge   subcuticular
suture

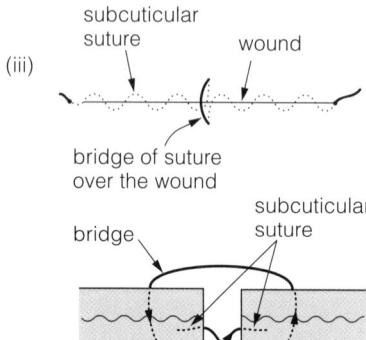

The bridge is inserted to ease
removal. Once cut, this allows
for two short sutures to be
removed instead of one long
one which may snap.

Fig. 9.15 Subcuticular suture *(cont.)*

(d) Finishing a subcuticular suture (nonabsorbable)

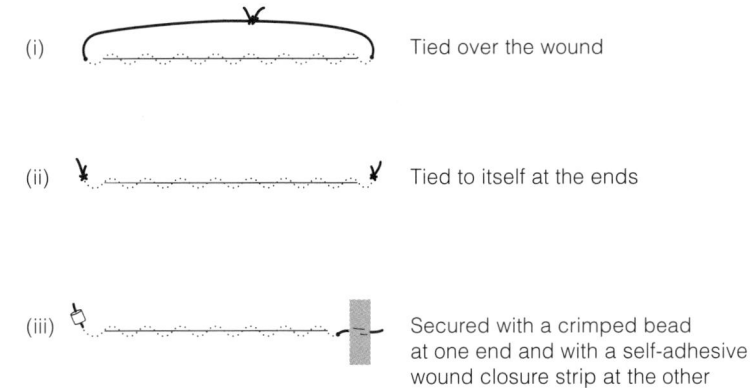

(i) Tied over the wound

(ii) Tied to itself at the ends

(iii) Secured with a crimped bead
at one end and with a self-adhesive
wound closure strip at the other

Fig. 9.15 Subcuticular suture *(cont.)*

Barron suture

The Barron suture (Fig. 9.16) is a special stitch that gives the advantages of both a horizontal mattress suture (eversion) and a subcuticular suture (low tissue ischaemia). It is used in situations where one side of the wound is likely to have poor blood supply and a normal suture may cause pressure ischaemia. Situations such as this occur when a flap of skin, with a narrow or distant base needs to be secured in position, such as in a pretibial laceration.

The insertion starts as a simple suture but bites only as deep as the dermis. As it exits into the wound a subcuticular bite is taken (horizontally) for 5–10 mm. At the exit point the needle is once again used to complete a dermal-level, simple suture. It is then tied as a horizontal mattress (Fig. 9.16).

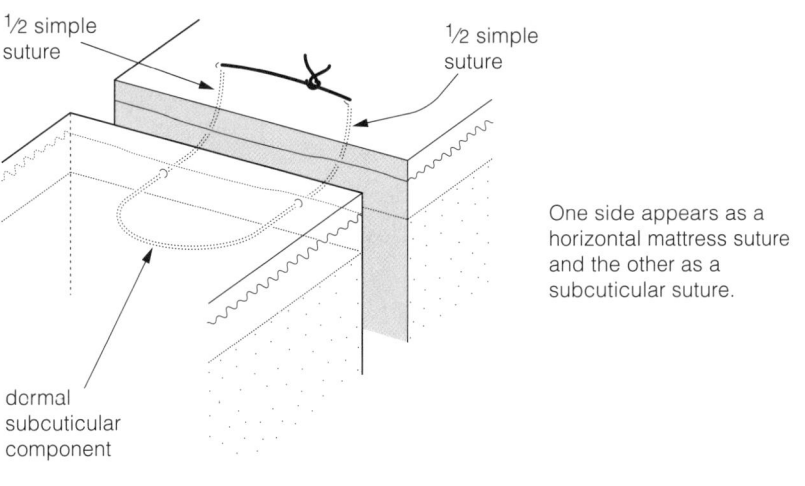

½ simple suture

½ simple suture

One side appears as a
horizontal mattress suture
and the other as a
subcuticular suture.

dermal
subcuticular
component

Fig. 9.16 Barron suture

Three-corner suture

A variation of the Barron suture, the three-corner suture (Fig. 9.17) is a combination of horizontal mattress and subcuticular suture. It is used in stellate lacerations or skin flaps where three (or more) arms of a wound come together. In the 'flattest' of the surfaces a simple suture is begun but inserted only as deep as the low dermis. The subcuticular part of the suture is then carried through the dermis at the apices of the other tissue components. To complete the suture, a dermal-depth simple suture bite is inserted parallel to the first part of the suture and the two ends tied (Fig. 9.15).

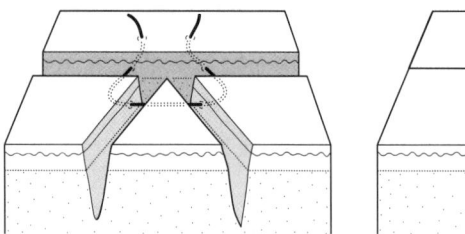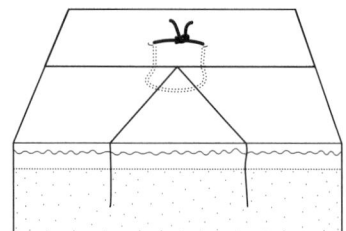

A variant of the Barron suture, the three-corner suture is used to hold the apices of stellate lacerations. The illustration on the right shows how it appears when tied.

Fig. 9.17 Three-corner suture

SUTURING IN PRACTICE

Basic skills in suturing relate primarily to closure of skin, connecting tubular structures, and suturing fascia and muscle. The practical examples and descriptions below provide an outline of the key principles involved when suturing these tissues and structures.

Skin

Skin closure is the main visible reminder for the patient of the surgeon's work. Following a few key principles during closure will improve the appearance of the skin scarring.

- Necrotic and foreign material should be excised or removed.
- Traumatic or contaminated wounds should be cleaned and irrigated.
- Skin edges should be handled gently with forceps and minimal pressure to reduce damage.
- Skin layers should be accurately aligned and apposed without tension or inversion.

Patient factors can also affect scar appearance. For example, scars are less obvious in older or wrinkled skin. They may heal poorly in oily or pigmented skin, anatomical areas that are under tension (e.g. over joints, sternal area), and in patients with poor nutrition.

Other technical points to remember are:

- Skin incisions made along relaxed skin tension lines ('Langer lines') will heal with a better scar. Incisions made perpendicular to skin tension lines heal with maximal scar contraction. When planning an incision it is useful to remember that these skin tension lines tend to run parallel to skin wrinkles and perpendicular to the underlying muscle.
- Wounds are often closed in layers to reduce tension on skin edges and reduce dead space.
- Knots of absorbable sutures should be buried if possible.
- Sutures removed within five days have a low risk of 'cross-hatching,' although wounds in some areas may need sutures for a longer time to reduce the tension directly on the scar (e.g. over joints).
- Monofilament suture reduces infection rate and tissue reaction. Surgical wounds are often amenable to a subcuticular suture, which can improve scar appearance.
- Small skin defects can be closed directly but larger defects may require more advanced techniques, such as skin grafting, advancement flaps or transposition or rotation flaps. These techniques are beyond the scope of this text.
- 'Dog-ears' are occasionally formed when closing a wound following an elliptical excision. This should be repaired at the time of suturing.

Tubular structures

Suturing tubular structures usually involves either anastomosis or closure of a defect. Specific concerns and techniques apply to individual tissue types; however there are some key principles. These are:

1. handle tissues gently to avoid damage at the suture line
2. the suture line must be tension free
3. ensure good blood supply at the suture line.

The specific application of these general principles is described below for bowel anastomosis, ureteric repair and arterial vein patch.

Bowel anastomosis

The aim of the anastomosis is to invert the mucosal layer and appose the tissue layers without causing ischaemia. Healing of gastrointestinal anastomoses relies on gentle tissue handling, adequate blood supply and lack of tension on the anastomosis. Silk was used for many decades, but it is now most common to employ a monofilament absorbable 4/0 or 3/0 suture, depending on surgeon preference. Anastomoses can be performed with continuous or interrupted sutures, in a single or double layer.

The essential steps in bowel anastomosis are:

1. Mobilise the bowel ends to allow minimal tension at the anastomosis while preserving good blood supply.
2. Place mesenteric and antimesenteric 'stay' sutures secured in artery forceps.
3. Insert posterior wall sutures 5–6 mm apart, including a large bite of the submucosa. There is no strength in the mucosa. Sero–submucosal or full thickness sutures can be used, but the surgeon should be consistent.
4. Insert the sutures on the anterior wall.
5. Check the lumen by palpating between finger and thumb to ensure that it is patent and of appropriate calibre.
6. Close mesenteric windows, being careful not to interfere with the mesenteric blood supply.

The most vulnerable points of this type of anastomosis are the 'corners' where the stay sutures are placed, and special care should be taken when changing from the posterior to anterior walls. These and any other points of potential weakness can be reinforced with a further suture at the end of the anastomosis.

Ureteric anastomosis

Ureters are narrow tubes, and a circular anastomosis is likely to form a stricture. To reduce the likelihood of this occurring, the ends of the ureter are 'spatulated' to widen the joined ends and create an elliptical anastomosis (Fig. 9.18) Full thickness 4/0 or 5/0 absorbable interrupted sutures are placed around the back wall. A double-J stent is often then introduced, running from renal pelvis to bladder to facilitate urinary drainage and support the anastomosis. The anterior wall is closed over the stent with further interrupted sutures. Non-absorbable sutures should never be used in the urinary tract since these will almost inevitably act as a nidus for stone formation. Drains are usually placed adjacent to urinary anastomoses.

Vascular anastomosis

Gentle handling of vessels is critical for the success of any vascular anastomosis. Any trauma to the vascular wall can cause endothelial injury, which may accelerate intimal hyperplasia or cause thrombus formation. For these reasons the vessel wall should not be grasped with forceps. Traction on the suture or gentle retraction of the vessel with forceps tips (without grasping) can display the area to be sutured. Fine, double-armed (needle at both ends) monofilament suture should be used. The suture material should never be grasped with instruments, as this may crush and weaken the thread.

When suturing, the needle is passed through the vessel wall from inside to outside, to minimise delamination of atherosclerotic plaque, which can cause dissection. The suture should be brought through to the wall of the vessel without dragging to minimise bleeding from stitch holes. All knots are hand tied on the outside of the vessel.

Fascial closure—anterior abdominal wall

Failure of an abdominal wall closure results in incisional hernia or, in total failure, acute abdominal wound disruption ('burst abdomen'). 'Mass closure' of the abdominal wall, with the suture passing through all the layers of the abdominal wall except the skin, is the most common method of closure. The layer with the most strength is the anterior layer of rectus sheath, and all sutures must include this layer. Closure in multiple layers has not been shown to have any advantage in strength or complication rate, and is now uncommon. Suture bites including muscle should be avoided, if possible. Commonly used sutures are slowly absorbable or non-absorbable monofilament. Looped sutures obviate the need for a knot at the beginning, but have no other advantage. A continuous suture distributes the tension along the wound. Excessive tension on mass closure sutures is a common fault that should be avoided because it results in increased postoperative pain and a greater likelihood of wound dehiscence due to ischaemia and cutting through of sutures. Placing a stoma or drain through the main incision should be avoided.

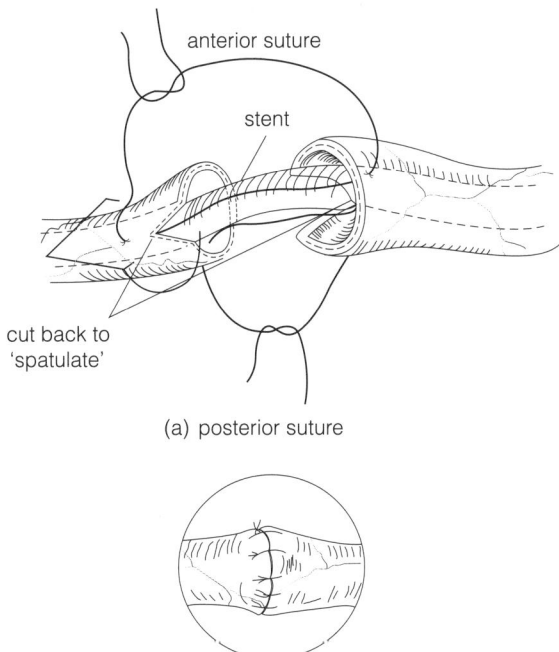

(a) posterior suture

(b) completed spatulated anastomosis

Fig. 9.18 Spatulated ureteric anastomosis

Muscle repair[1]

When a functionally important muscle is disrupted or lacerated, especially in a young person, early surgical repair is indicated. Torn ends are debrided so that healthy tissue can be apposed. Interrupted, absorbable mattress sutures are placed close together around the circumference of the muscle, including the muscle sheath when possible. The repair can be reinforced with locally available tissue e.g. fascia lata in the leg. Appropriate joints should be splinted, if possible, to reduce tension on the muscle repair.

Tendon repair

The purpose of tendon suturing is to approximate the ends of a tendon or to fasten one end of a tendon to other tendons or to bone, and to hold this position during healing. Tendons should have minimal handling to reduce reaction, scarring and adhesions. Grasping of the uninjured surfaces should be avoided. Tendon repair techniques are often designed to convert longitudinal tension into either oblique or transverse compressive force on tendon. Core sutures of braided polyester are commonly used to appose the tendon ends. Then fine monofilament epitenon sutures complete the repair.

Bone

Bone is occasionally sutured in order to fix a tendon to bone. The apposing surfaces of bone and tendon should both be scarified to hasten attachment. In one simple technique, a core suture is secured in the end of the tendon, and the two suture ends are threaded in opposite directions through a hole drilled transversely in the bone. The sutures are then tied tightly over the shaft of the bone. Alternatively, if the tendon is long enough, the end can be passed through the hole in the bone and secured to itself. After attaching the tendon, an attempt should be made to close the periosteum over it, or at least to suture the periosteum to its edges.

Solid viscera

Solid viscera, such as the spleen or liver, most commonly require suturing after trauma, either iatrogenic or accidental. Small lacerations can be managed with compression

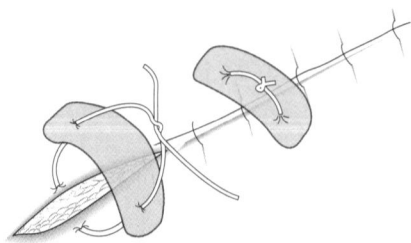

Fig. 9.19 Suturing solid viscera using pledgets

or application of haemostatic agents. Larger lacerations also require packing initially, to allow assessment of the injury. If suture repair is necessary, the preferred suture is an absorbable monofilament, swaged to a slim, blunt-tipped, round-body needle. The chance of sutures cutting through the parenchyma is minimised by placing large figure-of-eight stiches incorporating the capsule and the parenchyma, and tying them with minimal tension. Suture entry and exit points can be reinforced by pledgets to further security (Fig. 9.19). Pledgets can be made from synthetic material or biological material (such as anterior abdominal wall fascia).

STAPLING[2]

Principles

Stapling systems are designed as an alternative to suturing for specific purposes and tissue types. The staple height and closed configuration is selected according to the thickness of the tissue to be stapled.

There are three common classes of tissue staplers:

1. Skin staplers place individual staples closed in a rectangular configuration to approximate skin edges (Fig. 9.20).
2. Linear staplers deliver double- or triple-staggered rows of staples. They are available in various lengths and staple heights. The tissue can be divided, if necessary, along the edge of the stapler using a scalpel blade. Vascular linear staplers use fine, short (typically 2.5 mm) staples designed to ligate large-calibre vessels. Linear cutting staplers insert a parallel pair of double-staggered rows of staples (Fig. 9.21), and a blade within the instrument simultaneously divides the tissue between the two staple lines.
3. Circular staplers deliver a circular, double-staggered row of staples while simultaneously cutting out the disc of tissue inside the ring of staples (Fig. 9.22), creating a stoma between the two viscera to be anastomosed. Circular staplers are available in different calibres and often have a variable staple height.

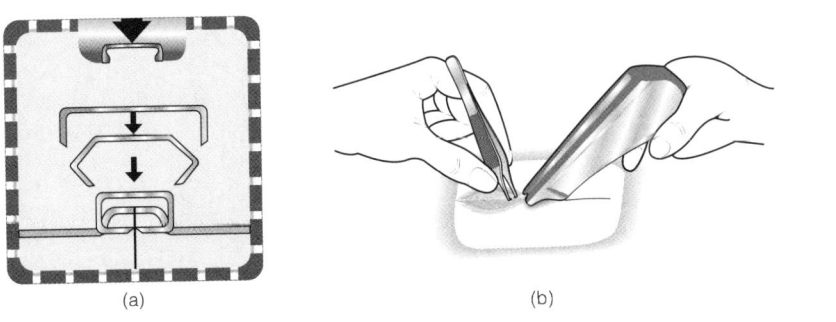

(a) (b)

Fig. 9.20 Skin stapler

Staplers have application in a wide range of procedures. Staplers should not be used on necrotic or ischaemic tissue. Illustrative descriptions of the use of staplers for skin closure, bowel anastomosis and in the respiratory tract are presented below.

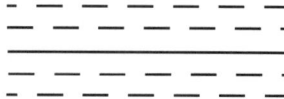

Fig. 9.21 Linear stapler

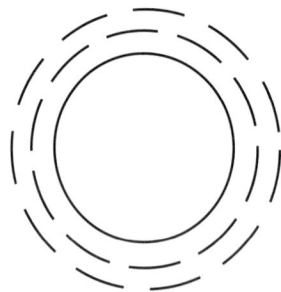

Fig. 9.22 Circular stapler

Skin

The principles of stapled and sutured skin closure are identical. Staples should be at least 5 mm anterior to underlying structures such as bones, vessels or other organs. Forceps are used to grasp and appose the skin edges. The stapler is then centred over the incision and fired. Staples are removed by unbending the staple, which is most conveniently achieved with a purpose designed staple remover (Fig. 9.23).

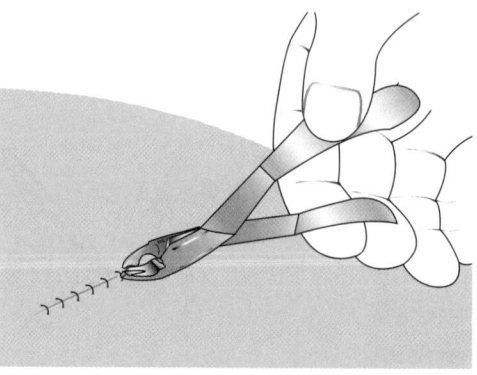

Fig. 9.23 Removing skin staples

Gastrointestinal staplers

Staplers can be used in various ways to create gastrointestinal anastomoses. To create a side-to-side anastomosis (Fig. 9.24), the bowel on either side of the mobilised segment is divided with a linear cutting stapler. This keeps the bowel ends closed to minimise peritoneal contamination. The two ends are aligned side by side, and the antimesenteric corner of each staple line is excised to allow one limb of the linear cutter to be introduced into each lumen (Fig. 9.25a). The stapler is closed and fired, creating a pair of staple lines joining the bowel walls, with a lumen cut between them by the knife blade in the instrument. Finally, the common opening is closed with a stapler or with sutures (Fig. 9.25b). Some surgeons oversew part or all of the anastomosis to promote haemostasis and add mechanical support.

A intraluminal stapler is used to create an end-to-end anastomosis (Fig. 9.26). Each open end of bowel is secured with a purse-string suture (Fig. 9.27), which is drawn tight around the protruding shafts of the stapler and of the anvil (Fig. 9.28a). The stapler and anvil are clipped together, and the device is closed and fired, creating two circular rows of staples, and cutting out the centre to create a lumen (Fig. 9.28b).

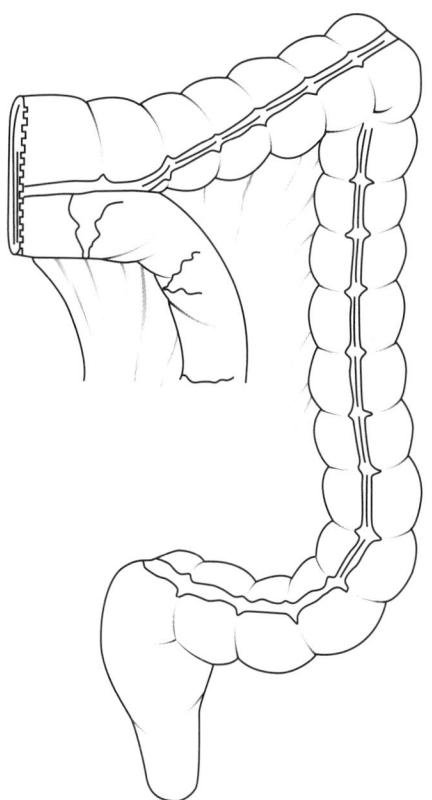

Fig. 9.24 Side-to-side anastomosis

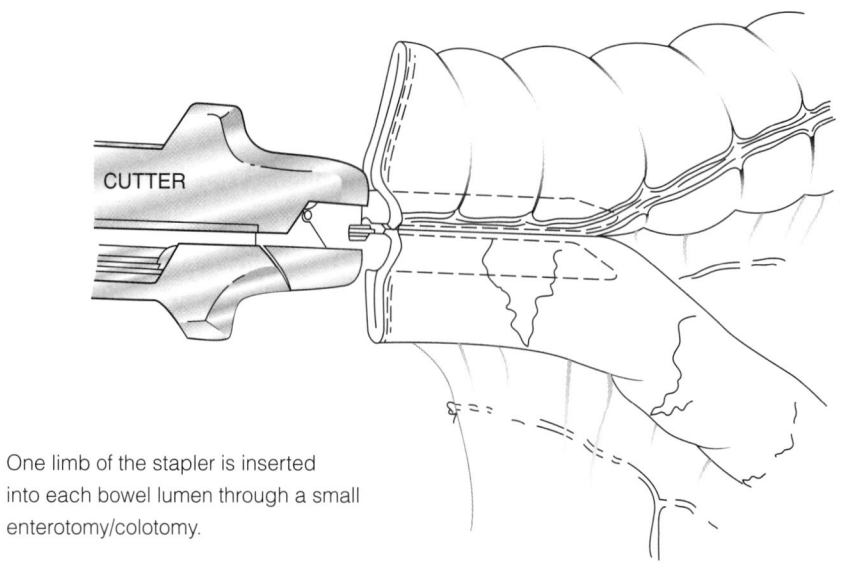

CUTTER

One limb of the stapler is inserted
into each bowel lumen through a small
enterotomy/colotomy.

Fig. 9.25a Stapler operation

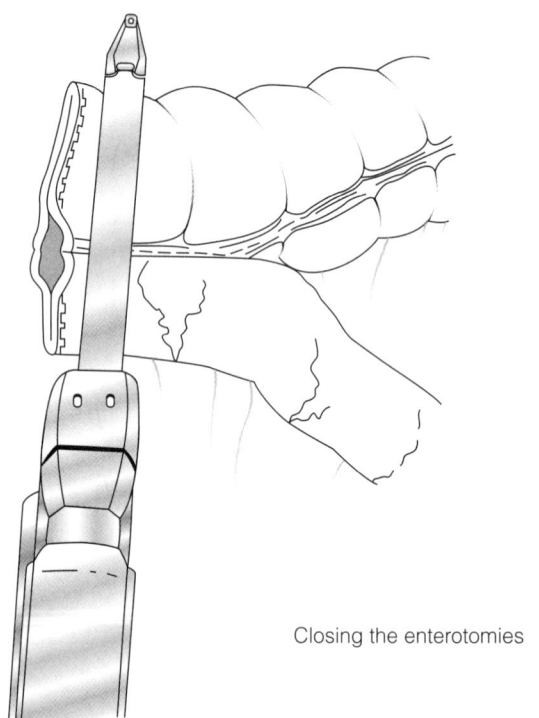

Closing the enterotomies

Fig. 9.25b Stapler operation

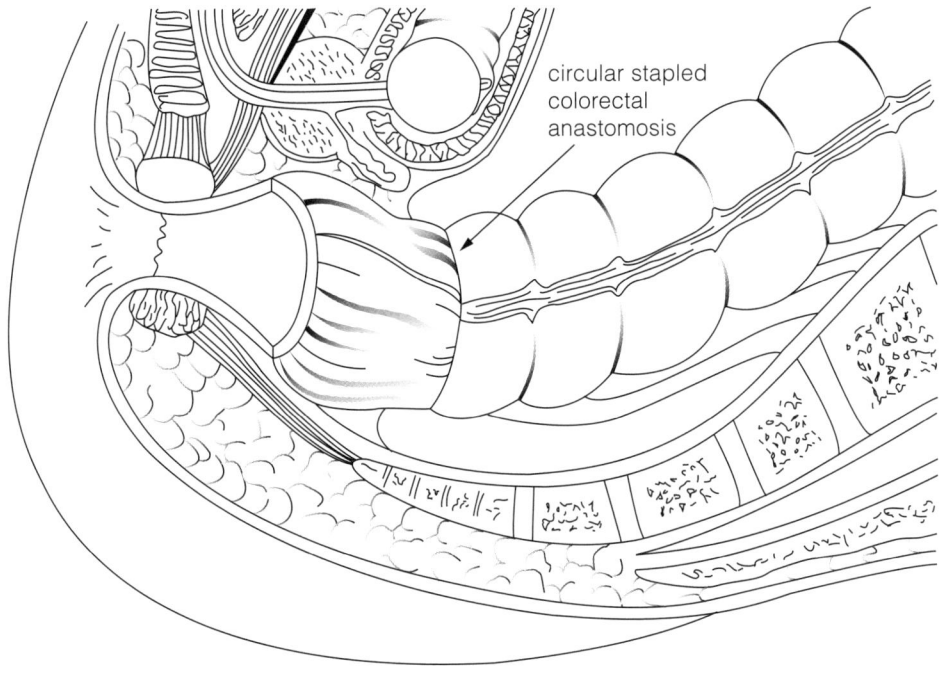

circular stapled
colorectal
anastomosis

Fig. 9.26 End-to-end anastomosis

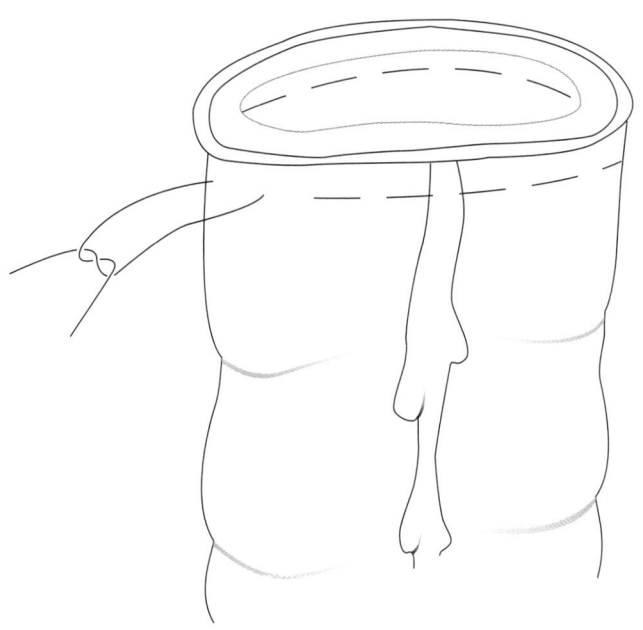

Fig. 9.27 Purse-string sutures securing bowel ends

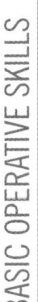

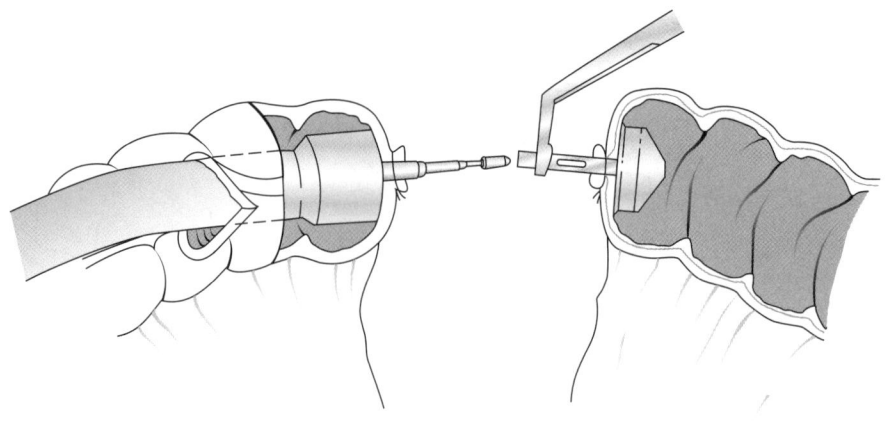

Fig. 9.28a Bowel stapled and cut

Respiratory tract

Staplers can be used for various applications in thoracic surgery, including division of bronchi and vessels. Linear cutter staplers can be used for non-anatomic pulmonary wedge resections. The portion of lung to be removed or biopsied is divided from the rest of the lobe by one or multiple firings of a linear cutter stapler. This usually creates an airtight seal.

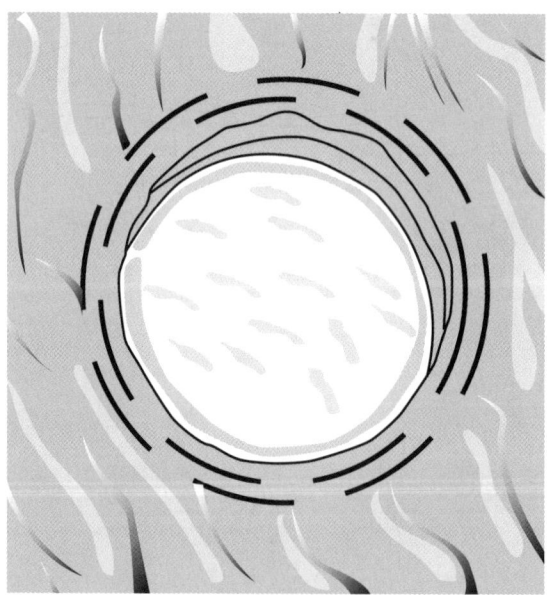

Fig. 9.28b Bowel stapled and cut

OTHER SURGICAL TECHNIQUES

Many special skills are required to perform surgical procedures safely. While some are unique to a single specialty, the great majority are used across all specialties. This section deals with many skills common to virtually every branch of surgery.

Tissue handling

Good tissue handling is a combination of common sense and adherence to the maxim 'first do no harm'. In Chapter 5 the different types of surgical instruments and their basic functions were introduced. Detailed knowledge of available instruments along with an appreciation of their structure and functional design is essential to handling tissue with minimal trauma.

The least-traumatic method of tissue handling should be selected according to the requirements of the procedure. For example, holding a loop of small bowel between fingers and thumb during division of adhesions will be less traumatic than using any type of forceps. In contrast, an orthopaedic procedure may require the use of very heavy graspers to achieve the surgical objective.

While it is important to select the most appropriate forceps for minimum tissue damage, gentle technique is also essential. For skin and fascia, toothed forceps are commonly used for grip, but with light pressure to minimise trauma. For bowel, non-toothed forceps are traditionally used; however, some surgeons use fine toothed forceps successfully with minimal damage. This highlights the role the surgeon has in tissue handling. Even with the most appropriate choice of instrument, significant damage is possible if care is not taken.

Incisions and excisions

A scalpel is the instrument traditionally used to incise skin (a basic introduction to the use of a scalpel is found in Chapter 5).

The scalpel should always be held so that the blade is perpendicular to the skin surface to ensure a neat vertical cut that will heal with the least scarring. There are two common methods of holding a scalpel (see Chapter 5), the *overhand grip* and the *pen grip* (Fig. 9.29). The overhand grip is used for larger, straight, sweeping incisions and the pen grip for finer, curved work and sharp dissection.

Smaller or curved incisions are often marked with a skin pen to ensure accuracy of placement, or adequacy of margins (e.g. skin lesion or mastectomy). Sometimes these marks are cross-hatched to facilitate accurate closure. This marking must remain when the skin is prepped and so should be made with a permanent marker. Red ink, or a degradable pigment, should be used to reduce the risk of this mark tattooing the skin if pigment is drawn down into the dermis during the incision.

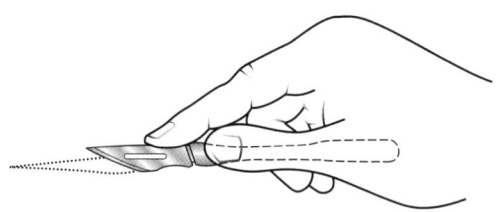

(a) The overhand or table-knife grip, used for long incisions.

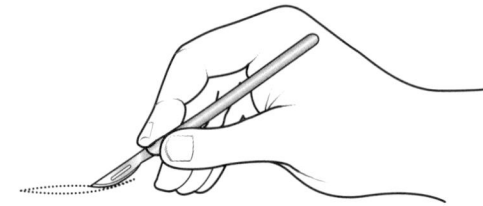

(b) The pen grip is used for fine incisions or excisions and for dissection with the scalpel.

Fig. 9.29 Holding a scalpel

The whole length of the blade, not just the tip, should be employed in cutting. For a long skin incision, such as that for a laparotomy, a larger handle and blade (e.g. size 4 handle and 22 blade) are required. Held in the *overhand grip* (Fig. 9.29a), like a dinner knife, the depth of cut is controlled by a combination of smoothly drawing the blade over the tissues and applying constant firm pressure with the forearm. With experience this can be controlled with great accuracy.

Traditionally, the majority of larger incisions are made with a scalpel, and this still holds in emergency situations. However, with concerns about sharps, it is now quite common to use the scalpel to divide only the epidermis and most, or all, of the dermis. Diathermy is then used to complete the incision to the desired depth.

For the finer and more precise incisions required in the excision of small skin lesions, the debridement of dirty wound edges and many plastic surgery procedures, a small handle and blade should be used (e.g. size 3 handle and 15 blade). This scalpel should be held in the *pen grip* (Fig. 9.29b) and most of the movement imparted on the blade comes from the hand and fingers. With this grip the surgeon's wrist can also be placed against the patient, an instrument or his or her other hand to steady the blade while cutting. The full length of the blade should still be used for the incision.

Let us illustrate the finer of these two techniques with excision of a skin lesion as the example.

Step 1

Plan an incision in the best possible line for closure. Mark an ellipse around the lesion to ensure adequate margins of excision (Fig. 9.30a).

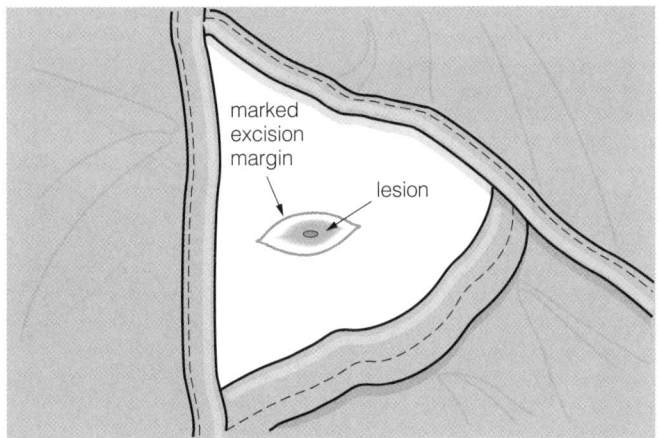

Fig. 9.30a Step 1

Step 2

Grasp the scalpel in a *pen grip* and make the first incision by drawing the scalpel smoothly along the more *dependent* of the two marked lines, keeping the blade perpendicular to the tissue (Fig. 9.30b). This tactic prevents blood from running over, and obscuring, tissues that have not yet been incised. The skin to be incised should be placed on stretch, preferably at right angles to the line of incision (Fig. 9.30b).

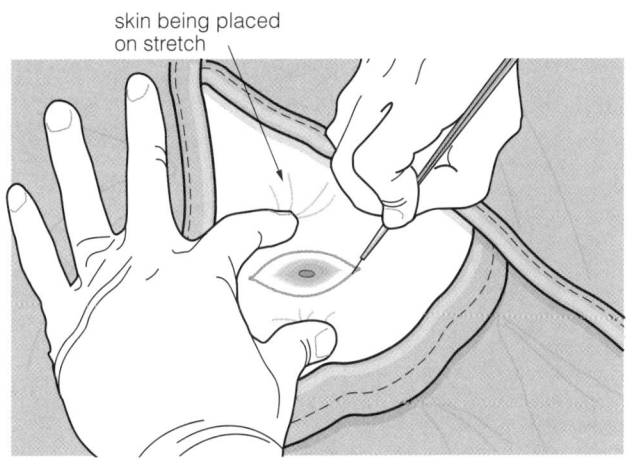

Fig. 9.30b Step 2

Step 3

Once the scalpel blade is through the dermis of the 'lower' margin, the upper incision can be made. A tissue forceps may need to be placed on the already cut edge to assist in providing tension to cut against (Fig. 9.29c).

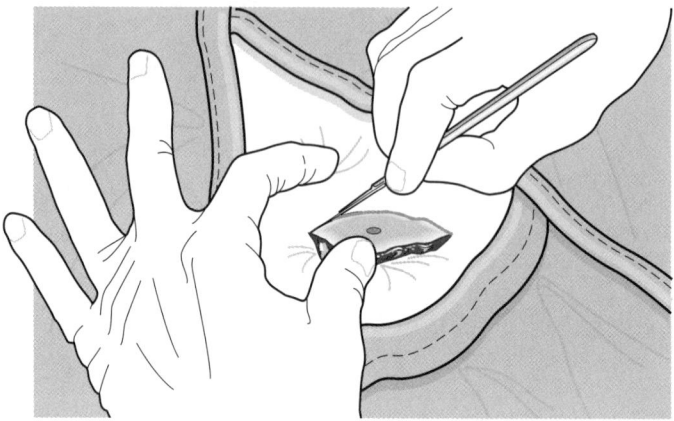

Fig. 9.30c Step 3

Step 4

Particular attention must be paid to completely incising one angled corner of the specimen. This can then be lifted with tissue forceps and the subcutaneous tissue (fat) dissected by knife, scissors or diathermy down to, and along, the plane of the deep fascia. This dissection should proceed almost vertically to its deepest extent as a shelving (V) incision may leave behind involved tissue (Fig. 9.30d).

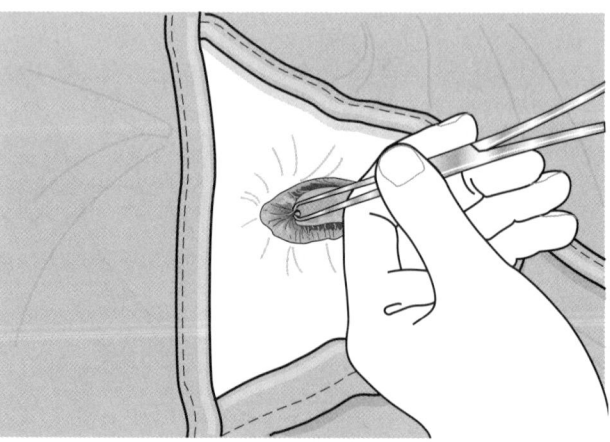

Fig. 9.30d Step 4

Step 5

During dissection of the specimen (step 4), or after complete removal of the specimen, haemostasis must be obtained. Diathermy or ligation are the commonest methods, although twisting vessels and pressure are also valid techniques (Fig. 9.30e).

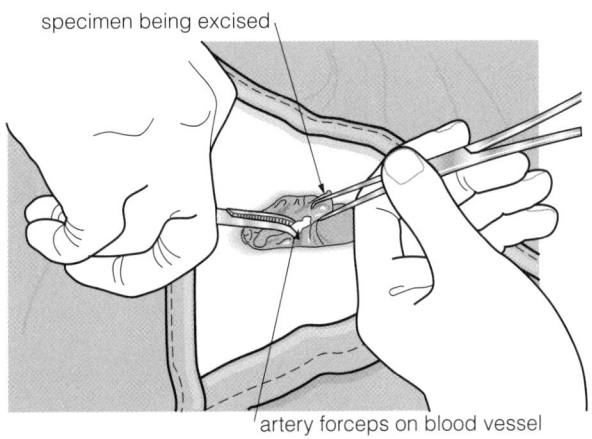

specimen being excised

artery forceps on blood vessel

Fig. 9.30e Step 5

Step 6

Closure is now effected using a combination of deep (if required) and cutaneous sutures (Fig. 9.30f).

In contrast to the above procedure, a mid-line abdominal, laparotomy incision is made by cutting down through all layers of the abdominal wall to the peritoneum. A combination of scalpel, diathermy and (sometimes) scissors are used for this task. The initial cut should be carried through the epidermis and dermis in one long sweeping motion of the whole blade (not just the tip) held in the *overhand grip* (Fig. 9.29a) which may be rehearsed in the air over the abdomen prior to commencing. Once through the skin, the fat and linea alba may be cut with scalpel, scissors or diathermy. The peritoneum is then lifted between two artery forceps and nicked with a scalpel blade. This allows viscera to fall away from the anterior abdominal wall with the inrush of air. Remnant tissue can then be cut with heavy scissors or diathermy.

In concluding this section it is probably wise to reflect upon the ease with which a scalpel cuts. It is razor sharp and will cut anything it is brought against

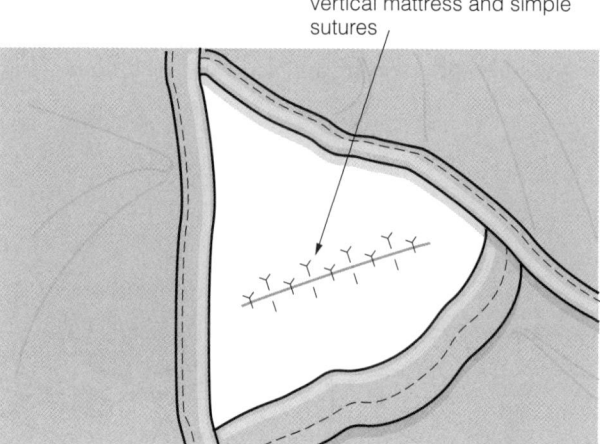

skin closure with alternating vertical mattress and simple sutures

Fig. 9.30f Step 6

under pressure or tension. This property makes the scalpel a potentially dangerous tool that can easily incise or divide a vital structure (e.g. peripheral nerve or vessel) inadvertently if appropriate care is not taken. This risk also applies to any body parts of the scrub team that the scalpel comes in contact with!

Following the simple rules in Table 9.2 will minimise this risk.

Table 9.2 Principles of safe incision

1.	Do not cut anything that you cannot actually see.
2.	If the tissue to be divided is superficial to a vital structure, insert an instrument or cutting guide between the structures.
3.	If dissecting near a known structure (e.g. nerve or vessel), cut in the line of the structure to prevent dividing it accidentally. This does not prevent incising it longitudinally but these injuries are usually much less serious.
4.	Plan (and mark) your incisions.
5.	If cutting in a deep cavity, time spent improving the access and exposure equates to time saved repairing a potential error.
6.	There is no substitute for excellent sharps technique in the prevention of penetrating wounds in the operator and scrub team.

BASIC DISSECTION TECHNIQUES

Dissection is the separation of tissues required to approach, identify and expose an underlying structure or lesion.

Dissection may be undertaken in a *blunt* or *sharp* fashion. Blunt dissection involves opening tissue planes and separating tissues by pushing, splitting, stripping, squeezing and so on, without actively cutting. Sharp dissection makes use of scalpels, scissors or diathermy to actively divide tissues in a very precise manner.

The process of dissection must be carried out with the maximum care for all involved structures. Good dissection requires a combination of abilities. An intimate knowledge of the relevant anatomy is vital, along with an understanding of the spatial relationships between structures. The structure of connective tissues must also be appreciated so that correct planes and lines of dissection can be identified and entered. Experience with surgical dissecting techniques is essential, as this will ensure that appropriate decisions are made regarding the best method of dissection. Tissue trauma must be minimised by the gentle handling of both tissues and structures and, finally, tension (distraction of tissue) must be used appropriately to define the planes and expose the best lines of dissection.

Genuine skill in the area of dissection, then, is generally regarded as one of the hallmarks of general surgical competence (Table 9.3).

Table 9.3	Essential elements for successful dissection.
•	An intimate knowledge of gross and three-dimensional anatomy
•	A knowledge of connective tissue structure
•	An understanding of tissue planes
•	Experience with various methods of dissection
•	Gentle tissue handling to minimise tissue trauma
•	The ability to use tension to display tissues and planes

Blunt dissection

The simplest form of dissection is to follow the tissue plane that has been entered by pushing apart the tissues with fingers, a gauze swab or blunt instruments. This form of dissection does not involve the division of tissues, merely their separation along planes of cleavage.

An important element in expert dissection is the appropriate use of tension. When a 'distracting' (pulling apart) force is applied to tissues across the line of planned division, they part with less direct force at the point of dissection. Tension also helps display the best line of dissection and simplifies the decision about which method of dissection to use. With excessive tension, tissues may be 'torn' apart at their weakest point (usually a plane or line of cleavage). Unfortunately, this is an *inexact and often uncontrollable method* which may result in damage to adjacent structures. It is best avoided if possible.

With fingers

With appropriate tension, the peeling away of layers by the insinuation of a finger or gauze peanut (pledget) on an instrument may be undertaken. The same effect can be achieved by the use of a hand-held swab, or with a blunt instrument such as the reverse end of a scalpel handle (Fig. 9.31a).

The second variation of splitting is when closed scissors (or any similar hinged instrument) are inserted between the fibres of a structure and opened to separate the fibres. This is particularly effective in the dissection of layers of the spermatic cord during inguinal hernia repair (Fig. 9.31b).

Blunt dissection can also be used to divide tissues without damaging vital structures contained within them. Once again fingers can be used for the techniques of pinching and finger fracture. *Pinching* involves the squeezing of tissues between the thumb and forefinger to separate them along natural cleavage planes or lines of least resistance. This may be done to separate adjacent adherent tissues or to break through tissues such as the mesentery, or the oedematous fat in the Calot triangle during open cholecystectomy for acute cholecystitis.

A variant of this technique, called *finger fracture*, is used to dissect through friable vascular organs such as the liver. It has the advantage that homogeneous cellular material is broken down without disrupting blood vessels or bile ducts. These can then be separately clamped, divided and ligated.

With instruments

Blunt division of tissues with instruments relates mainly to dissection through a tissue *in the line of its fibres*. This process is usually referred to as *splitting tissue*. Muscle, aponeuroses and the connective tissue surrounding 'longitudinal' structures (nerves, vessels, bones and tendons) are all amenable to division by this method.

Two main variations exist within the technique of splitting with instruments. In the first, a pair of scissors is held in the semi-open position. One blade is inserted through the tissue to be divided. The scissors are then pushed along the line of the tissue, separating adjacent fibres. The open scissors blades will passively divide any fibres at right angles to this plane. This method is particularly used for aponeuroses and connective tissues as described above.

The second variation of splitting is when the closed scissors (or any opening instrument of scissor type) is inserted between the fibres of a structure and then

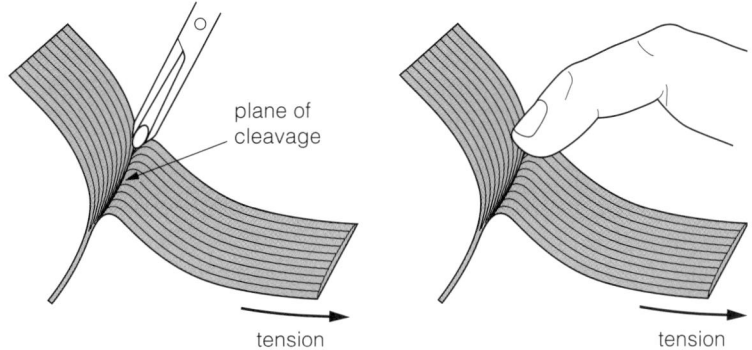

(a) Push method

plane of
cleavage

tension

tension

Tissue planes may be dissected by putting one element on
stretch (tension) and then pushing a blunt instrument (finger
or peanut swab) into the plane.

(b) Wipe method

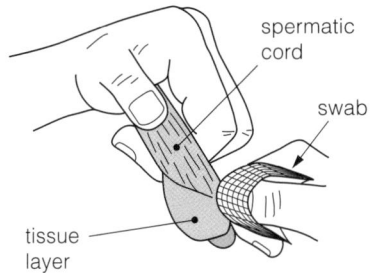

spermatic
cord

swab

tissue
layer

A gauze swab held
between the thumb
and forefinger of the
right hand is used
to 'wipe' away layers
of the spermatic
cord during a hernia
repair.

Fig. 9.31 Blunt dissection

opened to spread these apart. This 'spreading' manoeuvre may be performed in, or
across, the line of the fibres. Once commenced it may be enlarged further by the
use of retractors or fingers to spread the structure being divided more widely. The
opening of the abdomen for appendicectomy via a Lanz (oblique right iliac fossa)
incision employs both forms of this splitting technique (Fig. 9.32a, b).

Sharp dissection

Sharp dissection is the process of using a cutting instrument to divide tissues in order
to access deeper tissue planes or structures. The most common instruments used are
scalpels, scissors (dissecting patterns) and diathermy machines. All these instruments
will divide along planes and through tissues with reasonable ease. Problems with
cutting usually only occur when inappropriately small instruments are used for

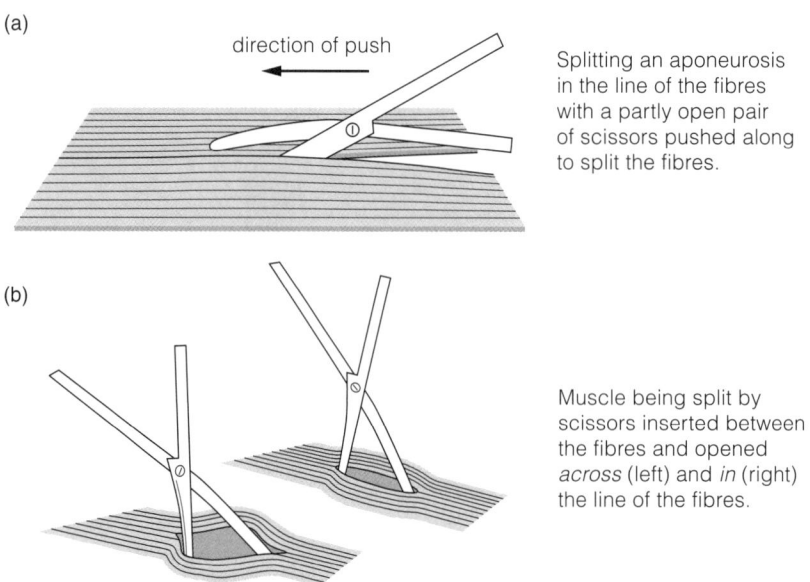

direction of push

Splitting an aponeurosis
in the line of the fibres
with a partly open pair
of scissors pushed along
to split the fibres.

(b)

Muscle being split by
scissors inserted between
the fibres and opened
across (left) and *in* (right)
the line of the fibres.

Fig. 9.32 Splitting tissue with scissors

bulky tissues or the instrument is actually blunt. It must also be remembered that most scissors are designed for use in either the left or right hand, making dissection technically challenging with the other hand.

The scalpel is an effective instrument for sharp dissection, but it requires skill to use effectively and safely, and is not commonly used as a first-line dissecting tool. When held like a pen the scalpel is a very precise instrument. However, it will only incise tissues cleanly if it can overcome the frictional drag of those tissues. If this is not achieved the tissues will pucker, drag and cut unevenly. The easiest way to overcome a problem with friction and drag is to provide stabilising tension either in the line of the incision or at 90° to it.

The main advantage of the scalpel is the minimal damage it causes to surrounding tissue. The cut it produces is clean and the depth to which it penetrates can be varied with pressure of the forearm. These benefits are often outweighed, however, by the potential it has for damaging deep structures in the line of incision. With this in mind the scalpel should be used sparingly and only in situations of extreme control or where no vital underlying structures exist.

Scissors are an excellent tool as they can be used for both sharp and blunt dissection, can dissect in planes and through structures and cause minimal adjacent tissue damage. The blades must be kept in contact while cutting or they will grab and crush the tissue to be incised. As the deep blade is often hidden from view all tissues should be thoroughly assessed for other structures (such as nerves, vessels or ducts) prior to performing the cut.

A number of energy sources are used to dissect tissues. See Chapter 7.

Monopolar diathermy, in the form of a single-bladed instrument or forceps, can be used to dissect along or through planes and tissues. In view of the cutting and heat-producing potential of diathermy it is advisable to insert an instrument, or even a finger, below the layers to be incised to protect adjacent tissues. Such a technique is particularly useful when cutting rectus abdominis in a Kocher incision (place an open packing forceps below it) or when incising linea alba after the initial scalpel incision (fingers are excellent here). When using this technique it is important to avoid direct contact or any arcing between the diathermy tool and any metal instrument, as this will result in inadvertent damage where the instrument is in contact with tissue.

Bipolar coagulation forceps incorporating a blade can be used to divide tissues and to seal and divide blood vessels with less heating of surrounding tissues.

Ultrasonic forceps coagulate and divide tissues, and the vapour produced can also help dissect tissue planes. Less heat is generated than with diathermy devices.

HAEMOSTASIS

Principles

Control of bleeding during an operative procedure is a basic skill, allowing optimal view for the surgeon and minimising the risk of postoperative complications such as infected haematoma and unplanned return to theatre to control haemorrhage. The prevention or reduction of bleeding from the operative site is known as *haemostasis*. There are two main principles in the process of haemostasis. The first is the *prevention of bleeding* and the second the *management of bleeding*.

While these processes may sound straightforward there are other factors such as experience, knowledge of techniques and a systematic approach to difficult situations which affect the potential outcome of haemostasis. The prevention and management of bleeding, then, relies not only on good technique but also on good clinical judgement. This is as true in the case of persistent ooze as it is in the handling of acute torrential bleeding.

Prevention of bleeding

Prevention of bleeding and its consequences begins *preoperatively* with the correction of anaemia and detection of clotting disorders. During the *intraoperative* phase the use of gentle and appropriate techniques of dissection and exposure, following tissue planes wherever possible, will reduce bleeding. Coupled with this, a strong anatomical knowledge will prevent inadvertent damage to major vascular structures.

Preoperative strategies

Coagulopathy should be actively sought in the at-risk patient (e.g. jaundice, liver disease, uraemia or anticoagulant therapy). This should be corrected with vitamin K (if related to hepatic causes) and/or clotting-factor-rich solutions, such as fresh frozen plasma or cryoprecipitate. Vitamin K should be commenced as early as possible during the clinical course for any jaundiced patients who may require surgery and in all jaundiced patients with deranged clotting. Intravenous clotting factors should be started in the immediate preoperative period, to maximise their efficacy, or commenced during the procedure if not obtainable before this.

Platelets are rarely required in the thrombocytopenic patient. They do not become active for some hours and normal clotting can still occur with platelet counts of as low as 40 ($\times 10^6$ mm^{-3}). If a patient is found to be thrombocytopenic the underlying cause should be found and treated.

In elective patients anticoagulation medications and platelet inhibitors must be managed to reduce the risk of bleeding. For example, aspirin should be ceased at least one week prior to operating and warfarin approximately 4–5 days prior. For patients who have ceased warfarin, an international normalized ratio (INR) check the day before surgery will confirm that clotting has returned to normal levels. If there is a pressing reason to remain on anticoagulants, surgery should be delayed until the anticoagulants can be stopped or the patient should be managed with heparin in the perioperative period. This allows closer titration of anticoagulation, easy reversal and the ability to use a rapidly acting antidote (protamine sulphate) if required.

Preparation of a preoperative cross-match (or group and hold serum) will facilitate the provision of blood should the need arise. Local haemorrhage may also be reduced by the use of a pre-incision injection of vasoconstrictors and tourniquets on limbs.

Intraoperative strategies

Careful incision of the skin with the use of diathermy to cut subcutaneous tissue will result in the coagulation of all but the larger vessels. Any bleeding vessels may then be grasped and diathermied. Alternatively, the use of accurate dissection with the application of artery forceps and vessel ligation is equally acceptable. Only curved artery forceps should be used in these situations. If inserted with the forceps tips facing upwards, a ligature may easily be slipped over the points and tied. Alternatively, the vessel may be dissected out and widely spaced ligatures placed around it before division. Any ligature too close to the point of division may slip at a later time and lead to unexpected bleeding (Fig. 9.33). For small vessels a twist of the artery forceps is often enough to seal the vessel. If a tie is

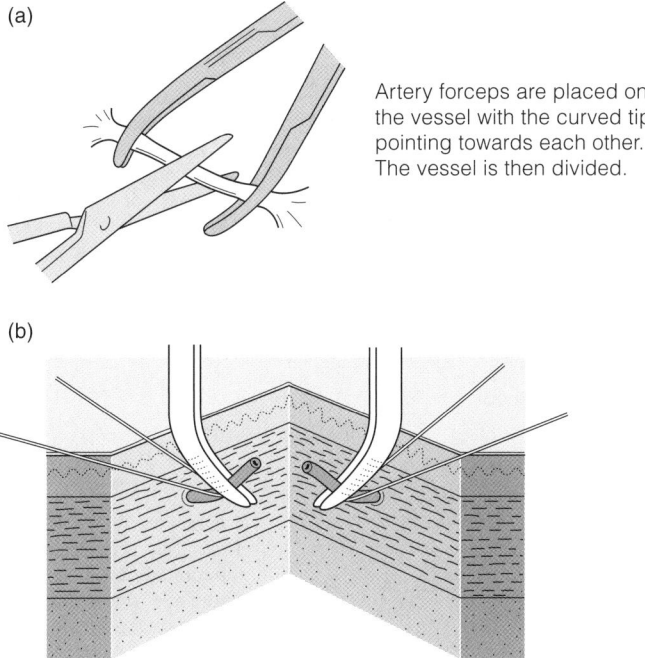

(a)

Artery forceps are placed on the vessel with the curved tips pointing towards each other. The vessel is then divided.

(b)

Threads are then placed around the vessel ends, behind the forceps, and the vessel ligated.

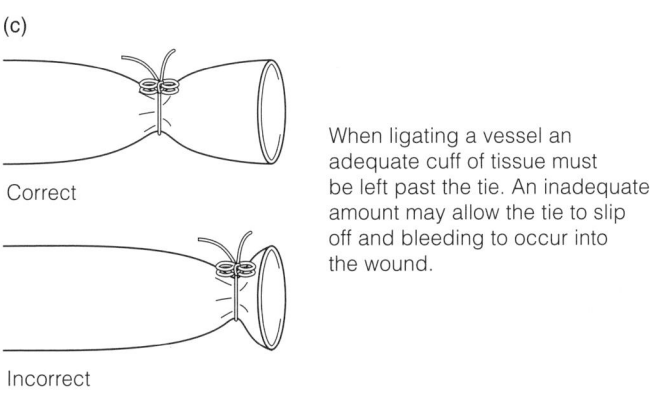

(c)

Correct

When ligating a vessel an adequate cuff of tissue must be left past the tie. An inadequate amount may allow the tie to slip off and bleeding to occur into the wound.

Incorrect

Fig. 9.33 Vessel ligation

not deemed adequate the vessel may be formally oversewn or transfixed with a heavy suture (Fig. 9.34).

Use of local anaesthetics with adrenaline, adrenaline solutions alone or octapressin will also reduce bleeding in these layers. In certain types of distal limb surgery an arterial tourniquet may be used. This will render the distal part of the limb totally ischaemic and prevent blood obscuring the operative field in any procedure where loss of vision may be disastrous. Unfortunately, a potential consequence of using an

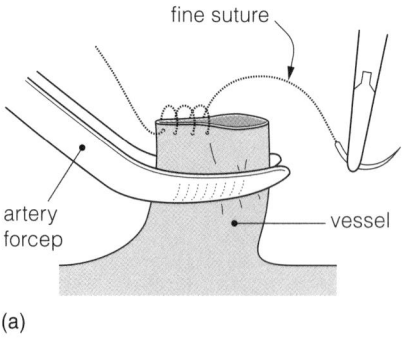

fine suture

Oversewing
A large vessel—especially if divided near to a main trunk—may need to be oversewn for security. This is often done for pulmonary vessels in thoracic surgery.

artery forcep

vessel

(a)

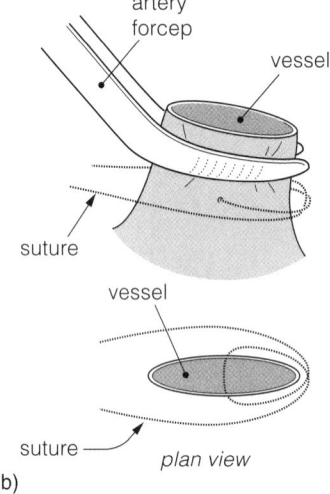

artery forcep

vessel

Transfixion
The suture is inserted through the middle of the vessel or pedicle. A single throw is placed on the tip side of the vessel, then the thread is brought back around to the other side. It is tightened as the artery forcep releases and a reef knot is tied.

suture

vessel

suture

plan view

(b)

Fig. 9.34 Oversewing and transfixion of vessels

arterial tourniquet is the difficulty in recognising potential bleeding points during the operation. The subsequent lack of adequate intraoperative haemostasis may lead to postoperative bleeding, haematoma formation and a potential for infection.

When operating on, or adjacent to, major vessels these should be dissected and controlled with a rubber sling or vascular clamps. This will provide the maximum safety if damage occurs. A sling can be lifted and tightened to occlude flow and a loosely positioned clamp may be easily closed (Fig. 9.35).

If control is not obtained and a major vessel is disrupted, the best way to gain immediate control is to apply direct pressure. This is usually done with a pack, although in some situations such as aortic rupture, special instruments have been designed for the purpose. If the bleeding is arterial, proximal pressure on the vessel is just as effective. Once controlled, the damage can be repaired in most instances. Occasionally, however, the vessel must be tied off or, if not visible, the whole area from where the bleeding originates may have to be oversewn (Table 9.4).

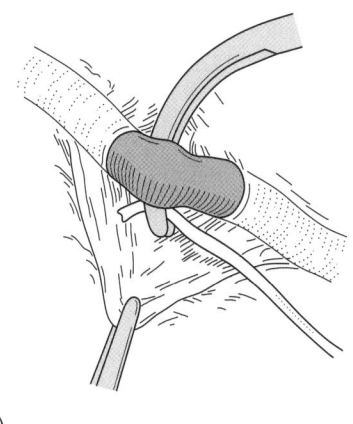

Inserting a silicon vascular sling: the right-angle forcep is used to dissect a tunnel behind the vessel and draw the sling through.

(a)

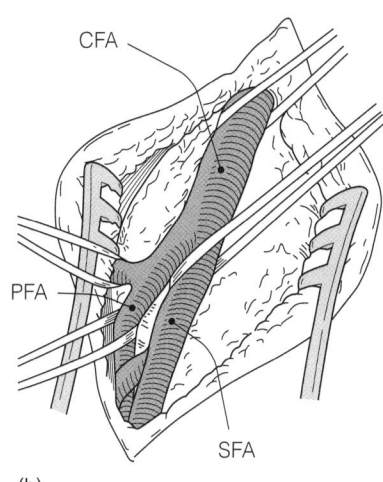

CFA

PFA

SFA

(b)

The right femoral artery complex with slings around the:

• common femoral artery (CFA)
• superficial femoral artery (SFA)
• branches of the profunda femoris artery (PFA).

The slings are inserted before applying the non-crushing vascular clamps.

Fig. 9.35 Vessel slings

Continued bleeding from a site where no individual vessels are found, or where the bleeders are too small and numerous to deal with (capillary oozing or venous bleeding), can be exceptionally difficult to control quickly. Initial pressure with a pack, combined with progressive diathermy as the pack is slowly removed, will often alleviate this situation. In more stubborn situations the application of haemostatic substances such as topical thrombin, gel-foam or haemostatic gauze may often help. If a large vessel or area of bleeding is observed it may be ligated, transfixed or oversewn. Sometimes a combination of packing and pressure is required to prevent massive bleeding, and on rare occasions these packs may be left in situ for several days before removal. This provides a tamponading effect and the packs can be removed at 48+ hours during a second-look laparotomy.

Table 9.4 | Methods of mechanical haemostasis

- Initial pressure with a pack
- Ligation, transfixion or oversewing of bleeding vessels or areas
- Progressive diathermy as the pack is removed
- Application of haemostatic substances (topical thrombin, gel-foam, haemostatic gauze)
- Packing and pressure left in situ for a period of time (tamponade)

Postoperative measures

Preventing postoperative hypothermia has been shown to reduce the risk of postoperative bleeding. Surgeons should always be alert to postoperative signs of blood loss, and should monitor blood components and coagulation profile when indicated so that measures can be taken early to replace blood being lost, correct coagulopathy and anticipate the need for reoperation if bleeding is excessive.

DEBRIDEMENT

Debridement is a term applied to the manual removal of foreign, dead, devitalised and contaminated materials from an open wound (Fig. 9.36). The objective is to reduce the chance of infection. The debridement process may be as simple as irrigating a minor wound with saline or may require general anaesthesia and extensive removal of tissue. The ultimate extension of this concept is the *en-bloc* excision of an entire contaminated wound to leave a fresh, surgically created wound, with no contamination, ready for primary closure!

There is no single technique of wound debridement, or any prescribed number of debridements required to declare a wound clean or fit for closure. The broad aim is to remove any material that may impair healing. At the time of initial debridement any tissue of uncertain viability may be left to declare itself and a second or even third debridement procedure planned to complete the process. In general, skin is pink, fat yellow, fascia white/silver and muscle red/pink. Any tissues of abnormal colour should be suspected of being dubiously viable or dead. Principles, therefore, must be followed to ensure consistent success in a variety of situations.

Steps in wound debridement

1. Gross contamination and foreign bodies should be removed with forceps. The wound should then be irrigated and scrubbed to remove surface debris. This is often done once the patient is anaesthetised but prior to prepping and draping.

(a)

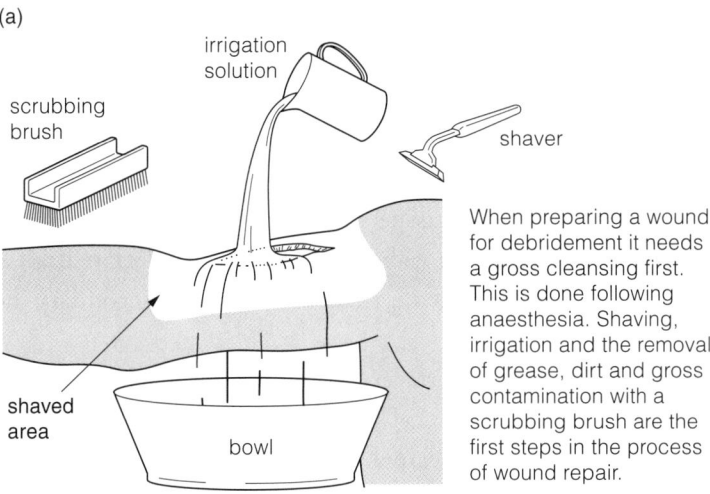

scrubbing brush

irrigation solution

shaver

shaved area

bowl

When preparing a wound for debridement it needs a gross cleansing first. This is done following anaesthesia. Shaving, irrigation and the removal of grease, dirt and gross contamination with a scrubbing brush are the first steps in the process of wound repair.

(b)

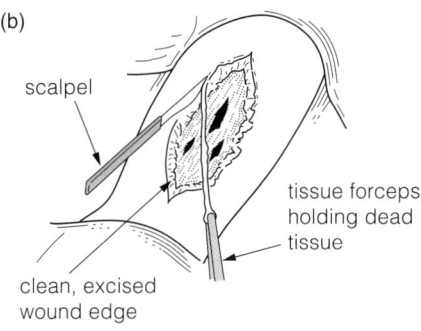

scalpel

tissue forceps holding dead tissue

clean, excised wound edge

Damaged skin, dead and devitalised tissues and foreign bodies are all removed as part of a process of sharp excision of the wound edges.

(c)

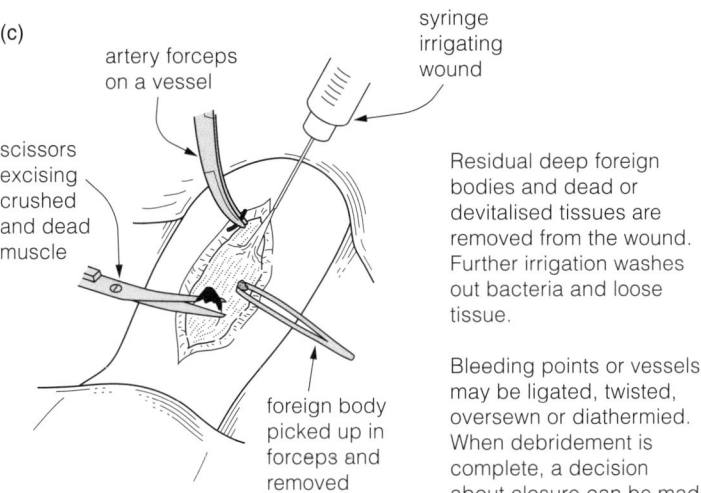

syringe irrigating wound

artery forceps on a vessel

scissors excising crushed and dead muscle

foreign body picked up in forceps and removed

Residual deep foreign bodies and dead or devitalised tissues are removed from the wound. Further irrigation washes out bacteria and loose tissue.

Bleeding points or vessels may be ligated, twisted, oversewn or diathermied. When debridement is complete, a decision about closure can be made.

Fig. 9.36 Debridement

2. The site is then widely prepped and draped. Tourniquets should be avoided except in the presence of major vascular trauma as they prevent the bleeding that confirms tissue viability but that needs to be controlled prior to closure.

3. All dead tissue must be fully excised.

4. Crushed or dubiously viable tissue should also be excised if primary closure is planned. Tissue of marginal viability may be left to declare itself if second-look debridement and delayed primary closure or secondary healing are planned.

5. The skin edges and deep surfaces should be cut back to bleeding tissue. This gives the double benefit of ensuring viability and providing vertical skin edges for a fine scar. A scalpel should be used to debride skin and this, or scissors, may also be used for soft tissues. The process involves a gradual trimming of tissues back to a clean and bleeding edge. It is important when cutting skin edges to provide good counter-traction so that only a fine sliver of damaged tissue is removed. Care should be taken to debride in the line of any longitudinal structures (e.g. limb arteries, veins or nerves) to avoid transection or damage. In small wounds a complete (*en-bloc*) excision of the entire lesion will provide surgically clean tissue for primary closure.

6. Further irrigation is used to wash out bacteria, residual foreign bodies and small non-viable tissue fragments. Normal saline is usually used for irrigation. Povidone iodine solution, antibiotics and other antiseptics are occasionally used but there is little evidence of their benefit; in fact, there is research evidence to suggest that these may all cause damage at a cellular level that impairs the healing process. The irrigant may be poured or squirted onto the wound and is usually caught in a kidney dish or gallipot to minimise spillage and mess. In small wounds a 10 ml syringe and #23 needle deliver irrigant at a near perfect pressure, when squeezed gently.

7. Adequate haemostasis is essential prior to completing the debridement but, especially if the wound is to be primarily closed, excessive diathermy or ligation can leave dead tissues and foreign (suture) material as foci for infection.

8. Once debridement is complete, the need for a second-look debridement should be determined and the appropriate mode of closure attended to. A low vacuum drain may help drain haematoma, seroma and pus from the wound if primary closure is attempted.

Debridement is a vital part of managing all traumatic or infected wounds. It has only a small role to play in major elective surgery but it is an essential skill required by all surgeons who treat wounds.

Table 9.5 | Principles of traumatic wound debridement

1.	Remove foreign bodies and gross contamination.
2.	Irrigate and scrub to remove surface debris.
3.	Wide prep and drape.
4.	Avoid tourniquets unless vital.
5.	Excise all dead tissue.
6.	Excise crushed or dubiously viable tissue if primary closure is planned or leave it to declare itself and plan a second-look debridement.
7.	Cut skin edges and deep surfaces back to bleeding tissue. Debride in the line of any longitudinal structures (e.g. limb arteries, veins or nerves) to avoid transection or damage.
8.	Further irrigate the wound to wash out bacteria, residual foreign bodies and small non-viable tissue fragments. Use normal saline, not povidone-iodine solution, antibiotics or other antiseptics as they may be tissue-toxic.
9.	Obtain haemostasis prior to completing the debridement.
10.	Decide whether a second-look debridement or formal closure is required.

BASIC ASSISTING TECHNIQUES

Surgical assisting is a learned skill and should not be regarded as a boring prelude to learning how to operate. It is physically and mentally challenging, and the best assistant is usually one who knows the operation intimately and who can anticipate each step. Anticipation and preparation will ensure a smooth-flowing sequence of steps, and this is the assistant's ultimate goal. The assistant must concentrate as hard as the surgeon on the task at hand. A good assistant will also, politely, point out any relevant surgical or anatomical features of a procedure that they feel the surgeon may have missed. The surgeon should guide general discussion during the procedure and relevant questions are best asked only at rest, or at low-stress points of the operation. If asked an opinion on the situation at hand it should be presented concisely together with the reasoning behind it. The philosophy of surgical assisting comes down to one phrase: 'A good assistant makes the surgeon perform a good operation.'

The assistant has two major duties: exposure of the operative field and the performance of surgical tasks.

Exposure relates to both the view and the physical access that the assistant creates for the surgeon. Retraction of tissues is the mainstay of this process and provides both an adequate view of the operative site and access for hands and instruments. Ensuring adequate exposure also involves appropriate light alterations, dabbing away of blood, suction, provision of traction for dissecting, and holding instruments and sutures. For some procedures a second assistant is needed to achieve all this. If available, the scrub nurse may also be able to hold retractors or perform some of these tasks. Unfortunately, perfect exposure for the surgeon may lead to no line of vision for the assistant, a trade-off that is sometimes essential for the success of the operation.

The surgical assistant must also be able to carry out many surgical tasks. These include tying sutures, applying or removing instruments, cutting, stabilising, providing counter-traction for dissection, closing wounds with sutures, and following sutures. An assistant who works with one particular surgeon will frequently find these things becoming an automatic part of the operative routine. All this must be done while resisting any temptation to try to replace the surgeon by performing parts of the operation. Dissection or the undertaking of any part of the procedure without an express request from the surgeon is not only bad manners; it may be detrimental to the patient and potentially litigiously problematic. The notes below provide some guidelines for assistants in the preoperative, operative and postoperative phases of a procedure.

Preoperative assistance

It is extremely useful for the surgeon if the assistant ensures the presence of correct medical images, appropriate reports and test results. Assistance in moving and positioning the patient is also much appreciated by the surgeon and theatre staff. Insertion of in-dwelling urinary catheters is often delegated to the assistant and it is of great benefit to be familiar with this procedure in both males and females.

Prepping and draping are usually done by the surgeon, but the assistant or scrub nurse may be required to do this on occasion. The exact pattern used is often a matter of the surgeon's personal preference and guidance is usually provided for assistants if they are required to do it. Once the patient is prepped and draped the operative field must be set up with diathermy, suction, light handles, self-retaining retractors and other instruments as directed.

Intraoperative assistance

Incision

Placing a pack on the skin and providing traction at 90° to the incision will assist the accuracy of this procedure. The pack may then be inserted into the edge of the wound and held with flexed fingers to compress bleeding points and provide further exposure and traction for incising. Resist the temptation to wipe with a pack: dabbing soaks up blood without disturbing clots on the ends of vessels but wiping disrupts these clots and causes bleeding. The pack can be slowly peeled away as the surgeon commences haemostasis. If an abdominal incision is being made, fingers or an instrument may be required to lift the peritoneum or anterior abdominal wall as the incision is continued superiorly and inferiorly.

Retraction

Retraction may be provided with tissue-holding forceps or purpose-built retractors. The art of retracting is to gently displace the tissues, without causing damage, while minimising energy expenditure so that the arm holding the retractor does not fatigue and lose exposure. If you feel the retractor is about to move, inform the surgeon who may wish to interrupt the procedure to prevent inadvertent damage and reposition the instrument. If a surgeon takes hold of the retractor, loosen your grip immediately to allow repositioning of the blade.

The assistant should move the retractor only if specifically told to do so, if a suggestion for better exposure is accepted or if it follows the pattern of dissection or suturing—for example, along the edge of a mastectomy wound. Any movement of the retractor must be delayed until the surgeon is not cutting or suturing. A loss of vision caused by movement of the retractor may result in accidental damage to a vital structure. Special precautions must also be taken with long retractors, especially those with a posteriorly angled lip. Any excessive pressure, or toe-in movements from lifting the handle, may cause damage to deep structures such as liver, spleen or mesentery (Fig. 9.37).

Good retraction does not necessarily involve excessive force. Merely preventing the ingress of tissues by having the retractor in the correct position is often enough to give excellent exposure. If this is not adequate the judicious raising of a hand,

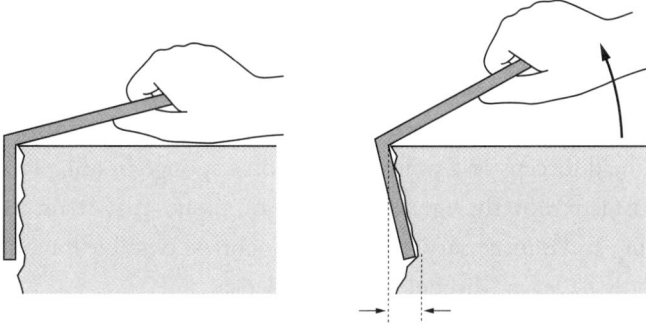

The effect of raising the hand with the bend of the retractor as a fulcrum is demonstrated. A significant increase in retraction is achieved with minimal increase in force. Care must be taken not to damage structures near the tip of the retractor.

Fig. 9.37 Retraction

with the bend of the retractor as the fulcrum, will often retract structures much further with less force. Care, as outlined in the previous paragraph, must be taken with this manoeuvre.

Table 9.6 summarises points to consider when retracting tissues.

Table 9.6	Points to consider when retracting tissues
1.	Gently displace the tissues without causing damage.
2.	Minimise energy expenditure and reduce fatigue so exposure is not lost.
3.	Retain exactly the position in which the surgeon placed the retractor.
4.	If the surgeon takes hold of a retractor, let go—he or she wants to move it.
5.	Only move the retractor if:
	• told to do so
	• your verbal suggestion to improve exposure has been approved
	• it follows the pattern of dissection, e.g. along the edge of a wound the surgeon is not cutting. Loss of vision may result in accidental damage to a vital structure.
6.	Be careful with the toes of long retractors as excessive pressure caused by pulling or 'toe-in' movements may damage deep structures.
7.	Good retraction does not necessarily involve excessive force. The judicious raising of a hand with the bend of the retractor as the fulcrum will often retract structures much further with less force (NB: point 6).

Tension

Firm and gentle traction of tissues at 90° to the line of incision or dissection will often provide the surgeon with an obvious line or plane to follow. It will generally focus the greatest force on this line, thereby allowing those tissues to be divided most easily. The tension will also distract the tissues manually and assist with their physical separation. Application of tension may be achieved with retractors, hands, tissue forceps, hand-held forceps or a swab mounted on a sponge-holding forceps (*swab-on-a-stick*). Unfortunately, overly vigorous traction on tissues may result in uncontrolled tearing, bleeding and unnecessary damage. The gentlest possible force should be used and this can only be learnt through long experience.

Following

Holding the suture thread for the surgeon during suturing is termed *following*. It serves two main purposes. When a surgeon is creating an anastomosis, transfixing a vessel or vascular pedicle, oversewing bleeding sites or closing tissues, there is often a need to maintain tension in the thread. This prevents suture slip and therefore laxity or gaps in the sutured tissue. It also keeps loose thread from encroaching on the tissue to be sutured and out of the surgeon's way, as well as lifting and presenting these tissues for the next suture bite.

The correct technique for following a suture involves certain practical considerations. When taking the suture from the surgeon, it should be pulled only at the same pressure and angle at which it was given. This will prevent inadvertent ischaemia by over-tightening the stitch, keep the tissues best displayed, and keep the surgeon's line of view clear.

The suture should be held '60/40', that is, 40% of the suture between the assistant's hand and the last stitch and 60% between the hand and the needle holder. This allows enough laxity for the surgeon to insert the next suture without excessive suture obscuring the view or tangling with the next bite. As the suture is pulled tight after each bite the assistant should allow the thread to run gently through the fingers. As it nears the end, following the thread all the way down to the tissue being sutured before release will keep the tension on the previous bite and allow this bite to sit in good position.

The thread should be observed carefully to prevent tangling or catching on instruments or other fixed structures (known as 'locking up'). Locking up the thread may cause breakage or damage to tissues as it is pulled tight.

Tying and suture skills

The assistant must occasionally tie sutures, especially when the surgeon's hands are engaged in critical retraction or when the angle is unfavourable for the surgeon to tie. More commonly, the assistant will be required to steady and present an artery forceps for tying around. To do this well, the handles or arms of the instrument should be held in a comfortable position that presents the tips of the instrument for the thread to be slipped around. The instrument should not be pulled upwards as this may tear the vessel or tissue being tied, allowing it to retract and present further difficulties to control.

As the surgeon begins to tie, the forceps should be angled to allow the easiest access for tightening the knot. While doing this the assistant's hand and arm should be kept out of the surgeon's line of sight. When (and only when) asked, release the forceps slowly and gently and remove them from the surgeon's line of sight. If asked to *ease and squeeze*, gently release the forceps, leave them in position and reapply them once the first throw of the knot has been tightened. This manoeuvre allows control to be retained on the structure being tied and a second tie to be applied for further security if required.

When cutting sutures the scissors should be stabilised on the other hand, or another steady point, and the thread cut with the tips of the blades. This will ensure that no adjacent structures are cut and that the suture is trimmed to precise length. In general, a tag end of 3–6 mm should be left, depending on the size of the suture. Any longer than this and it may tangle with another stitch or present a foreign body for infection. Any shorter and the knot may unravel, leading to potentially disastrous consequences.

Haemostasis

Blood in the operative field is a great distraction to the surgeon. It obscures the view and makes any manoeuvre hazardous. There are several methods for removing pooling blood prior to obtaining adequate haemostasis.

A sucker may be used to remove blood from the operative field. The most common is the Yankauer sucker, but other styles and sizes are available depending on the procedure. These are usually connected to high-pressure suction from the wall suction inlet, via a collecting bag system. It is a very rapid method of removal but has the disadvantage that it may dislodge a clot and actually worsen a bleeding problem. Suckers are described in more detail in Chapter 5.

As an alternative, the *swab-on-a-stick*, a gauze swab wound around a sponge-holding forceps, is effective for small amounts of bleeding such as that on the bowel edge during an anastomosis. It is used to dab bleeding in these small areas and doubles as an effective retractor or as an instrument to put tension on tissues being dissected.

The placing of a pack into a bleeding wound will soak up free blood, tamponade bleeding while *in situ* and pull out any free clot when removed. The disadvantage of this is that the flow of the operation must cease while the pack is in place. It is a very effective method, however, for cavity bleeding such as in the pelvis.

Wound closure

The process of wound closure involves most of the skills described above, including tissue retraction, following the suture, assistance with tying and blood removal. The one special skill is in the insertion of skin staples. There are many methods of insertion but one of the commonest requires both surgeon and assistant to pick up adjacent edges of the wound with toothed forceps. They both evert the edges and hold them together while the staple is inserted. This process is then repeated about one centimetre further on until the whole wound is closed. Alternatively, the surgeon may pick up both wound edges together with a heavy forceps in one hand and insert the staples with the other.

Postoperative assistance

Once the incision is closed, the area is washed and dried, a dressing is applied and drains are secured with dressings and tape. The assistant should remain sterile and assist with these procedures. Assistance in moving the patient is, once again, greatly appreciated by all staff. The surgeon or assistant should take responsibility for all catheters and drains during this procedure. One or both should then follow the patient into recovery to ensure all is well. It is only when the patient reaches the recovery room safely that the 'true' traditional assistant's job is at an end.

REFERENCES

1. Canale, ST. Campbell's Operative Orthopaedics. 9th ed. Mosby-Year Book, 1998.
2. Feil W , Lippert H, Lozac'h P, Pallazzini G, Amaral J. eds. Atlas of Surgical Stapling. Heidelberg: Johann Ambrosius Barth Verlag, 2000.

FURTHER READING

Dudley DG. The Surgical Assistant. Surgery, Gynecology and Obstetrics, 1962 Aug;115:245.

ETHICON. Wound Closure Manual, USA: Johnson & Johnson Co., 1994.*

Kyle J, Smith J, Johnston D, eds. Pye's Surgical Handicraft, 22nd ed. Oxford: Butterworth–Heinemann, 1992. Chap. 10, Assisting at Operations.

Kirk RM. Basic Surgical Techniques. 4th ed. Edinburgh: Churchill Livingstone, 1994. Many of the chapters deal, in greater depth, with the topics covered in this chapter.

Thompson RVS. Primary Repair of Soft Tissue Injuries. Melbourne: Melbourne University Press, 1969. Chap. 6, Lacerations without Skin Loss.

Thompson S. Super Suturing. Australia: Davis and Geck, 1991.*

Zederfeldt H, Hunt T. Wound Closure—Materials and Techniques. USA: Davis and Geck, 1990.*

(* These three books may be available through the appropriate company representatives that service your hospital or area.)

CHAPTER TEN
WOUND MANAGEMENT

Mercutio: *No, 'tis not so deep as a well, nor so wide as a church door; but 'tis enough, 'twill serve.*

William Shakespeare (1564–1616), *Romeo and Juliet*, III i 97

INTRODUCTION

The assessment and management of wounds is a cornerstone of surgical practice. The primary objective is to maximise the chance of uncomplicated wound healing while optimising recovery of function. The same principles apply under the strict aseptic conditions of theatre as in the emergency department or on the battle field. An appropriate assessment of the wound directs the decision making and techniques required in the management phase. It is necessary to understand how the wound was caused and the ramifications of the mechanism of injury. Selection of appropriate wound management techniques also depends on an understanding of how wounds heal and the factors that may affect healing.

ASSESSMENT OF WOUNDS

Type of wound

The decision-making process in wound management must begin with assessment of the wound itself and consideration of the ramifications of how the wound was made. By necessity, the site of the wound and the amount of tissue loss will also impact on the management, but details of this will be left to more specialised texts (see Further reading).

One schema by which wounds may be classified is shown in Table 10.1. This provides four classes of wound and relates to a combination of situation, mechanism, contamination and likelihood of infection (Fig 101). The lower a wound is rated (on a scale of 4), the more likely that primary closure will be possible.

Reclassification of a wound is possible by either complete excision in a sterile environment, thereby converting any wound to type 1, or by extensive debridement and copious irrigation with conversion to a type 2 at best.

Type 1 wounds (clean) are essentially those made in an operating theatre or other sterile environments where no contaminated tissues are breached. These include procedures on the body walls and all non-contaminated deep tissues (e.g. thyroid gland, blood vessels, brain and bones). They suffer minimal contamination by airborne particles and heal with negligible risk of infection. Primary wound closure (see later) is the method of choice. Contaminated wounds can sometimes be converted to type 1 by complete excision of the original wound in all planes.

Type 2 wounds (clean contaminated) are minimally contaminated wounds such as clean and tidy incisional wounds inflicted by a sharp cutting implement in a non-sterile environment or sterile surgical wounds where a non-infected tract (e.g. biliary, small bowel, bronchial tree) has been opened with minimal macroscopic contamination. The risk of wound infection is still low and these wounds should be closed primarily after some form of wound toilet. Some type 3 and 4 wounds can effectively be converted to type 2 by wide debridement and copious wound irrigation.

Type 3 wounds (contaminated) are those untidy and contaminated wounds created in a dirty environment, those wounds in operative procedures where an infected tract (e.g. infected bronchial tree or infected urological tract) or a dirty tract (e.g. large bowel or rectum) is opened or wounds in procedures where gross and widespread contamination from a non-infected tract occurs (e.g. abscess). These wounds may require wide debridement and copious irrigation (i.e. conversion to a type 1 or 2 wound) before delayed primary or even primary closure. They have a significant risk of wound infection.

Type 4 wounds (dirty) are infected, contaminated or devitalised wounds, open wounds of duration greater than 12 hours or operative wounds in areas of gross septic or faecal contamination. They should never be closed unless confidently converted to a type one or two wound. Infection rates are high and the risk of gas gangrene or other necrotising infections exists.

Table 10.1 The four-tiered system of wound classification

Classification	Cause	Comments
1. Clean	• Elective surgical wounds, e.g. hernia surgery or breast biopsy	Low wound infection rate approximately <2% Routine primary closure
2. Contaminated—tidy	• Low-velocity traumatic incisions • Clean and sharp with local damage • Contamination minor and brief • Minor intraoperative contamination, e.g. — kitchen knife/clean glass cut — small bowel or bronchial tree opened intraoperatively	Wound infection rate 1–5% Routine primary closure after some debridement and irrigation
3. Contaminated— untidy	• Low-velocity lacerating, tearing or bursting wounds • Ragged and contused with gross local damage • Contamination apparent and prolonged • Major intraoperative contamination • All high-velocity injuries, e.g. — crush injuries — garden tool injuries — large bowel, infected bronchial tree or infected urinary tract opened intraoperatively	Wound infection rate 5–25% May be closed after wide debridement and copious irrigation or may require delayed primary closure

4. Dirty/Infected

- Wounds with signs of infection such as erythema, cellulitis or pus
- Grossly contaminated wounds
- More than 12 hours after injury
- Severe tissue damage and excessive ischaemic tissue, e.g.
  — severe crush injuries
  — penetrating abdominal trauma with hollow visceral perforation
  — 'war wounds'
  — cloth, shrapnel, faeces etc. in wound

Wound infection rate near to 50% if the wound is closed

May be closable after total excision or wide debridement and copious irrigation but often requires healing by delayed primary closure or secondary intention.

WOUND MANAGEMENT

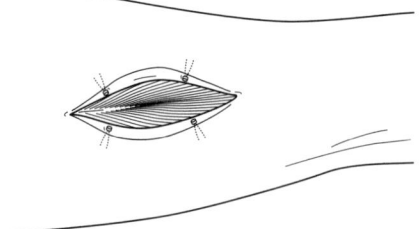

Type 1 wounds are surgically created in a sterile environment.

(a) Type 1—clean wound

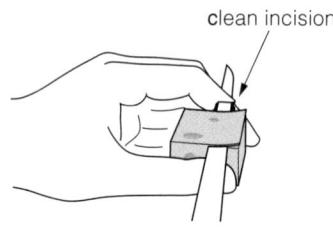

clean incision

Type 2 wounds are created with a sharp instrument, are cleanly incised and minimally contaminated.

(b) Type 2—clean contaminated wound

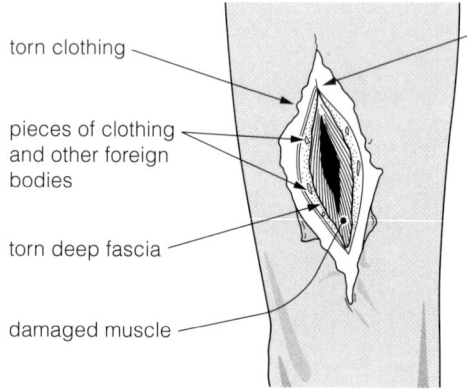

skin surface

torn clothing

pieces of clothing and other foreign bodies

torn deep fascia

damaged muscle

Type 3 wounds are created with tearing or incision and are contaminated. There is no frank infection and minimal dead tissue. Type 3 wounds may become Type 4, over several hours, if left untreated.

(c) Type 3—contaminated wound

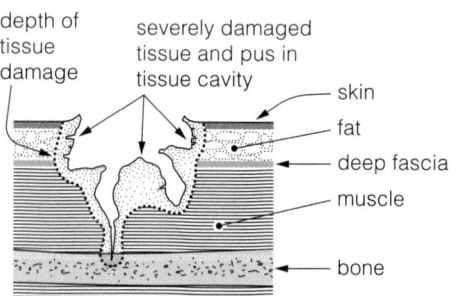

depth of tissue damage

severely damaged tissue and pus in tissue cavity

skin
fat
deep fascia
muscle

bone

Type 4 wounds have severely damaged tissues with devascularisation and (often) gross contamination. Infection also constitutes part of this classification and may be a primary or secondary problem.

(d) Type 4—infected wound/grossly contaminated wound

Fig. 10.1 Wound types

Mechanism of injury

The mechanism of injury impacts greatly on the decisions made during wound management and specific information regarding this must be elicited. When the patient is unable to describe how the injury occurred, the appearance of a wound will often provide clues to the cause. Blunt trauma, penetrating trauma, thermal injury, chemical injury, electrical injury and injury by ionising radiation are the six major mechanisms of injury. For completeness, all six are dealt with but in reality the most commonly treated wounds are caused by blunt trauma, penetrating trauma or heat. An appreciation of their effects and ramifications are essential for good wound management practices.

Kinetic energy injury – closed (blunt)

This is a very common form of injury and results from either an object striking a person or a person striking an object. The essential component of this injury mechanism is deceleration with a subsequent transfer of kinetic energy. The two variants, however, have significantly different ramifications.

In the case of an object striking a person the major injury is usually localised to the region of impact. Take the example of a cricket ball striking the forehead. As the ball first strikes, the skin of the forehead is compressed and may burst open as a stellate laceration. Blood vessels and underlying tissue also burst with subsequent haemorrhage and contusion (Fig. 10.2).

The energy transfer continues through the tissues resulting in deformation or fracturing of the underlying bone. Further propagation of energy, combined with the bony deformation or fracture, may cause disruption of underlying brain tissues, blood vessels and meninges. Bleeding, contusion and possibly soft tissue fracture are common sequelae. Spikes of bone may even penetrate the underlying tissue causing further injuries (Fig. 10.3). Finally, the forced compression of the brain against the back of the cranial vault, and its subsequent recoil, may result in damage to the occipital lobes (contre-coup injury) (Fig. 10. 4).

When a moving person strikes an object (e.g. the ground after a fall from a roof), there are several mechanisms of injury. The first is the direct strike of body parts causing localised blunt injuries, as above, at one or multiple sites. Equally important is the effect of deceleration on the rest of the body. Internal organs, such as the aorta, liver, mesentery and others, which are only partly fixed to the body wall, may continue to move after the body wall has stopped. This may result in tearing of structures at points of attachment, such as in the upper descending thoracic aorta, or compression against decelerated tissues, such as the liver against the abdominal wall (Fig. 10.5).

Another consequence of body deceleration is the abnormal deformation of bones and joints. For example the mid-point of the lower limb may be stopped by an object such as the dashboard of a car, but the lower portion continues to move resulting in

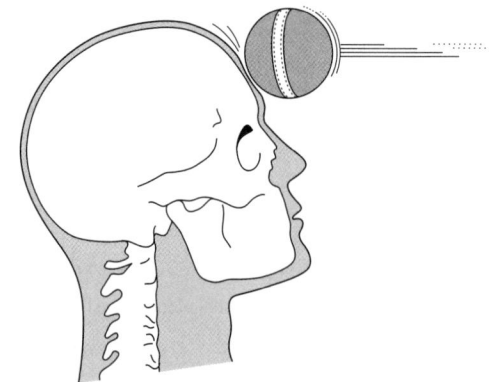

(a) Cricket ball strikes forehead compressing the skin and subcutaneous tissues and causing them to burst.

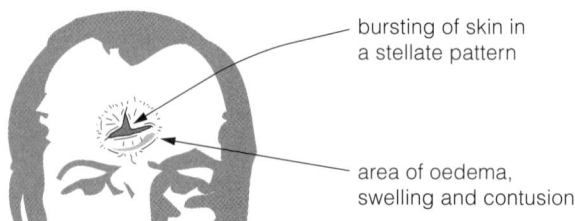

bursting of skin in a stellate pattern

area of oedema, swelling and contusion

(b) The burst laceration is usually stellate and raised due to both oedema and haematoma/contusion.

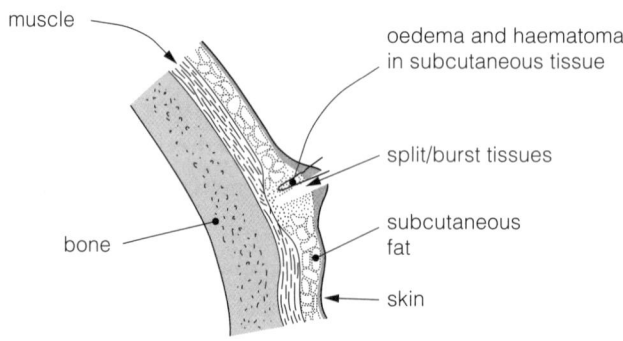

muscle

oedema and haematoma in subcutaneous tissue

split/burst tissues

subcutaneous fat

bone

skin

(c) Cross-section of burst/lacerated tissues showing oedema and haematoma.

Fig. 10.2 Surface contact injury with transfer of kinetic energy

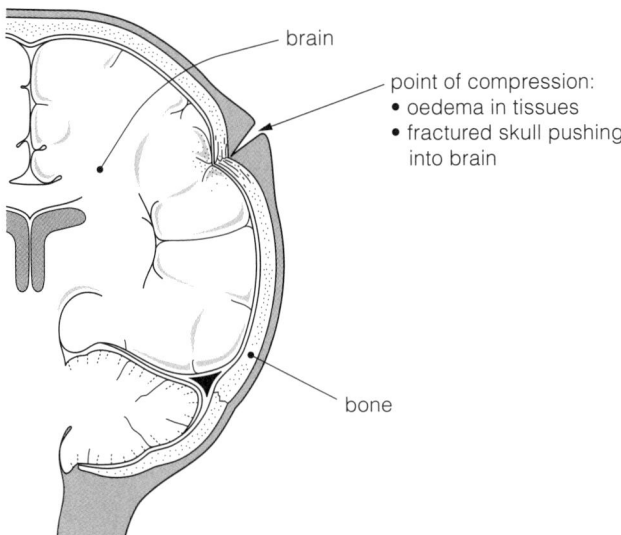

Fig. 10.3 Skull fracture compressing brain, causing haemorrhage and cerebral damage

Contre-coup brain injury occurs at the point opposite impact. At the point of impact the brain is compressed and the opposite pole of the brain experiences a negative pressure leading to injury here as well.

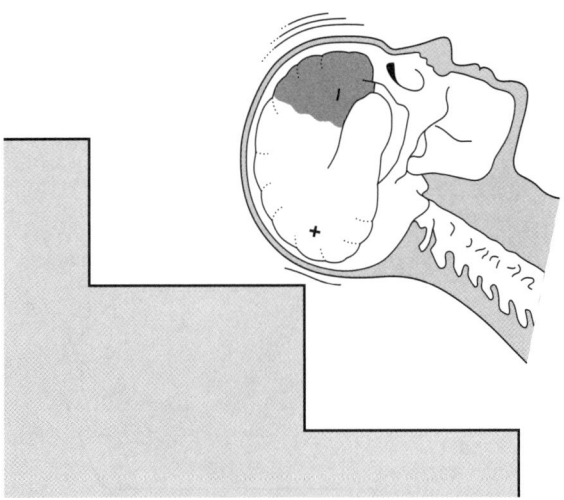

Fig. 10.4 Contre-coup brain injury

a fracture to the tibia and fibula (Fig. 10.6). Hyperflexion or hyperextension of the spinal column is also commonly related to deceleration trauma and this can lead to a variety of fractures and spinal cord damage (Fig. 10.7).

In many cases of blunt injury, such as in that suffered by the driver of a motor vehicle involved in a head-on collision, there is a combination of the two mechanisms. Direct compression of the epigastrium by a steering wheel, seat belt

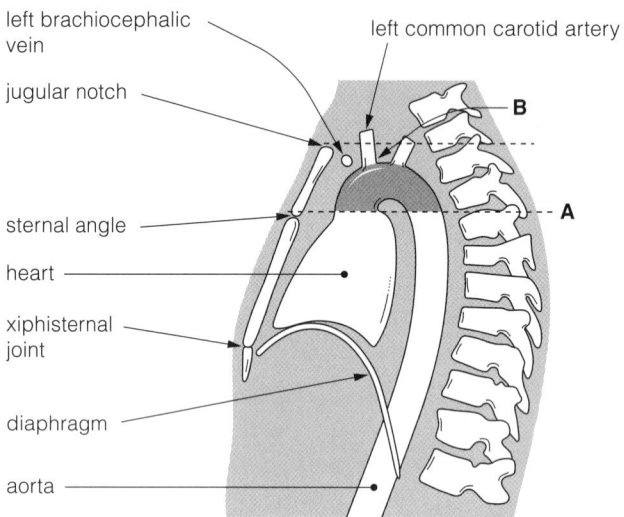

The aorta below point **A** is *fixed* to the posterior wall of the thorax. It is semi-fixed at the great vessels **B**. When the body decelerates and the free part of the aorta (shaded) continues to move, it may partially or completely tear.

Fig. 10.5 Thoracic aorta (a lateral view of the chest)

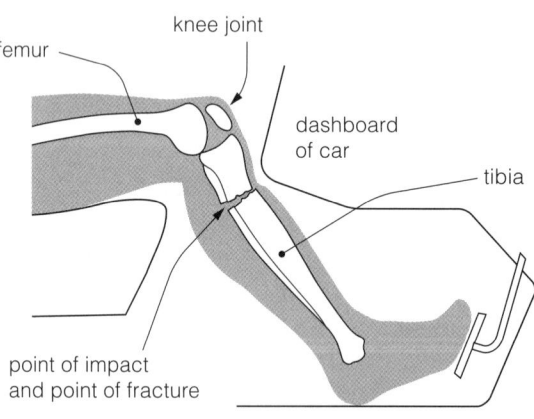

Fig. 10.6 Fracture occurring at the point of impact, where the distal part of the limb continues to move after the proximal part stops

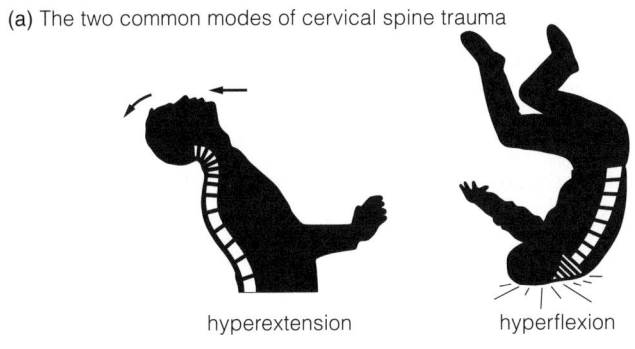

(a) The two common modes of cervical spine trauma

hyperextension　　　　　hyperflexion

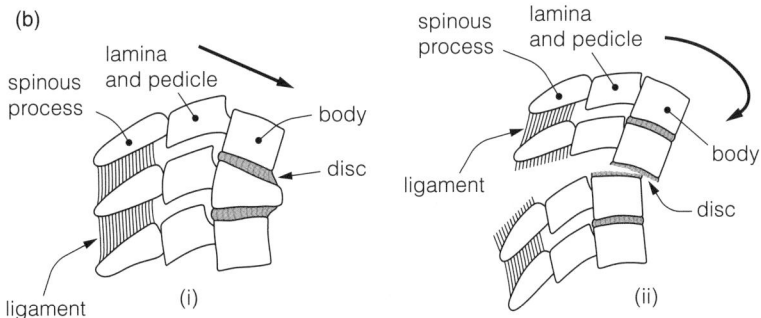

(b)

spinous process

lamina and pedicle

body

disc

ligament

(i)

spinous process

lamina and pedicle

body

disc

ligament

(ii)

Hyperflexion may cause a wedge fracture of the vertebral body (i) or complete ligamentous and intervertebral joint disruption with partial or complete dislocation (ii). Cord damage is common in both scenarios.

(c)

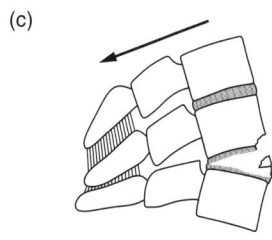

Hyperextension causes ligament disruption and vertebral body fractures anteriorly, and potential posterior dislocation.

(d)

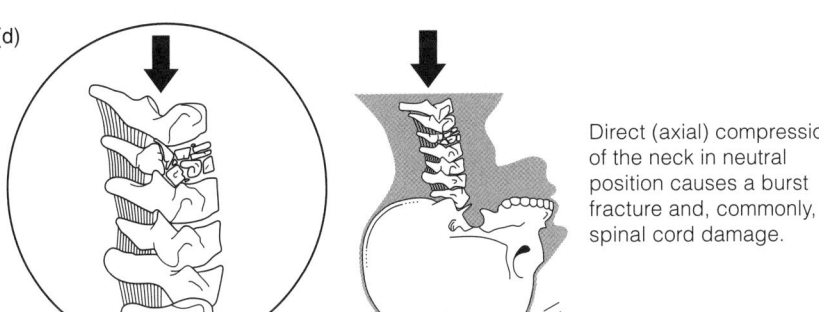

Direct (axial) compression of the neck in neutral position causes a burst fracture and, commonly, spinal cord damage.

Fig. 10.7 Cervical spine hyperflexion and hyperextension leading to spinal cord damage

or airbag may result in rupture of the pancreas, duodenum, stomach and spleen with spinal hyperflexion and fracture, potentially leading to spinal cord damage. The deceleration of the rest of the body may result in thoracic aortic rupture, cervical spine hyperflexion with further spinal cord trauma and long bone fractures.

While many of the features described above relate to major trauma, a set of basic principles emerge for this type of injury. Whether major or minor it can be said that blunt injuries:

- burst tissues raggedly
    — contuse tissues
    — lead to contamination by any material between the impact and the tissue
- cause compression or deformity to deeper structures
- may be associated with injuries to other body parts.

It is these principles, then, that must be borne in mind when assessing injuries of this type.

Kinetic energy injury – open (penetrating)

Penetrating wounds may be caused by something as simple as standing on a nail or as complex as multiple high-velocity bullet wounds. The main differentiating factor is the energy of the injury. Low-energy wounds result from anything up to the impact of a small-calibre bullet, such as a .22 calibre, and mainly cause damage in the line of the penetration (Fig. 10.8). Higher-velocity projectiles transfer much more energy and are more dangerous as they cause wide cavitation due to the pressure wave that is created during their passage through tissue (Fig. 10.9). Cavitation causes damage to, and devascularisation of, nearby tissues. While somewhat variable, the average diameter of the cavitation is about thirty times the diameter of the projectile.

Most penetrating wounds seen in the emergency department will be low-energy and accidental puncture or incision wounds, which are frequently contaminated. Unless obviously superficial it must be assumed that all deeper structures in the line of the wound are involved. Examination of distal motor and neurovascular function may suggest which structures are damaged but partial injury to these may not be detectable. For example a three-quarters-lacerated tendon will function normally with gentle examination but will rupture a week later when stressed. In general, then, exploration to exclude damage to deep structures and to perform wound toilet is mandatory in these wounds.

High-energy/velocity projectile wounds will not be dealt with in this chapter.

Thermal energy injury

Thermal injuries may be caused by either heat or cold. Dry heat or friction causes a 'burn', moist heat causes a 'scald', prolonged exposure to a cold wet environment causes 'chilblains' or 'trench foot' and actual freezing of tissues by cold causes 'frostbite'. While similar in outcome the pathophysiology of heat and cold injuries differs greatly.

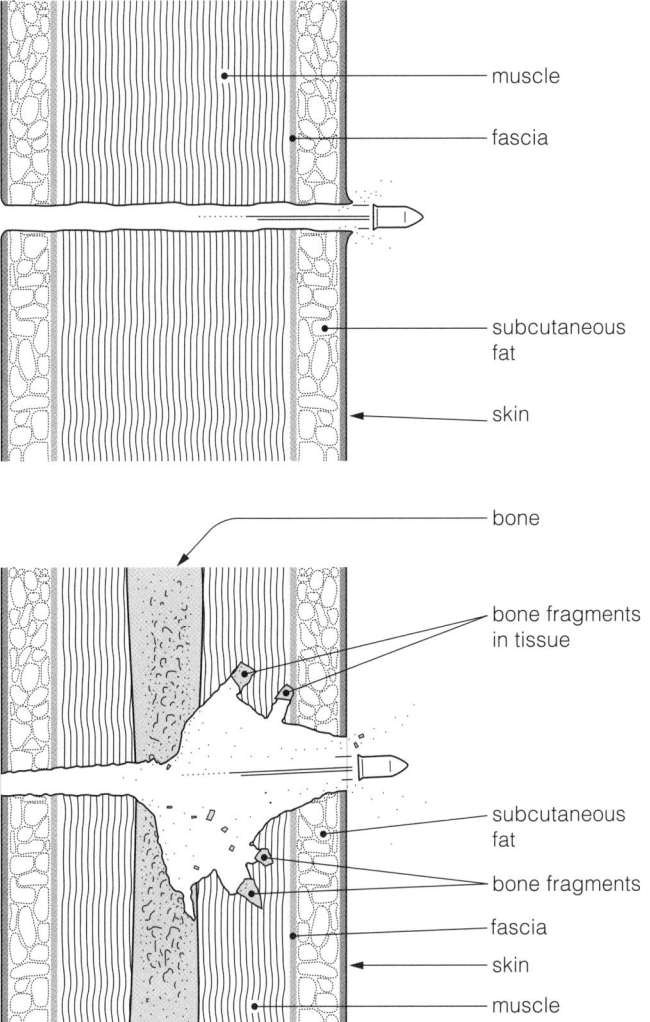

muscle

fascia

subcutaneous fat

skin

bone

bone fragments in tissue

subcutaneous fat

bone fragments

fascia

skin

muscle

Damage is caused in the line of penetration only. This can be worsened if a bone is fractured and the bone fragments cause damage, or if the bullet itself fragments.

Fig. 10.8 Tissue injury caused by low-velocity penetrating trauma

Heat injury

The pathology of a heat injury (burn or scald) is a coagulative necrosis of epidermis and dermis to a variable depth. The depth of this necrosis is the basis for burns classification and the descriptive terms of *first-degree* (superficial), *second-degree* (deep) and *third-degree* (full thickness) (Fig. 10.10 and Table 10.2).

A superficial or first-degree burn involves part or all of the epidermis. It is caused by a mild heat source such as the sun or short exposure to a more immediate heat

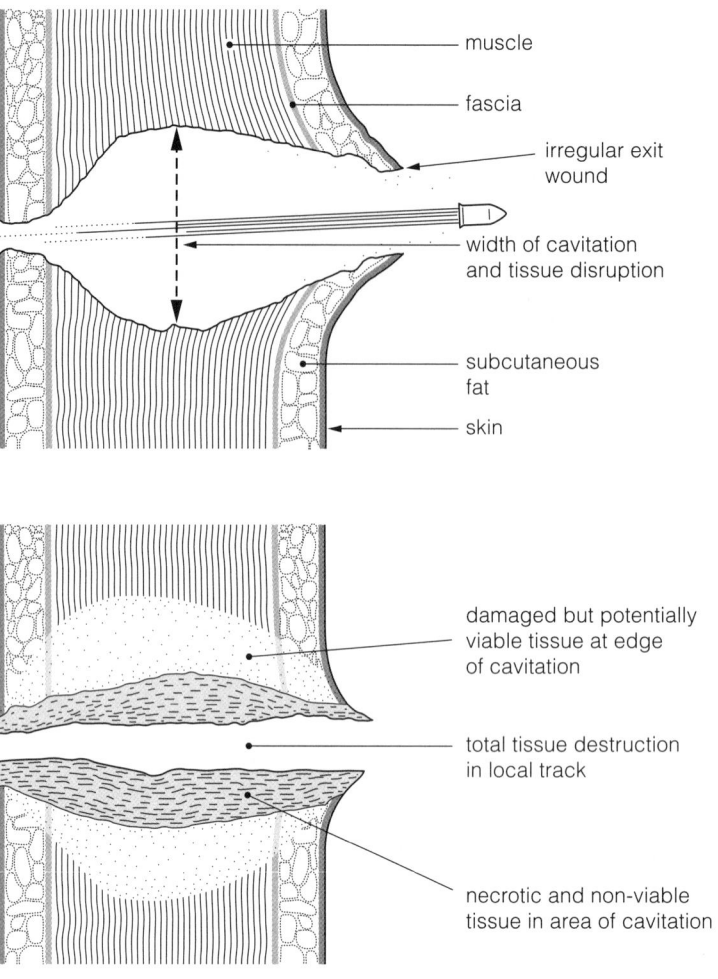

muscle

fascia

irregular exit
wound

width of cavitation
and tissue disruption

subcutaneous
fat

skin

damaged but potentially
viable tissue at edge
of cavitation

total tissue destruction
in local track

necrotic and non-viable
tissue in area of cavitation

There is widespread damage due to tissue
cavitation with high-velocity projectiles.

Fig. 10.9 Tissue and organ damage caused by high-velocity penetrating trauma

source such as a flame or steam. The injury is always intensely erythematous due to underlying vasodilation and the epidermis is either dry or has small blisters. Involved skin is painful and tender and retains all sensory functions. Infection is rare and healing occurs within a week with no scarring.

A deep or second-degree burn necroses a variable depth of dermis, but not so deeply that it destroys all structures that contain epidermal cells. It is caused by sustained contact with a heat source or chemical. Hair follicles and glandular structures (sebaceous and sweat) are left partially intact and it is the cells lining these, as well as the edges of the burn, that provide the basis for re-epithelialisation. The area appears pink and mottled due to the depth of necrosed

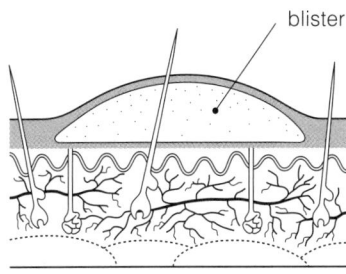

blister

Superficial, or 1st degree, burns affect only the epidermis and result in blistering. These heal themselves in most cases.

(a) Superficial burns

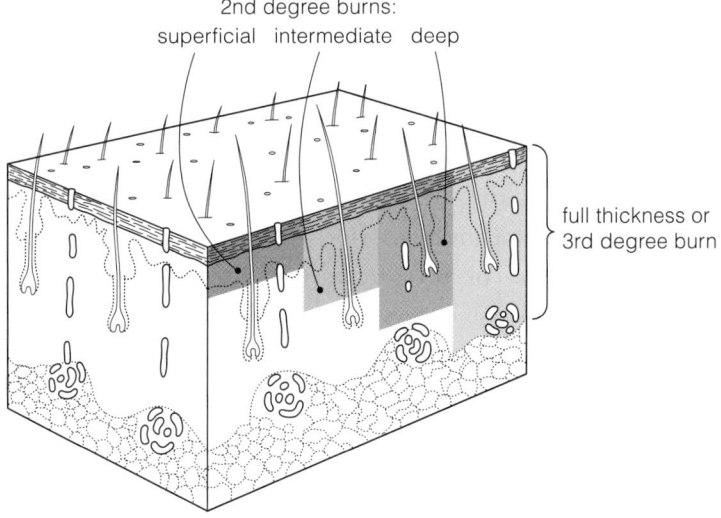

2nd degree burns:
superficial   intermediate   deep

full thickness or 3rd degree burn

(b) Deeper burns

The deeper the burn the less likely it is to heal. All but the deepest 2nd degree burn will heal. Deep 2nd degree and 3rd degree burns usually require skin grafting.

Fig. 10.10 Burn thickness (depth)

tissue overlying the dilated vessels below the burn. Large blisters and copious fluid loss in regions of de-epithelialisation are common. These injuries are intensely painful but, if deep, may lose pinprick sensation. Healing is much slower than for a first-degree burn and there is a moderate risk of infection. Scarring is also common and more severe second-degree burns will require pressure garments or special dressings to reduce this. Occasionally skin grafting is required but most will heal autonomously within two to five weeks. Rehabilitation may be required, as may revisional scar surgery.

A full-thickness or third-degree burn necroses the entire dermis and variable amounts of deeper tissues. Prolonged exposure to the heat source or chemical, extremely high temperatures or high-voltage electrical contact are required to cause this level of destruction. All epithelium-containing elements are destroyed and therefore spontaneous healing cannot occur. The burn looks pale and marbled due to the depth of injury and vessel thrombosis within it. There is little or no pain (unless there is a zone of lesser degree burn around it) and all sensory functions of the skin are lost.

Tissue burnt this severely is not distensible and, especially if it is a circumferential burn on a limb or torso, underlying tissue pressures may rise due to accumulating inflammatory oedema. If the increase is great enough to prevent blood flow (and hence oxygen delivery) limb compartment syndrome occurs. In the torso, a lack of skin stretch may restrict ventilatory capacity. This situation requires urgent incision of the burned area (escharotomy) and sometimes of the underlying deep fascia (fasciotomy) to relieve or prevent a compartment syndrome or to improve ventilation.

In all third-degree burns the risk of infection is high. Complete excision of the burn followed by skin grafting is routinely used to achieve rapid healing but scarring is common. The use of pressure garments, revisional scar surgery and rehabilitation is very common.

The patient with cutaneous burns must be examined closely to exclude other injuries. Blunt and penetrating trauma may occur as part of the situation that led to the burn and signs of this must be looked for specifically. There are also special types of burn, such as respiratory burns, ocular burns and genital burns, which require the intervention of a specialised practitioner. Assessment of the amount of skin surface area that has been burnt is approximated by the 'rule of nines' (Fig. 10.11). Children have a different surface area to mass, as indicated in (Fig. 10.11) and require specialist management for fluid resuscitation and pain management.

Cold injury

The final effect of cold injury is very similar to that caused by heat: tissue necrosis. Unlike heat, however, it is not a coagulative process from the start. As with heat injury there are levels of severity but they are not classified as strictly as burns (see Table 10.3).

Mild cold injury is called 'pernio' or 'chilblains'. These occur on exposed body parts exposed to a dry source of cold that is above freezing point. Local ulceration, blistering and haemorrhage may occur. The area usually appears cyanosed.

Exposure to a wet cold source that is above freezing point, such as immersion of feet in cold water for one to several days, results in the phenomenon of 'trench foot'. 'Immersion foot' is a similar injury caused by prolonged (days to weeks) exposure to water that is not cold enough to cause trench foot. The affected regions appear

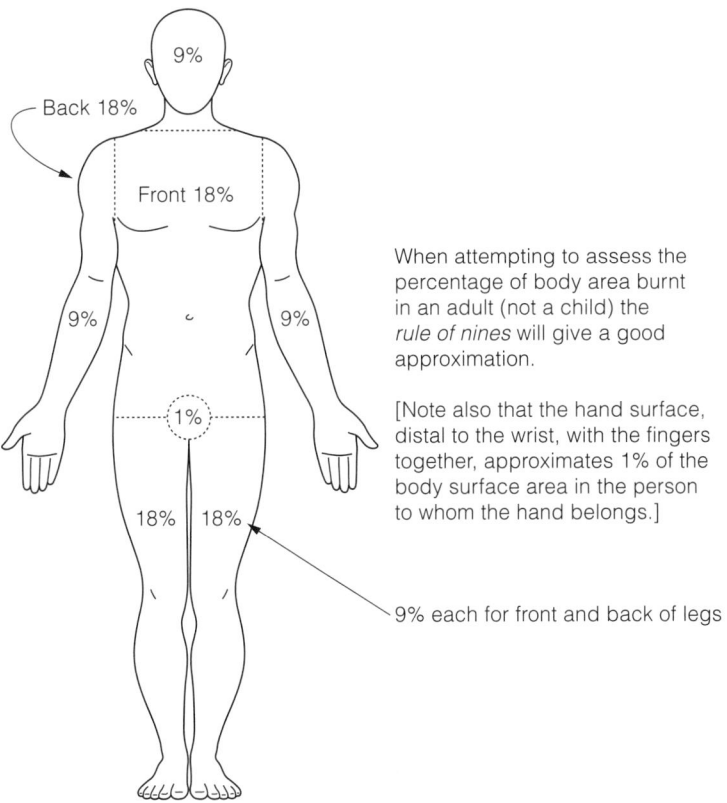

When attempting to assess the percentage of body area burnt in an adult (not a child) the *rule of nines* will give a good approximation.

[Note also that the hand surface, distal to the wrist, with the fingers together, approximates 1% of the body surface area in the person to whom the hand belongs.]

9% each for front and back of legs

Fig. 10.11 Rule of nines

gangrenous and are usually anaesthetic. The pathology of both is very similar and is due to microvascular endothelial injury, capillary stasis and vascular occlusion. Superficial gangrene may appear impressive but deep tissue loss is usually minimal.

'Frostbite' is caused by actual freezing of body tissues. The extent of damage is increased by the rapidity and duration of freezing. Pathologically, the injury of frostbite is caused by the combination of freezing and subsequent thawing. Intracellular ice crystallisation, cellular dehydration and microvascular thrombosis begin the process, which worsens as the tissue is reheated. There are four levels of frostbite severity (see Table 10.4). Thawing tissue loses protein-rich fluid, which increases tissue pressure. Local vasoconstriction also increases (paradoxically) to be at its greatest when tissue temperature reaches 15 °C. Both these factors may worsen tissue damage.

Warming is an essential part of treatment but this, at least in the short term, may appear to worsen the injury. Hence, early surgical intervention is not recommended as significant amounts of potentially viable tissue may be removed. Once it is certain that all salvageable tissue has recovered then the smallest possible debridement of tissue may be undertaken. In the long term any of the more severe cold injuries can

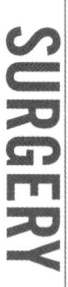

Table 10.2 Characteristics of burns

	First degree (superficial)	Second degree (partial thickness)	Third degree (full thickness)
Cause	• Ultraviolet light (sun) • Short-term exposure to steam, radiant source or hot object	• Longer exposure to steam, hot liquid or object, radiant source or chemical	• Prolonged exposure to hot liquid or object, radiant source or chemical • Contact with high-voltage electricity
Depth	• Epidermal	• Low to mid dermis	• Deep dermis and subcutaneous tissues
Appearance	• Erythematous • Blanch to touch • Dry or small blisters	• Mottled pink • Large blisters or weeping areas	• Dry and pale with vessel thrombosis (marbled) • May be charred • Deep tissue loss or wet necrosis with chemicals or electricity
Sensation	• Painful with intact pressure and pinprick	• Very painful with intact pressure sensation but potential loss of pinprick if quite deep	• Anaesthetic surface with no intact sensation
Course	• Heal spontaneously within 10 days • Minimal infection risk • Minimal scarring	• Most heal spontaneously but occasionally require grafting • Moderate infection risk • Within 2–5 weeks • Minimal to severe scarring	• May require escharotomy, fasciotomy and surgical management of damaged deeper structures • Always requires skin grafting • High infection risk • Healing time related to severity and scarring • Severe scarring common
Outcome	• Normal tissue	• Skin discolouration • Occasional contractures and unsightly scars • Scar reducing pressure garments or dressings sometimes required • Some rehabilitation of limbs and patient may be required	• Flexure and other contractures commonly require surgical treatment • Long-term use of pressure garments • Rehabilitation need based on severity and extent

Source: Compilation assisted by information from *Sabiston's Textbook of Surgery*, 18th edn. Philadelphia: WB Saunders Co., 2005.

Table 10.3 Characteristics of cold injury

	Chilblains	Trenchfoot	Frostbite
Cause	• Exposure to dry cold above freezing • Vascular cause	• Exposure to cold, wet conditions • Vascular cause	• Freezing of tissues • Ice crystals, dehydration and vasospasm
Depth	• Superficial	• Superficial tissues with occasional deep tissue involvement	• Any depth of tissue but is classified according to four levels (see Table 10.4) • Recovery may occur in much of the involved tissue
Appearance	• Small ulcers, blisters and bleeding with local cyanosis	• Macerated and gangrenous tissues widespread on foot and lower leg	• Dry, desquamated, pale, grey and gangrenous appearance
Sensation	• Painful with intact normal sensory function	• Anaesthetic initially • Long-term paraesthesia, cold intolerance and pain with weight bearing may occur	• Anaesthetic initially • Long-term paraesthesia, cold intolerance and pain with weight bearing may occur
Course	• Rapid healing	• Slow healing of most tissue with some superficial (and occasionally deep) tissue loss	• Slow recovery of affected tissue depending on severity • Final demarcation usually much less than initially apparent injury
Outcome	• Normal tissue	• Some tissue loss and scarring	• Variable tissue loss by surgical debridement after final demarcation

Source: Compilation assisted by information from *Sabiston's Textbook of Surgery*, 18th edn. Philadelphia: WB Saunders Co., 2005.

Table 10.4 | Frostbite injury

Four levels of frostbite severity based on appearance after thawing

First degree

- Very superficial freezing
- Hyperaemia, oedema and minimal necrosis

Second degree

- Partial thickness injury
- Hyperaemia, rapid oedema and large blisters
- Necrosis present
- Sensation intact

Third degree

- Full-thickness skin injury
- Pale with slow onset oedema
- Eventual necrosis
- Sensation lost

Fourth degree

- Full skin thickness and deep tissues
- Limb infarction
- Requires amputation

lead to paraesthesia, cold intolerance, muscle weakness, pain on weight bearing and acrocyanosis. Further discussion regarding the treatment of thermal injury may be found in specialised texts.

Chemical injury

Many chemical agents cause damage to living tissues and have this effect through a number of mechanisms. These include heat liberation from exothermic chemical reactions, liquefaction by strong alkalis and acids, delipidation by petrochemicals and vesicle formation by various gases. The severity of damage is related to factors such as the amount of chemical, its concentration and the duration of contact. Initial treatment is by copious and prolonged irrigation with water. In a very few instances, specific solvents or antidotes are required but this decision should be left to specialist treatment facilities. At times early excision is required to minimise local damage.

Certain special cases also occur. In the case of gas exposure respiratory damage may occur and should be suspected. Chemical ocular injuries also need copious irrigation and early consultation with an ophthalmologist.

Electrical injury

Electrical current causes direct tissue injury by conversion to thermal energy at the site of entry and along planes of conduction. This has clinical applications in the use of surgical diathermy (see Chapter 7). This phenomenon is a function of 'current density' (i.e. current flow per unit of cross-sectional area). Unlike direct heat injury, however, the deeper tissues cool more slowly than the superficial tissues and are more liable to sustain a greater injury.

The entry wound is usually heavily charred and at low voltages (less than 1000 V) the increased electrical resistance created by this will prevent further current flow. At high voltages this is not true and the current will continue to flow, causing damage to deeper structures.

The major injuries from high-voltage shocks occur in limbs, with muscle and other deep tissue being effectively 'cooked' by the liberated heat. This leads to myoglobinuria and renal failure, which may be further compounded by failure to correctly appreciate the amount of fluid resuscitation required. Hyperkalemia may also occur as a consequence of tissue damage and acute renal failure. Increases in tissue pressure will lead to a compartment syndrome and this requires urgent fasciotomy to preserve blood flow to any viable local and distal tissue.

Other consequences of high-voltage shocks include cardiac arrest and rhythm disturbances, central and peripheral neurological injury, visceral injury, spinal compression fractures, joint fracture or dislocation and late haemorrhage. These should be watched for and the patient frequently reassessed during their inpatient stay.

Ionising radiation injury

While ionising radiation is an uncommon source of acute injury, an understanding of the biologic basis of radiation damage completes knowledge of the major mechanisms of tissue injury. In essence, radiation emits energy as it passes through tissue. The amount of energy released varies with the type of radiation source and the tissue being traversed. This energy ionises molecules and starts a chain of biochemical events that leads to damage to DNA, RNA, cellular fibres and membranes. The effects of this include cell death, chromosomal rearrangements and point mutations. These changes are variably reversible. Individual cells appear to be more sensitive if they divide frequently (e.g. haemopoietic stem cells) and less sensitive if they do not (e.g. nerve cells).

Local tissue effects of radiation endarteritis, with progressive devascularisation and fibrosis, impair the transfer of nutrients to irradiated regions. This affects wound healing and increases the rate of wound breakdown in these areas. Late manifestations of radiation injury may include radiation-induced malignancies, radiation osteonecrosis and underlying organ damage (e.g. heart, lungs and gut). Very high doses of radiation, such as received in nuclear explosions or accidents, cause widespread proliferative cell death. This in turn breaks down host barriers, such as the gut, and defences, such as the immune cell system, and leads to eventual demise of the organism.

THE PATHOLOGY OF WOUND HEALING

Understanding the type, mechanism and ramifications of a wound is the first component of the ability to manage it effectively. A sound knowledge of wound healing and factors that affect this, in the individual patient, are equally important for the adequate assessment of a traumatic wound.

Wound healing

The repair of any soft tissue relies on:

1. the body generating capillaries and collagen on both sides of the wound;
2. this collagen cross-linking with wound-edge collagen and new collagen;
3. the wound contracting in size;
4. the unaligned, cross-linked collagen maturing into regularly arranged bundles (a scar) to provide the healed wound with strength; and
5. epithelial regrowth across the defect.

While the actual process is identical no matter how the wound is managed, three modes of wound healing are described. First intention healing, or primary closure, describes the reparative process with the wound closed and the edges brought together (Fig. 10.12). Second intention healing describes repair when the wound is left open and it slowly heals from the base up (Fig. 10.13). A combination of these two methods, delayed primary closure, relies on the wound initially remaining open, beginning granulation and the edges subsequently being closed together to speed the healing process.

Second intention healing

A description of the healing process of an open wound supplies the basic description of the healing for all wounds. At the beginning of this process, the open defect fills with clot and exudate. Drying of the surface provides a crust to cover the moist depths of the wound. In the moist region collagenolysis and digestion of tissue by phagocytic white blood cells are the body's own form of wound debridement. Subsequently capillary loops grow from the edges of the wound into a matrix of white blood cells, mucopolysaccharides and fibroblast, which produce collagen. This is called granulation tissue. Specially differentiated actin- and myosin-containing fibroblasts (myofibroblasts) aid the healing process by causing wound contraction. Gradually the collagen, which is both types one and three, cross-links

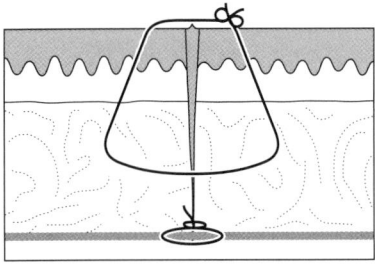

(a) All layers approximated with sutures and narrow gap filled with fibrin.

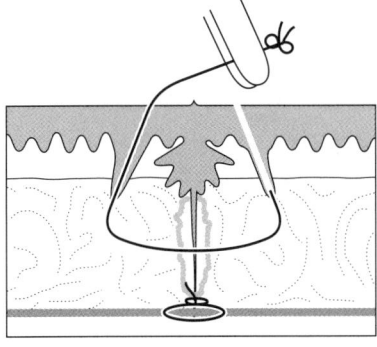

(b) Removal of skin sutures several days later. Epithelial growth into dermis at suture tracks and wound.

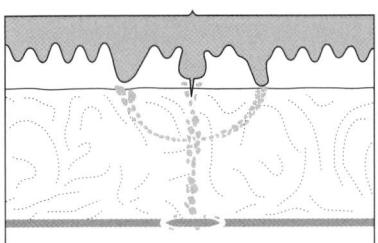

(c) Weeks later the epithelial plugs are disintegrating and fine scars develop in the wound and suture tracks. Absorbable sutures disintegrate.

Fig. 10.12 First intention healing, or primary closure

and forms the basis of the scar. Epithelium migrates from the edges of the wound to cover this tissue. Over a period of six to twelve months the collagen in the scar realigns (matures), type three collagen is lost and more type one is laid down, the scar thins and the hyperaemic, capillary rich, scar tissue pales as vessels diminish in size and number.

First intention healing

First intention healing occurs by virtually the same processes, but only in that minute gap between the accurately opposed wound edges. Fibrinous adhesion between the surfaces occurs by about 24 hours but there is little strength until true healing begins. As in other wounds, granulation tissue grows in and collagen is laid down.

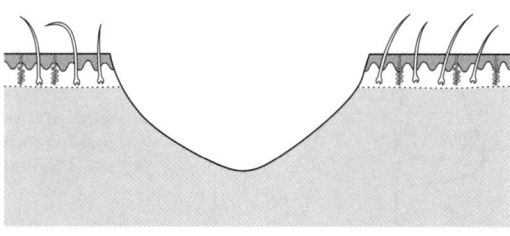

(a) Initial wound

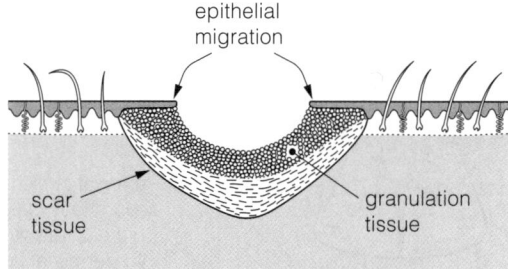

(b) Simultaneous development of granulation tissue and epithelial migration. Wound contraction causes the gap to reduce.

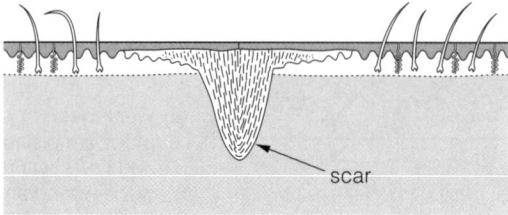

(c) Final result is scar contracture and epithelial cover devoid of skin appendages or rete ridges.

Fig. 10.13 Second intention healing

Contraction, scar formation, re-epithelialisation and scar maturation also occur. The difference between first and second intention healing is, therefore, quantitative rather than qualitative.

Factors influencing wound healing

The factors that affect the healing of wounds can be divided into three categories: local, general and technical. If we look at each of these categories in relation to the healing process, the effect of each factor must be to cause mechanical disruption, necrosis, reduction in local collagen, an inhibition of new collagen formation or a combination of these. The outcome may range from a minor wound infection through to non-healing and major dehiscence of the wound.

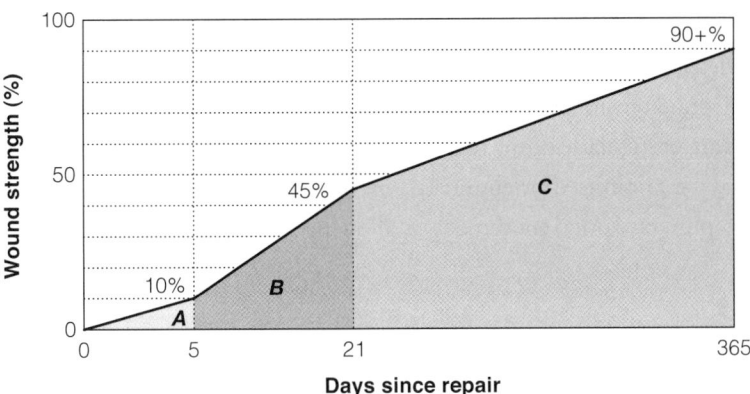

A *Lag phase Days 1–4*. Inflammation and phagocyte debridement. Initial collagenolysis (may be marked in bowel) and assembly of components for collagen synthesis. Strength mainly dependent on sutures.

B *Proliferative phase Days 5–21*. Fibroblasts lay down a collagen lattice in a ground substance.
Rapid increase of wound strength to about 30–50%.
Period during which sutures are usually removed.

C *Remodelling phase Days 22–1 year*. Process of constant absorption and replacement of collagen in the wound along lines of stress. Strength increases to virtually 100% over this period.

Fig. 10.14 Healing processes and wound strength

Local factors

Ischaemia

Ischaemia is the lack of blood (and hence nutrients and oxygen) supply to living tissue. In a healing wound this may be due to:

- inadequate vascular inflow to the tissue because of vessel ligation, peripheral vascular disease or generalised hypotension;
- the presence of dead tissue at the wound edge;
- overly tight or closely spaced sutures preventing flow through capillaries at the wound's edge; or
- tension on the wound edges leading to high tissue pressures and increased tension on sutures thereby preventing flow.

Individually, or in combination, these factors reduce blood flow at the healing edges of the wound. This reduces white blood cell and fibroblast inflow, oxygen and nutrient supply and capillary ingrowth. The end result is failure of healing, with subsequent wound disruption, wound infection or frank necrosis of wound edges.

Ischaemia is prevented by ensuring tissue is loosely apposed and that sutures are not tied tightly. The need for excessive tension in closure should prompt consideration of grafting or healing by second intention.

Tension

If a tissue defect requires excessive amounts of force to draw the edges together, there is significant wound tension. Wounds in areas of poor skin mobility or with large amounts of skin loss are particularly prone to this. The resulting ischaemia inhibits wound healing. Tension may be minimised or eliminated by the use of grafts and flaps, post-operative splinting to prevent wound movement or allowing healing by secondary intention.

Dead space

The presence of a cavity deep in the wound allows for collection of blood and serous fluid, which provides an ideal culture medium for bacteria and predisposes to infection. Attention to accurate wound closure or placement of a drain will reduce wound dead space.

Foreign bodies and contamination

The presence of extraneous foreign material, dead tissue or a large amount (inoculum) of bacteria all increase the risk of infection and wound disruption. Wounds in 'dirty' regions (e.g. groin and natal cleft), long duration of contamination, bacterial virulence and antibiotic resistance compound this problem. Prevention is by adequate debridement, wound lavage and the use of appropriate antibiotics in certain circumstances.

Wound infection

Wound infection is more likely in contaminated wounds, ischaemic wounds and those in which haematoma or fluid collections have occurred. With the accompanying local inflammatory response, collagenolysis increases and tissue pressure elevates. These can combine to cause further ischaemia and impair the healing process. Prevention or early treatment of wound infection by a combination of antibiotics and drainage or debridement can save major wound and patient complications.

Haematoma

The presence of a wound haematoma predisposes to infection and wound complications. Inadequate haemostasis, bleeding due to the relaxation of vessel spasm, late bleeding in wound infection or patient anticoagulation by drugs or disseminated intravascular coagulopathy are the major reasons for haemorrhage. A close attention to haemostasis and relevant patient factors will minimise the risk of this.

Local trauma

Damage to tissues may contuse and render them partially or totally ischaemic. This may provide a nidus for infection. Local trauma also increases the inflammatory response in a way similar to sepsis, thereby promoting collagenolysis (especially related to gastrointestinal anastomosis). It may also increase the rate of sepsis. Care in operative management and wide debridement will minimise this.

Chronic tissue factors

Local tissue problems such as chronic lymphoedema, chronic ischaemia, venous hypertension and past scarring can all contribute to poor wound healing. Little can be done for these conditions other than use of assiduous techniques and optimisation of other factors.

Sutures

Tightly tied sutures can cause pain, ischaemia and wound edge necrosis. Certain suture materials, such as silk, cause an increased inflammatory response and may increase wound infection rates and collagenolysis. Sutures may also 'cut out'. Gentle but firm knots and minimal wound tension will minimise this factor.

Irradiation

With the modern trend of preoperative irradiation in certain disorders (e.g. rectal cancer and prophylaxis for heterotropic ossification), tissue healing may be impaired due to the fibrosis and microangiopathy associated with this treatment. Post-operative radiotherapy may also increase the incidence of wound complications.

Conclusion

As can be seen from the descriptions above, all local factors can contribute directly to poor healing. Interestingly, each may also contribute to creating or worsening other factors. Resolution of only one of these, then, may have far-reaching implications in reducing or preventing the effects of a wide range of other adverse factors, thereby preventing an adverse wound outcome.

General factors

The following general factors may all play a part in retarding the healing of any wound because of their effect on local factors as well as their endogenous effects on collagen synthesis and immune function. Individually, they may only present a minor problem but many patients present with a number of these factors and do, predictably, quite poorly.

The factors include:

- age and medical conditions, e.g. diabetes, renal failure, hepatic failure, respiratory failure, immunodeficiencies and obesity
- anaemia or blood loss
- shock, hypovolaemia, hypoxia

- weight loss, malnutrition (including vitamin C and A, zinc, protein deficiencies)
- major infections, septicaemia
- advanced malignancy
- steroid use.

Many of these factors are partially remediable in the perioperative period and particular attention should be paid to identifying and reversing as many of them as possible. In the more severely unwell individual this may require assistance from of medical, anaesthetic and intensive care specialists.

Technical factors

Wound evaluation and surgical techniques are skills dependent on the individual practitioner. Adequacy of initial instruction and appropriate amounts of supervised experience are the only ways to develop the skills to deal appropriately with wounds. In general they reflect the clinical ability and judgement of an individual at a given time and therefore may differ for the same person over time.

Conclusions

As many of these factors as possible should be identified and addressed, in order to maximise the rate of healing achieved in adverse conditions. This will usually, but not always, lead to a successful patient outcome. Failure to identify reversible factors by inadequate assessment and understanding of the injury often results in adverse outcomes.

THE SURGICAL MANAGEMENT OF WOUNDS

Before undertaking the responsibility of wound assessment and management, an understanding of wounds, wound healing and factors affecting wound healing is mandatory. Assuming this knowledge, this section aims to provide a basic format for the evaluation of a small, peripheral, traumatic wound and the principles involved in its management. With experience, you will be able to modify these to suit your own practice and individual situations as required (Fig 10.15).

Evaluation of more severe wounds, burns of any type and critically injured patients will not be dealt with here. This type of global assessment is the province of formal trauma education systems such as the Royal Australasian College of Surgeons Early Management of Severe Trauma (EMST) course.

Wound evaluation

The evaluation of minor traumatic wounds is based on three main tasks:

1. ascertain the mechanism of injury
2. examine the wound site
3. decide on the method of repair.

The first is to ascertain the mechanism of injury by taking an accurate history. In knowing this mechanism, especially the causative implement and angle and depth of penetration, potential sites of concomitant or occult injury can be predicted. Symptoms of deep structure damage such as anaesthesia with nerve damage, inability to move digits with tendon damage and pain on movement symptomatic of deep compartment penetration must be specifically enquired after. At the same time, factors that may affect the choice of repair or the healing process should be sought.

Secondly, an assiduous examination of the wound site and deep tissues, if possible, will allow classification of the wound type and give further clues to the amount of damage suffered by underlying structures. This process must include testing for distal motor and sensory function and vascular competence prior to anaesthetic administration. Examination of involved and adjacent bones and joints, seeking restrictions or excesses of movement in both passive and active ranges, may suggest joint, bone, ligament or tendon damage. Obvious deformity will suggest fracture. If foreign body, bone or joint damage are suspected, an X-ray is required

Thirdly, a decision regarding the method of repair must be made. This must take into account wound severity and the structures involved, wound size and skin loss and factors that may affect healing. If the wound is a minor type 1 to 3 injury with no deep involvement and minimal adverse factors, repair may be undertaken in the emergency department by an appropriately experienced practitioner.

Large amounts of skin loss, actual or potential involvement of any major structures, uncertainty regarding depth or extent of damage, type 3 or 4 wounds, inexperience, inadequate facilities, the presence of any adverse factors or the potential need for complicated rehabilitation all mandate further assessment by an experienced practitioner or in-patient surgical team (see Table 10.5). Acceptable conditions for formal exploration and repair are usually found only in the operating theatre. Optimum lighting, good equipment, experienced assistance and absolute anaesthesia (whether regional or general) provide the surgeon with an environment where all injuries can be dealt with appropriately and so contribute to a potentially improved outcome for the patient.

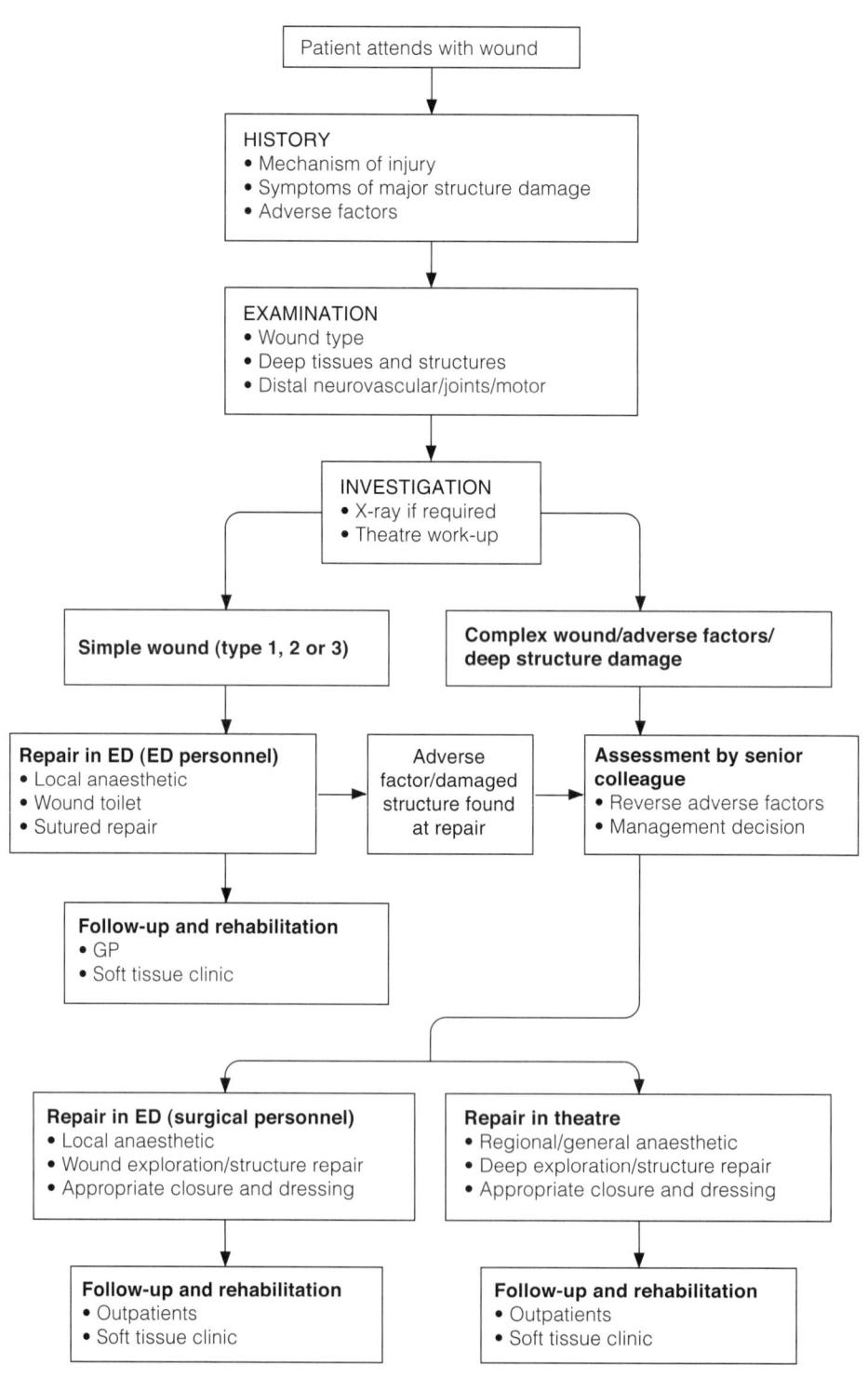

Fig. 10.15 Management of a minor wound

Table 10.5	Criteria for seeking expert assessment of wounds
1.	Inexperience
2.	Large skin loss
3.	Demonstrated deep structure injury
4.	Suspected or potential deep structure injury
5.	Large or complicated wound
6.	Type 3 or 4 wounds
7.	Inadequate facilities for repair
8.	Adverse factors — local
	— general
	— technical
9.	Rehabilitation required

Principles of treatment and repair

In repairing an acute traumatic wound there are many basic principles that should be considered. These begin in the decision-making phase and may continue until complete healing of the wound.

Before repair

Closure

Confirm that the decision to close the wound is the correct one. If there is any doubt regarding skin loss, injuries to other structures, contamination or any other adverse factors, seek the advice of a senior colleague before proceeding. Debridement, stabilisation and non-closure of the wound are acceptable and often represent optimal management.

Explanation and consent

One of the most effective methods of medico-legal protection is good communication. In obtaining consent for the procedure, four main areas should be discussed:

1. the procedure to be carried out and any other treatment required
2. the alternatives to your treatment plan
3. the benefits of your treatment plan
4. the risks of both your treatment plan and the alternative plans.

Further discussion should also describe the planned outcome, ongoing treatment needs, follow-up and plans for rehabilitation. Explanation of potential problems in the post-operative period, how to recognise them and when to re-present for reassessment are also important for each patient.

Antibiotic prophylaxis

Antibiotics are thought to make a difference in visibly contaminated and infected wounds and must be given as soon as possible after injury. Penicillin derivatives such as flucloxacillin or dicloxacillin provide staphylococcus cover and penicillin V provides cover for streptococcus and some clostridial species. Erythromycin and cephalexin are oral alternatives for staphylococcus and streptococcus. Enteric flora require broad spectrum cover such as penicillin or cephalosporin plus gentamicin, and metronidazole.

Tetanus is an infection by the anaerobic, spore-forming, gram-positive bacillus *Clostridium tetani.* It enters the wound as spores and incubates in the warm anaerobic environment of devitalised tissue in a wound. Tetanus-prone wounds are those that have deep contamination from any external source. Inevitably the greater the contamination and the more devitalised the tissues, the greater the risk.

Immunisation against tetanus is now widespread and it is rarely a problem. If the patient has not had a booster in more than five years, one should be given. If not immunised for more than ten years, a full re-immunisation should be undertaken. In these patients, or patients with an uncertain status, passive immunisation with anti-tetanus immunoglobulin may be required until active immunity is re-acquired.

Tetanus, and other clostridial or synergistic infections, such as gas gangrene and necrotising fasciitis, are life-threatening. Diabetes, immunosuppression, peripheral vascular disease and carcinoma may all predispose to these. Adequate debridement, provision of immune prophylaxis, antibiotics and open treatment of wounds by dressing and repeat debridement are some of the measures required to prevent necrotising infections.

The repair

There is a set of minimum requirements for safe repair of soft tissue wounds in the emergency department. Adequate light, instruments, anaesthesia, resuscitation facilities and a sterile field are all required. The following considerations bear special mention here but are also dealt with more fully in other chapters. A summary of the factors required for good management is found in Table 10.6.

Anaesthesia

If a wound is small or superficial, adjacent infiltration of local anaesthesia or a peripheral nerve block are usually adequate. Xylocaine is a rapid acting anaesthetic for short-term local anaesthesia. Further information regarding local anaesthesia is found in Chapter 11.

Table 10.6 | Factors in wound management

•	Antimicrobials
	— antibiotics
	— tetanus prophylaxis
•	Anaesthesia
•	Haemostasis
•	Debridement and irrigation
•	Wound closure
	— method
	— materials
•	Immobilisation

Wound preparation and the sterile field

Local anaesthesia is best administered early so that gross decontamination with soap and water, antiseptics and a scrubbing brush can be performed before prepping. Skin around the wound site should be widely shaved and prepared to allow wound extension and skin graft harvest if required. As with any surgical procedure a sterile field is mandatory. This is achieved by preparing the wound with antiseptic solutions of povidone iodine or chlorhexidine. Alcohol-based prep solutions should be avoided due to their irritant potential and fire risk. Sterile towels are draped over the unprepared regions and operating table to prevent contamination. Further information is provided in Chapter 4.

Debridement

Any contaminated wound requires the debridement of dead, contaminated and devitalised tissues, foreign bodies and contaminating bacteria to prevent infection and necrosis. Excision of the wound margins to various levels must include bone, fascia, muscle, fat, foreign material and skin. Copious irrigation will also help reduce the volume of bacterial inoculum and further prevent infective complications. Remove as much skin and tissue as necessary to create a 'clean' wound; 1–2 mm is usually adequate for skin edges and enough contaminated wound tissue to create clean, freely bleeding surfaces but protecting vital structures (nerves, arteries etc). Skin edges should be incised perpendicular to the skin surface to ensure the greatest likelihood of a fine linear scar. Debridement is also discussed in Chapter 9.

Haemostasis

Tissue that bleeds will generally heal whereas ischaemic tissue may provide a seat for infection and prevent healing. Uncontrolled wound bleeding, however, may cause a wound haematoma and predisposes to infection and non-healing. All major vessels in the wound should be ligated or electrocauterised. After debridement back to bleeding tissue, the minimal use of diathermy and ligatures may be necessary to restore haemostasis.

Closure

A decision must be made as to the best method of closure for a wound. In clean wounds, or contaminated wounds that have been converted surgically to clean ones, direct suturing in layers allows first intention healing. If there is any doubt as to the viability of tissue, or the risk of infection, closure should not be performed. In this scenario the wound may either be left open and allowed to granulate, healing by secondary intention, or an ongoing course of wound debridement and secondary closure may be used. This final method is called delayed primary closure. Deep structures such as bone, vessels, nerves or tendons may also require specialised repair or fixation prior to soft tissue or skin closure. Skin grafts and flaps are not considered here.

Choice of suture material

This is discussed in Chapter 6.

Dressings and splints

The rate of epithelialisation of a wound is doubled if a moister occlusive dressing is used instead of allowing the wound to dry.[1] When the wound is very exudative, the dressing must be absorbent to prevent maceration of the surrounding skin. Selection of the appropriate dressing for a wound must take these two sometimes conflicting principles into account. Priority is given to removal of potentially infected exudate. Vacuum assisted dressing systems can be helpful in managing large or exudative wounds. If there has been repair of a deep structure, such as a tendon, nerve, vessel or bone, or if the wound is in a mobile region, the wound site should be immobilised with a splint.

After repair

The discharge routine from the emergency department should include the provision of slings or crutches where appropriate, the prescription of antibiotics and analgesics and arrangements for follow-up and rehabilitation, the one invariable need of all injuries; although variable, it must be planned and executed in all instances. Explanations of best posturing and allowed movements, normal course of healing, variants to be expected during this time, problems to return for and who to consult also need to be discussed. Appropriate work certificates should also be provided at this time.

CONCLUSIONS

For any practitioner who plans to manage traumatic wounds, an understanding of wound type, mechanism and healing are vital. Strict adherence to the basic principles of wound evaluation, debridement and repair will inevitably lead to a high rate of both cosmetic and functional wound healing. Unfortunately a failure to perform an adequate assessment of both the patient and the wound, or a neglect of the principles of repair, may condemn the patient to a protracted and unsatisfactory course of management.

REFERENCE

1. Winter GD. Formation of the scab and the rate of epithelization of superficial wounds in the skin of the young domestic pig. Nature 1962; 193:293–4.

FURTHER READING

Friedin J, Marshall V. Illustrated Guide to Surgical Practice. Melbourne: Churchill-Livingstone, 1984. Chapter 1: Wounds – healing and management.

McGregor A, McGregor I. Fundamental Techniques of Plastic Surgery. 10th ed. Edinburgh: Churchill-Livingstone, 2000. Chapter 1: Wound management.

New Zealand Guidelines Group. Managment of Burns and Scalds in Primary Care. Wellington: Accident Compensation Corporation, 2007. Availble at: http://www.nzgg.org.nz/guidelines/0139/Burns_full.pdf

Sabiston DC Jr. ed. Sabiston's Textbook of Surgery. 18th ed. Philadelphia: WB Saunders, 2008. Chapter 8: Wound healing; Chapter 22: Burns.

Thompson RVS. Primary Repair of Soft Tissue Injuries. Melbourne: Melbourne University Press, 1969. Chapters 1 to 10.

CHAPTER ELEVEN

A GUIDE TO LOCAL ANAESTHESIA

My heart aches, and a drowsy numbness pains
My sense, as though of hemlock I had drunk,
Or emptied some dull opiate to the drains
One minute past, and Lethe-wards had sunk:

John Keats (1795–1821), *Ode to a Nightingale*

INTRODUCTION

Neurones transmit electrical impulses. Motor nerves take impulses generated in the brain and conduct them to a muscle to initiate a contraction. Sensory nerves conduct in the reverse direction, from a receptor in the periphery to the brain, allowing perception of a stimulus. The objective of local anaesthesia is to prevent perception of all sensory stimulation in the periphery, both noxious and non-noxious, by blocking impulse conduction along sensory nerves.

BASIC PHYSIOLOGY

Nerve cell conduction relies on a process of local depolarisation and repolarisation across the cell membrane, which progresses from the point of stimulus origin along the nerve cell axon to the next synapse. Cellular depolarisation is caused by a rapid movement of sodium ions into the cell from outside. Repolarisation of the cell occurs as potassium ions exit the cell. Finally, equilibrium is restored by special 'membrane pumps' which return the translocated ions back to their original position inside or outside the cell (see Figure 11.1).

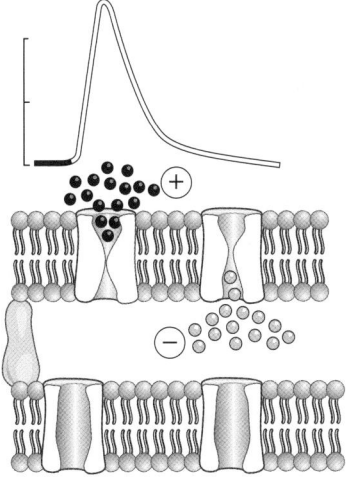

(a) Resting potential—positive outside the cell and negative inside.

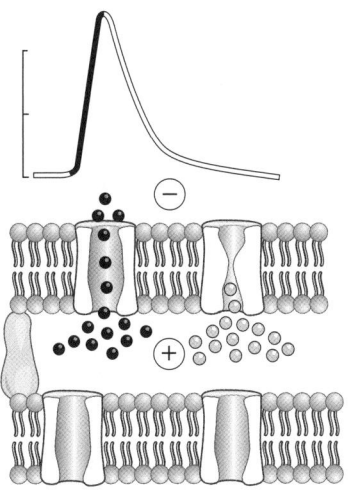

(b) Threshold potential is reached, sodium channels open and positively charged (Na+) ions flow into the cell depolarising the membrane.

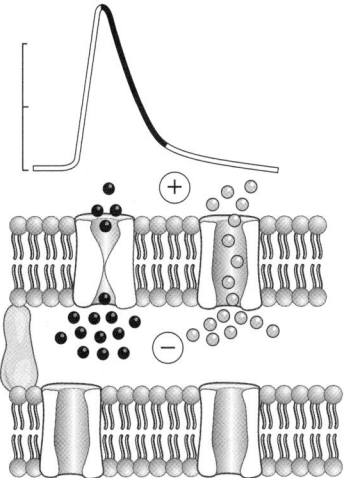

(c) Potassium channels open and positively charged ions (K+) flow out of the cell to repolarise the membrane back to resting potential level.

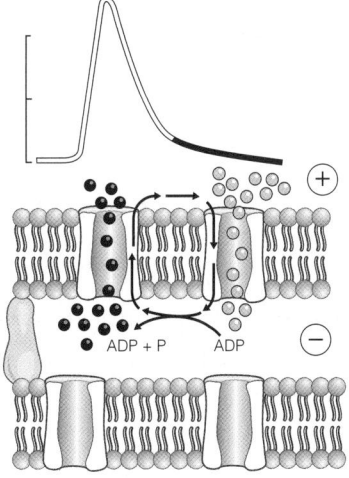

(d) An active transport mechanism transports sodium out of the cell and potassium back in. This restores the correct balance of ions inside and outside the cell while maintaining resting potential.

Fig 11.1 Nerve depolarisation

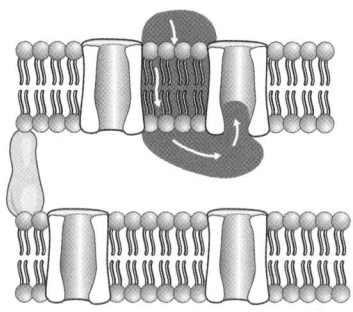

(e) Local anaesthetic enters the nerve cell via the cell membrane and blocks the ion channels from within the cell. This prevents conduction of impulses along the nerve. Anaesthesia occurs in the region supplied by the sensory axons of the blocked nerve.

Fig 11.1 Nerve depolarisation *(cont.)*

Local anaesthetics are a heterogeneous group of substances that prevent electrical conduction along neurones. As they are poorly water soluble and are bases, the active anaesthetic is in the form of a hydrochloric salt. They act by transiently 'blocking' sodium transport channels in the cell membrane. This prevents initial depolarisation of the cell, and is referred to as 'membrane stabilisation'. The result is an inability of the neurone to reach the 'threshold potential' at which it depolarises to create an action potential. As a consequence, the conduction of electrical impulses is interrupted and the neurone's function is temporarily impaired or halted. Sensory neurones are more sensitive to this process than are motor neurones. The overall aim of local anaesthesia is to block local or regional sensory neurones with minimal effect on motor function. In acidic environments, such as due to inflammation, sepsis or ischaemia, effectiveness is often reduced. A classic example of this is minor surgery for acute skin sepsis.

There is a wide spectrum of procedures, from simple excision (skin lesions) to major surgery such as craniotomy that can be performed under local anaesthesia. Local anaesthetic can be administered in a variety of ways, ranging from topical application, through direct infiltration of tissues, to injection around peripheral nerves, spinal nerve roots or the spinal cord (see Table 11.1). In general most practitioners will only ever use local anaesthetics for the repair of minor wounds or local excisions. Pre-emptive local infiltration prior to incision augments general anaesthesia, and can reduce analgesic requirements intra- and postoperatively. The more advanced uses of local anaesthetic generally remain within the province of the specialist anaesthetist.

LOCAL ANAESTHETICS AND DOSAGES

Two distinct families of local anaesthetic exist, esters (of various substances) and amides. The latter are more commonly used in day-to-day practice. Esters, such as tetracaine, are mostly used for spinal anaesthesia or topical application. The main difference between the two lies in their metabolic degradation. Esters are hydrolysed in plasma by pseudocholinesterases and amides are metabolised by the liver. Both types act to block sodium channels in the cell membranes of neurones.

The most frequently used local anaesthetics in non-specialist anaesthetic practice are lignocaine, bupivicaine, ropivicaine and prilocaine. Each has specific properties that make it most appropriate in certain circumstances and all are available in a variety of concentrations. EMLA (Eutectic Mixture of Local Anaesthetics) is a mixture of lignocaine and prilocaine used for topical skin application. Local anaesthetic agents may be combined with adrenaline or ornipressin to cause vasoconstriction and delay absorption.

The safe dose of any local anaesthetic can be affected by many factors and so may vary considerably between individuals. It is usually calculated in terms of a 'milligram per kilogram body weight' dose. An exact volume for administration can then be calculated by knowing the concentration of the anaesthetic solution. The main factor in deciding dosage regimes is the known toxicity profile of an individual drug. This usually has a fixed maximum value that should only be exceeded by experienced personnel.

The required rapidity of onset and duration of action are factors that may affect the choice of drug. These parameters are also dependent on site of administration, pH of the tissues and the co-administration of vasoconstrictors. The faster amide anaesthetics, prilocaine and lignocaine, start working within minutes whereas esters, such as procaine and tetracaine, may take up to 18 minutes to commence their action. Similarly, duration varies greatly.

LOCAL ANAESTHETIC TOXICITY

Toxicity

As with all drugs local anaesthetics have the potential to harm the patient through both known adverse actions and unexpected reactions. The non-allergic effects are usually dose related. Toxicity is directly related to the blood concentration of the anaesthetic. Overdose is the most common cause of toxicity; inadvertent intravenous administration or unexpectedly rapid absorption are the other major causes. A partial accidental intravenous dose causes transient toxicity, but an absolute overdose will

Table 11.1 Local anaesthetic uses

Method	Mechanism	Site of action and extent	Advantages	Disadvantages	Examples
Topical administration	A lipid-soluble cream, containing local anaesthetic, is applied to the skin. It is absorbed and blocks dermal neurones	Local tissues Up to several millimetres deep	Simple and effective	Shallow penetration	Local anaesthetic cream applied to the skin prior to an injection in children
Local infiltration	Local anaesthetic is flooded into the tissues and blocks all small nerves in the region	Minor sensory nerve branches and receptors Area of infiltration and subsequent diffusion	Simple and effective Adrenaline adds haemostasis and prolongs effect Hydro-dissection	End-artery risk with adrenaline Obscured view Rapid offset with no adrenaline	Local injected around a skin cancer before excision
Nerve or plexus block	Local anaesthetic injection around a major nerve or nerve plexus diffuses around and into the nerve to block all fibres	Neurones of large nerves The entire distribution of all nerves infiltrated Does have motor effect as well	Very effective with long action and no other anaesthesia needed	May fail and require GA Toxicity with accidental IV injection	Median and ulnar nerve blocks to anaesthetise the hand Brachial plexus block in the axilla to anaesthetise the arm
Intravenous block	Intravenous injection of local anaesthetic in an exsanguinated limb under arterial tourniquet. Back flow through the veins into capillaries and ECF leads to tissue level anaesthesia	All nerve tissue within the limb The entire limb below the tourniquet Motor and sensory effect	Rapid and effective Simple technique	Potential toxicity Exsanguination and ischaemia Special equipment required Occupies two doctors	Bier's block in the reduction of a Colles fracture

Centrineural block	Injection of local anaesthetic into the spinal column to anaesthetise at a central level **Epidural**—outside the dura, bathes nerve roots in their dural sheath **Spinal**—into the subarachnoid space to bathe the spinal cord and nerve rami inside their sheaths	**Epidural** – on the spinal nerve roots **Spinal**—directly on the spinal cord and nerve rami Multiple dermatome levels as the local anaesthetic diffuses along planes	Rapid and very effective Simple to administer Postoperative analgesia too	Failure rate and patient discomfort Injury to spinal cord CSF leak or haematoma Bacterial inoculation or abscess Sympathetic blockade Respiratory effect with high spinal	Spinal anaesthetic for the internal fixation of proximal femoral fractures. Placement of an epidural catheter for a major abdominal procedure.
Cavity administration	A catheter is placed into a wound or cavity (e.g. pleura) for intermittent or continuous administration of local anaesthetic as an analgesic	As far as the anaesthetic diffuses or spreads in the cavity	Simple and can be effective	Failure rate and patient discomfort Bacterial inoculation	Placement of a catheter into shoulder joint following surgery.

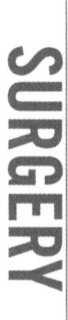

Table 11.2 Common anaesthetics and their properties

Drug	Dose (plain)	Dose (with adrenalin)	Onset (min)	Duration (h)	Comments
Lignocaine	2–4 mg/kg	7–9 mg/kg	5–10	1–2 (plain) 2–3 (adrenaline)	Commonly used as rapid onset with sufficient duration for short procedures
Bupivicaine	2.5 mg/kg	2.5 mg/kg	10–15	3–4 (plain) 3–5 (adrenaline)	Slower onset with less motor blockade More cardiotoxic than lignocaine and can precipitate arrhythmias
Prilocaine	5 mg/kg (400 mg max/day)	5 mg/kg (400 mg max/day)	5–10	1–2 (plain) 2–3 (adrenaline)	Rapid onset but much reduced toxicity Can be used IV (Bier's block) Methaemoglobinaemia at high doses
Ropivicaine	200 mg total	N/A	1–15	2–6	No better or longer with adrenaline Less cardiotoxic than bupivicaine

Note: The doses in this table are approximate only and should not be used in place of the appropriate product information. Review the product information for each drug before prescribing.

Source: Compilation assisted by Astra Pharmaceuticals product information literature.

produce chronic uptake from the tissues, and hence sustained toxicity. A surgeon administering local anaesthetic must be alert for the signs of toxicity. There is often warning of impending toxicity as the effects are usually evident in the central nervous system first.

The first signs of toxicity are dizziness and nausea, with perioral tingling, followed by confusion, loss of consciousness, grand mal seizures and cardiovascular collapse. With bupivicaine, cardiovascular collapse is likely to occur at the same time as central nervous system toxicity.

True allergic responses may occur but these are most commonly found in the ester group of anaesthetics. Any allergy may also relate to preservatives or other chemicals within the vial. If there is any doubt a properly supervised skin test should be performed (see Table 11.3).

Table 11.3 Reactions to local anaesthetic agents

Classification	Signs and symptoms
Neurological—early	Mouth and tongue numbness, tinnitus, anxiety, tremor and twitching, dizziness, confusion, drowsiness
Neurological—late	Fitting, coma, respiratory arrest, death
CVS	Hypotension, myocardial depression, cardiac arrest
	Cardiac arrhythmias with bupivicaine
Respiratory	Tachypnea or respiratory depression
Allergic	Nausea and vomiting, urticaria and anaphylaxis

Source: Compilation assisted by information from: *Sabiston's Textbook of Surgery.* 15th ed. Philadelphia: WB Saunders Co., 1977, and *Introduction to Regional Anaesthesia*, 2nd ed. Fribourg: Mediglobe SA, 1995.

Contraindications and precautions

There are some particular contraindications to specific local anaesthetic administration. These include known hypersensitivity to the anaesthetic, use of bupivicaine for regional intravenous anaesthesia and the use of prilocaine in anaemia or methaemoglobinaemia. The use of adrenaline-containing solutions in end-artery sites such as the fingers, toes and penis is also not recommended as the vasospasm may lead to ischaemic necrosis of the part.

Other situations in which local anaesthesia must be administered with extreme caution include patients with shock, hypotension or hypoxia as these potentiate the toxic effects. Patients with pre-existing heart block or dysrhythmias are also more at risk from the cardiovascular side effects. Caution should be exercised in the presence of liver disease, epilepsy or respiratory impairment.

Tips to prevent toxicity include never exceeding the recommended dose, choosing the agent with the lowest toxicity, careful and accurate administration in small aliquots and aspirating to ensure that the needle has not accidentally been inserted into a vessel. When high doses of local anaesthetic may be used, patients should be fasted and have intravenous access. Full resuscitation facilities should be available. Finally, any patient undergoing an intravenous (Bier's) ischaemic limb block should have two doctors in attendance; one to perform the procedure and one to administer and control the anaesthetic.

Management of toxicity

The earliest signs of toxicity are usually central nervous in origin but any situation, up to a cardiac arrest, may be the first indicator of a problem (see Table 11.3). Prevention is better than treatment but the administering doctor should be able to perform emergency life support and access assistance rapidly if required. Experienced assistance, brought most promptly by calling a cardiac arrest code, should be sought if there is any evidence of potentially significant toxicity. Full CPR and the management of an arrest will not be dealt with here.

When toxicity is suspected, the first step is to ensure an adequate airway and administer oxygen by mask. Intubation and ventilation are rarely required. If a convulsion occurs and persists for more than 20 seconds it should be controlled with an appropriate agent such as diazepam 5–10 mg by slow intravenous injection. Hypotension may require administration of a vasopressor. Intravenous administration of 100 ml of 20% lipid emulsion can rapidly reduce the blood concentration of local anaesthetic and may curtail toxic reactions.

ADMINISTRATION METHODS

There are many techniques by which local anaesthetics can be used to achieve anaesthesia (see Table 11.1). The major method used by non-specialist practitioners will be local infiltration but the others are discussed for completeness. The descriptions are not extensive and information regarding further reading material can be found at the end of the chapter.

Topical anaesthesia

Gel or cream forms of local anaesthetics are used very effectively on both mucous membranes and the skin. Lignocaine spray may also be used on the pharynx or respiratory tree for endoscopic purposes; lignocaine gel may be squirted into the urethra for painless catheterisation or instrumentation. EMLA creams are used for an hour under an occlusive dressing to numb cutaneous sensation. This has particular application for minor split skin grafting and for injections or intravenous cannulation in children.

The major advantages of this method are its simplicity and effectiveness. Unfortunately the penetration of anaesthesia is superficial and slow so it is only applicable for cutaneous work.

Local infiltration anaesthesia

The main use of local infiltration is minor surgery, where the advantages of this method include ease and effectiveness. The slower absorption and dissipation of anaesthetic solutions containing adrenaline prolongs anaesthesia, postoperative analgesia and hence patient comfort. Haemostasis is augmented by the adrenaline. Unfortunately the presence of adrenaline puts end-artery locations at risk of ischaemia, while its absence means more rapid offset of analgesia.

In some situations, hydro-dissection by the injected fluid volume can simplify dissection, but sometimes the operative site, or lesion, may be obscured due to large volumes of injected fluid.

Local infiltration is ineffective in infected tissues because amide-based drugs are unable to penetrate nerve fibres.

Nerve blockade

In this method of anaesthesia the local anaesthetic is injected, after anatomical localisation, directly onto a nerve or nerve plexus. This blocks the transmission of both sensory and motor impulses along the nerve. Blocks such as this are commonly used in limb, hand and foot anaesthesia. Digital and major nerve blocks, such as median, ulnar or posterior tibial are particularly effective in distal limb surgery. Instructions for each are found in the local anaesthetic texts available in most emergency departments or from companies that produce the agents. Brachial or other plexus blocks may be very effective but should only be performed by specialist anaesthetists trained in these techniques.

Regional blocks are exceptionally effective and patients often require no other anaesthetic during their procedure. The long acting agents used also provide excellent postoperative analgesia. Failure, however, effectively commits the patient to a general anaesthetic and all its risks. There is also a risk of damage to nerves and adjacent structures during insertion of the needle. Toxicity may occur due to inadvertent intravenous anaesthetic administration, especially in brachial plexus blocks.

Intravenous (Bier's) block

Intravenous anaesthesia is uncommon and only really applicable to limb surgery. After exsanguination and application of two tourniquets the local anaesthetic prilocaine is injected into a distal limb vein. The volume used fills all veins below the tourniquet and flows back into the capillary bed and extra-cellular fluid. This bathes peripheral nerves in local anaesthetic and provides complete motor and sensory blockade. Once completed, the tourniquets are sequentially deflated for slow controlled release of the prilocaine, which rapidly clears from the extracellular fluid of the limb.

This technique is particularly useful for fracture manipulation and distal limb surgery. It is rapid, simple and effective and may be performed in the emergency department. Toxicity is always a potential problem due to intravenous administration of the anaesthetic. Prolonged exsanguination and hence ischaemia may compromise the limb. Two doctors are mandatory for safety reasons and special equipment, including a dedicated arterial tourniquet, is required.

Centrineural anaesthesia

The mechanism of a centrineural block is administration of local anaesthetic into the subarachnoid or subdural space of the spinal column. This fluid bathes both the spinal cord and nerve roots in the subarachnoid space (spinal anaesthesia) or the durally sheathed nerve roots in the extra-dural space (epidural anaesthesia). This provides widespread anaesthesia in the areas supplied by the neural levels affected.

The solutions of local anaesthetic required for these procedures are generally either more or less dense (heavier or lighter) than cerebrospinal fluid (CSF), so spread is controlled by gravity and the curve of the spinal canal. Spinal anaesthetics are a 'single-shot' technique and find use in orthopaedics, urology and abdominal surgery. Epidural anaesthetics usually have a catheter inserted so that a mixture of anaesthetic and analgesic can be continually infused both intra- and postoperatively. The opiate component is used to block spinal pain receptors.

These two techniques are simple to perform, in experienced hands, and provide excellent operative anaesthesia and postoperative analgesia. Inherent in the techniques, however, is the risk of injury to adjacent structures such as nerve roots, the spinal cord and the dura. Dural puncture is planned in spinal anaesthesia but damage from the much larger epidural needle can cause significant CSF leakage and severe headache. Failure of the technique requires general anaesthesia and can be the cause of inadequate postoperative pain relief.

Hypotension from sympathetic nerve blockade is the most common complication of these procedures and requires adequate intravenous fluid administration, and often vasopressor drugs to correct. Similarly, respiratory compromise from a high spinal is also possible but uncommon. Bacterial inoculation with subsequent abscess formation and paraplegia is devastating but rare. Risks are increased in immune-compromised patients, and epidural use for more than 48 hours. Epidural haematoma is another rare cause of this major neurological complication. The risk of this is increased by use of epidural catheters in patients with a bleeding disorder or in those who require postoperative heparin therapy.

Cavity infusion analgesia

While technically a method of postoperative analgesia, this method of local anaesthetic administration should be mentioned. Catheters may be placed in a wound or cavity (e.g. pleural space or joint cavity) to allow bathing of the tissues in local anaesthetic. It is a simple technique but suffers from its lack of reliability. Fluid accumulation may provide a nidus for infection and introduction of bacteria through the catheter is a potential problem.

A GUIDE TO LOCAL INFILTRATION TECHNIQUE

This section will describe some basic principles of administration for infiltration of local anaesthetics. Specific techniques of nerve blockade will not be discussed as these can be found in the appropriate reference texts and are basically an exercise in surface anatomy.

Timing

Injection of the local anaesthetic prior to scrubbing allows adequate time for it to act before the first incision is made; the longer this interval, the more likely that adequate anaesthesia will be achieved. Bupivicaine, one of the slowest-onset anaesthetic agents, always requires this pause.

The skin should be prepared with an alcohol swab or antiseptic solution on a gauze swab first.

Dilution and mixing

If a large area is to be infiltrated, dilute the anaesthetic in normal saline to increase the volume without risking toxicity. Bicarbonate solution is sometimes used as this will also reduce stinging and speed the onset, as both are worsened by solution and tissue acidity. Two agents may be used, combining the short onset of action of one, and prolonged duration of action of the other. An example of this is lignocaine plus bupivicaine, used in carpal tunnel decompression. Users of this combination must be aware that dose-related toxic effects are additive.

Needle

Unless otherwise indicated, a #25 (orange) or #23 (blue) needle should be used for infiltration. These are fine enough to minimise discomfort but long enough to reach an adequate depth. The needle should never be bent or pushed into the hub, as breakage will necessitate operative exploration for the remnant.

Aspiration

Before injecting any substance the needle must be aspirated to ensure that inadvertent intravenous placement has not occurred. This is a potential cause of toxicity.

Infiltration technique

Sufficient width of infiltration must be provided for adequate debridement and skin excision. Both dermis and underlying tissues should be infiltrated; marking both the lesion and the extent of infiltration will facilitate the operation. If there is a clean open wound, injection through the virtually insensate subcutaneous fat will minimise patient discomfort (see Fig 11.2).

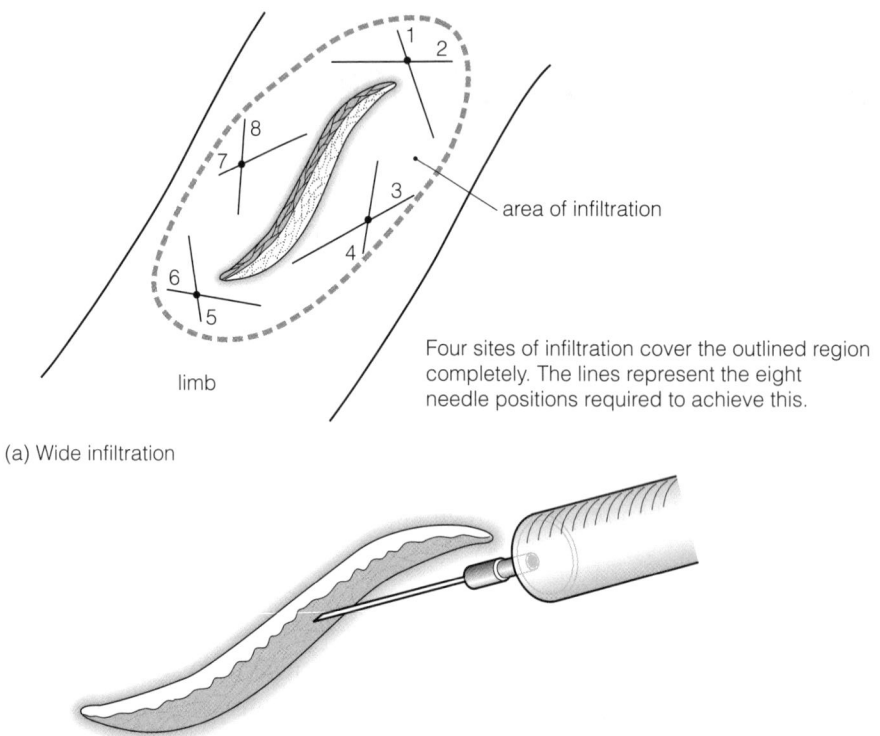

area of infiltration

limb

Four sites of infiltration cover the outlined region completely. The lines represent the eight needle positions required to achieve this.

(a) Wide infiltration

(b) Infiltration directly into subcutaneous fat results in less pain. This can only be done if there is minimal contamination.

Fig 11.2 Techniques of local anaesthetic infiltration

Pressure

Firm pressure on the site of infiltration will both stop bleeding and help diffuse anaesthetic further through the local tissues. This reduces the difficult problem of lesions obscured by local anaesthetic blebs and increases the width of infiltration by diffusion.

FURTHER READING

Various publications available through or from the product representatives are excellent and up-to-date resources.

CHAPTER TWELVE
MANAGEMENT OF JOINTS

The elephant hath joints, but none for courtesy; his legs are legs for necessity, not for flexure.

William Shakespeare (1564–1616),
Troilus and Cressida, act 2, sc. 3, l. 105–6

ASPIRATION OF JOINTS

Joints are aspirated or injected for diagnostic and therapeutic reasons. Aspiration is performed to identify suspected inflammation, infection or blood. Aspiration of blood in trauma followed by injection of local anaesthetic will relieve the pain of an acute haemarthrosis, for example, a radial head fracture in the elbow. The presence of fat globules in the aspirate of a haemarthrosis indicates an intra-articular fracture.

Joint injection
Joints are injected with diagnostic agents such as radiological contrast or local anaesthetic, or with therapeutic agents. Therapeutically the most commonly used injectate is cortisone (usually mixed with local anaesthetic) to treat degenerative or inflammatory conditions. Other agents include chemotherapy drugs (for tumours or chemical synovectomy) and visco-supplementation (hyaluronic acid derivatives) for the treatment of osteoarthritic joints.

KEY POINTS IN THE ASPIRATION OR INJECTION OF JOINTS

1. Use strict aseptic technique to avoid iatrogenic septic arthritis.
2. Do not attempt access to a joint through a contaminated site, an area of skin breakdown, erythema or where frank sepsis is present.
3. Know the surface anatomy of joints, especially in relation to the position of the articular surface, and use this knowledge to plan the safest and most direct route into the joint.
4. Be aware of extra-articular structures that should not be penetrated by a needle inadvertently. The site of joint entry should be away from neurovascular bundles, e.g. nerves and vessels anterior to the hip joint, and should avoid tendons and ligaments, with minimal transgression of muscles.
5. Imaging modalities such as fluoroscopy, ultrasound and CT scan may be required to confirm entry into a joint, for example hip, subtalar or facet joints.

Preparation

All required tools and agents should be prepared and set up in a sterile field, with strict adherence to aseptic technique. Materials required include:

- Skin preparation
- Drapes
- Select syringes of appropriate size. Use a large syringe if large volumes are anticipated, or a small one for a small volume joint or a small volume of therapeutic agent.
- Needles should be long enough to reach the joint, with a large enough bore to easily inject or aspirate the suspected fluid. Viscous fluid requires a large bore.
- A container large enough to hold the expected volume to be aspirated. Volumes can be large in knee and shoulder (especially if associated with a rotator cuff tear).
- Dressings.
- Agent for injection and drawing up cannula. Non-sterile packaging should not be opened onto the sterile field, and an assistant should be available to help with drawing up of the agent using sterile technique.
- Containers and culture swab sticks (with transport medium) to transport specimen to pathology for microbiology, histology and glucose estimation. These items may not be sterile and should be available outside the sterile field.

The patient should be positioned in a comfortable position with the point of entry to the joint easily accessible. Marking the surface anatomy with an indelible marker helps with joint location and entry after skin preparation. The area is prepared and draped with the same care and adherence to aseptic technique as is used for a surgical operation. Local anaesthetic may be infiltrated into the skin prior to insertion of the aspiration needle.

Suspected septic arthritis

If septic arthritis is suspected, aspiration of the joint should be performed in an operating theatre so that immediate operative debridement and washout can be performed if pus is encountered.

What to send to the laboratory?
- Fluid in sterile container
- Culture swabs of fluid in transport medium.

What to request?
- Urgent microscopy and gram stain (ask the laboratory to look for crystals).
- Culture and sensitivities.

When to act?
- Immediately
- Pathology staff on-call should to be 'called in' to perform the microscopy and gram stain and commence culture procedures.

Special consideration is required for a suspected infected total joint arthroplasty/ replacement where isolation of the pathogen is critical to management. Frequently the offending organism is of low virulence and may not be considered pathogenic if isolated elsewhere. Isolation of the infecting bacterium, knowing its virulence and determining its antibiotic sensitivity will help immensely in determining treatment options and will significantly affect the management of an infected joint replacement.

Microbiological recommendations for aspiration of suspected infected arthroplasties:
- No antibiotics for 7 days.
- Clean off skin with alcohol and allow skin to dry (consider doing the procedure in the operating theatre).
- Collect specimen in sterile container.
- Do not use blood culture bottle.
- Also collect 10 ml of saline from joint washout.
- Label specimen as joint fluid.
- Send promptly to laboratory labelled 'URGENT' infected prosthetic joint fluid'.

- Request the following tests:
  — microscopy, culture and sensitivity
  — add lysed blood agar plates
  — incubate aerobic/anaerobic for 10 days
  — antibiotics sensitivity test for *all* isolates.

REDUCTION OF DISLOCATIONS

A *dislocation* is the complete disruption of a joint so that the articular surfaces are no longer in contact. *Subluxation* is a disruption of the joint where there is partial loss of contact between the articular surfaces. Both may be associated with significant soft tissue injury (capsular and ligamentous injury) and require manipulation for relocation.

Management of joint dislocation

The clinical features of a dislocation are

- pain
- loss of normal contour and relationship of bony points.
- loss of motion
- abnormal attitude – the position the limb is held in may be diagnostic.

When faced with a joint dislocation it is important to take a proper history and perform a thorough physical examination of the patient. The history of the injury will help in the identification of associated injuries, as there are well-recognised injury patterns. Physical examination must include the neurovascular state and associated injuries. Look for and recognise associated injuries of nerves (higher incidence than in fractures), arteries (intimal tears are common, particularly in knee dislocations), skin, muscle and bone (fracture). These must be recognised and documented prior to any form of manipulation. This has important therapeutic and medico-legal implications.

Preparation for reduction

An X-ray should be performed prior to any attempt to re-locate the joint. This is to confirm the dislocation and define any associated fractures. It might be acceptable in some circumstances to reduce a frank dislocation if the limb shows clear neurovascular compromise.

Radiographic findings are an indispensable part of the examination. Their omission may lead to catastrophes. They must be interpreted in the context of the physical examination. A good example of this is the frequently missed posterior dislocation of the shoulder, where abnormal X-ray signs are subtle but examination demonstrates the marked limitation of motion.

A pre-reduction identification of a fracture may change the management and will help determine whether a fracture noted on post-reduction X-rays is iatrogenic.

Prior to attempting a joint reduction using sedation, appropriate monitoring and intra-venous access should be established. Appropriate resuscitation equipment needs to be available, in case of overdose of a sedative or analgesic or after the relocation of the dislocated joint, when there is a dramatic reduction of the painful stimuli and a patient may cease breathing under the influence of the pharmaceutical agents used.

Reduction

To relocate the joint, it is important to achieve good patient and muscle relaxation. This can be achieved by:

- Calming the patient with a non-threatening explanation of the planned reduction procedure and reassurance by the person relocating the joint in a quiet controlled manner.
- Performing the reduction in a quieter area and removing extraneous stimuli (not in the bright and busy centre of an accident and emergency department).
- Reducing the amount of muscle force the patient can generate by stopping the patient from gripping either the side of bed or the hand of another person.
- Pharmaceutical means:
  — muscle relaxants such as:
    o benzodiazepines, which also have a sedative action (e.g. diazepam or midazolam). The shorter acting agents are better as they make it less likely that the patient will stop breathing, as described above.
    o suxamethonium. This is normally used in the context of a general anaesthetic.
  — analgesia, usually an intravenous narcotic.

These should be delivered intravenously so they have a reliable and rapid onset of action. Oral and intramuscular routes of drug administration are slow and have variable onset of action.

Various techniques have been described in the reduction of dislocations. Most involve the use of traction and reversal of the mechanism of injury.

In the shoulder the most common mechanism of dislocation is abduction and external rotation. Hence the manoeuvre used to reduce the shoulder involves gentle traction, abduction and external rotation.

Causes for failure of reduction

There are many causes for failure of reduction:

- Incorrect diagnosis. Failure to recognise the injury is a fracture not a dislocation.

- Incorrect technique. The direction of dislocation has not been appreciated, as in anterior versus posterior dislocation of the hip. Each type of dislocation requires a different technique for its reduction.
- Inability to overcome muscle spasm or pain. Rather than use more force, it is better to achieve appropriate muscle relaxation by giving the patient an anaesthetic—regional or general—and a muscle relaxant. Remember the use of suxamethonium (short acting non-depolarising agent) requires patient ventilatory assistance.
- Tissue interposition, either bone as in a fracture dislocation or soft tissue, which may include joint capsule, infolded ligaments, tendons, muscle, nerves, arteries. Open reduction may be required to remove the offending tissue.
- Joint space filled by fluid, blood in an acute injury or synovial and exudate in chronic dislocations. Evacuation of the joint cavity, by aspiration, may be required before the joint can be relocated.

Post-reduction

After reduction, an X-ray should be performed. This is to confirm a concentric reduction. A further examination should be performed to look for associated injury such as fractures (their presence and position) and any neurovascular injury that may have been caused by the intervention. This is good medico-legal practice.

The joint should then be splinted to reduce pain and prevent re-dislocation.

In most cases the joint does not need to be held rigidly but should be prevented from being able to achieve the position in which the dislocation occurred. In the case of anterior dislocation of the shoulder that was caused by abduction and external rotation, a sling will hold the arm in internal rotation and adduction. For most interphalangeal joint dislocations the direction of dislocation is dorsal so excessive extension must be prevented. An extension-block splint or buddy strapping to the normal finger alongside will prevent re-dislocation. This allows for early mobilisation, rehabilitation and more rapid return of function.

A detailed knowledge of sequelae of dislocation and possible late complications is required for the successful management of the dislocation and return of optimal function.

Recognised late complications need to be addressed, including:
- Heterotropic ossification (the incidence is increased with certain associated injuries such as a head injury and certain joints such as the elbow and hip).
- Avascular necrosis (most common in hip dislocations). The incidence increases dramatically the longer the joint remains dislocated.
- Stiffness, which may be due to intra-capsular adhesions, capsular fibrosis or extra-capsular pathology (e.g. heterotropic ossification). These mechanisms can cause permanent loss of range of movement and fixed contractures.

Treatment of specific joint dislocations is beyond the scope of this book. Their treatment may be complex and involve operative open reduction and ligament reconstruction. Many excellent publications detailing their management exist.

FURTHER READING

McRae R. Orthopaedics and Fractures. Injury 1999; 31:4:278.

Saunders S, Longworth, S. Injection techniques in Orthopaedics and Sports Medicine: A Practical Manual for Doctors and Physiotherapists. 3rd ed. Churchill-Livingstone, 2006.

Solomon L, Warwick D, Nayagam S. Apley's System of Orthopaedics and Fractures. 8th ed. London: Hodder Arnold, 2001.

Wheeless Textbook of Orthopaedics; Data Trace Internet Publishing, 2008. Available from: http://www.wheelessonline.com.

CHAPTER THIRTEEN
FRACTURE FIXATION

*There never was a bone-setter got so much custom—man an'child, young an'old—
there never was such breakin' and mendin' of bones known in the memory of man.*

Joseph Sheridan Le Fanu (1814–1873 BC)
The Ghost and the Bone-setter (1838)

INTRODUCTION

Fractures are a frequent cause of visits to hospital emergency departments. You need to know how to immobilise the fracture to give it the best opportunity to heal while allowing the limb to retain its proper conformation and articulation.

SPLINTING AND IMMOBILISATION

Multiple techniques are available to hold, splint, immobilise, rest and protect musculo-skeletal tissue.

In this chapter we will only consider the most common and widely available product, plaster of Paris. It has been used for almost 200 years and remains an excellent material. It is very safe if used correctly but can do considerable harm if the correct application and technique are not followed.

Although seen as predominantly used in orthopaedics, plaster is used in many other surgical specialities, e.g. plastic, ENT, maxillofacial, neuro- and vascular surgery.

Standard 'plaster' consists of a bandage impregnated with anhydrous calcium sulphate, which, when hydrated (dipped in water), undergoes an exothermic reaction that produces a crystal structure with excellent mechanical properties.

The method of application is important for the plaster to achieve its desired function. It must be constructed to obtain a functional length and strength.

The plaster must be long enough the support or hold the 'body part' but not to immobilise more joints or tissue than is necessary. The general rule for fracture management is to immobilise the joint above the fracture, and the joint below the fracture (there are exceptions to this rule, but it constitutes a safe practice).

The plaster should be strong enough to support the body part and not disintegrate. The strength may be achieved and increased by several techniques.

1. *A complete or encircling cast:* This is much stronger than a plaster slab. It requires considerable skill to be applied well and should only be applied by trained personnel. A complete cast accommodates swelling poorly and may become too tight, causing a compartment syndrome. A poorly applied cast can lead to serious complications. For safety, appropriately supportive plaster slabs should be used in the acute injury setting or immediate postoperative phase. If you are experienced a split full cast may be acceptable.

2. *More layers of plaster:* In general 6–8 layers of plaster applied in the correct manner give sufficient strength. More layers provide greater strength, but at the expense of increased weight.

3. *Cold water:* Wetting plaster in cold water provides a finer crystal structure with a slower setting time and greater strength. Wetting plaster bandage in hot water produces faster setting times but the crystals are larger and consequently the plaster is weaker. The use of cold water is recommended to slow setting times and increase your chances of achieving an appropriately moulded plaster. Using hot water can in some circumstances cause a burn to a patient.

4. *Smoothing the plaster:* This makes for a professional appearance but more importantly removes air bubbles from the construct. This increases structural strength.

5. *Structural modifications:* The formation of ridges (guttering) or the use of cross struts or stirrups increase strength and may decrease the amount of plaster required.

6. *No movement while the plaster is setting:* Movement while the plaster is setting breaks the crystal formation and weakens the plaster. Strength will be greatly increased by ensuring no movement until the plaster has set sufficiently to withstand movement.

The plaster is set when:

- it is warm
- it is hard
- tapping produces a solid sound.

The general principles that apply to a plaster slab when applied to a limb in the acute setting are:

1. Avoid using encircling material sleeves especially the elastic type such as tubi-grip. These may cause a compartment syndrome in their own right.
2. Use of wool crepe (soft fluffy padding, e.g. webril, velband, softban) is required for padding, to accommodate swelling and to stop the plaster sticking to the hairs.
3. Dip plaster in water and squeeze out excess water. Squeezing the layers together with your fingers allows bonding between the layers.
4. Application of the plaster slab, smoothing (to reduce the air bubbles and increase the structural strength), addition of structural modifications (ridges, cross struts or stirrups).
5. Hold plaster slab to limb by bandage (beware of bandaging too tightly).
6. Do not move limb until plaster has set.

INSTRUCTIONS FOR PLASTER CARE

Patients should be given written advice on coping with their plaster on discharge.

1. Keep the limb raised as much as possible: arm in sling, foot on pillow on a stool when sitting or on pillows in bed.
2. Exercise fingers or toes frequently.
3. Do not push any object under (even for an itch!).
4. Do not wet your plaster.
5. Do not go near sand (beach or playgrounds).
6. Do not cut your plaster.
7. Contact the hospital for:
   pain that is not relieved after elevating the limb (above the level of your heart)
   marked swelling
   marked blueness or whiteness
   numbness, pins and needles or loss of sensation.
8. Your cast will take 48 hours to dry to full strength.

COMPLICATIONS

Several problems can arise from immobilisation. It is important to follow good practice to minimise the likelihood of these occurring.

Pain under plaster

Pain from a limb to which a plaster has been applied is common.

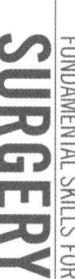

There are many possible causes. There is expected pain due to the underlying condition for which the plaster was applied (fracture, operation or to rest soft tissue). Then there is unexpected pain, such as complication of the original pathology, wound breakdown or infection, or pain due to complications from the plaster itself, such as compartment syndrome, localised pressure or friction areas, or extreme positioning. These conditions must be suspected and treated appropriately to avoid serious complications.

All possible adverse complications need to be considered, excluded or treated before additional analgesia is administered.

A child with an uncomplicated forearm fracture immobilised in a good plaster should not require narcotic analgesia.

Compartment syndrome

Any bandages or plaster that encircle a limb may cause a compartment syndrome. This is where perfusion of the muscle compartment is insufficient for cellular metabolism. If this is not reversed, cell death will ensue; the first tissue affected is muscle. Good distal perfusion or a palpable pulse does not rule out a compartment syndrome.

The hallmark symptom is increasing pain unrelieved by appropriate analgesia. The classic signs on examination are paraesthesia and excessive pain on passive stretching of the muscles of the relevant compartment.

Appropriate management of a suspected compartment syndrome entails:
1. Elevation of the affected limb.
2. Release of encircling bandages or plaster. This must be the entire length of the plaster or bandage and to the skin. *A plaster has not been split properly until you can see skin from end to end.*
3. If symptoms are unrelieved and you suspect compartment syndrome, urgent fasciotomy is indicated.
4. In an ambivalent case it is reasonable to measure compartment pressures using a compartment pressure monitor. If the pressure differential between the compartment pressure and diastolic BP is less than 30 mmHg then fasciotomy is indicated.

Pressure sores

The plaster slab may cause pressure problems, most commonly by thumb and finger imprints on the slab as it is setting or by poor padding over bony prominences. Patients can also cause pressure sores by 'balling up' the under-cast padding when they push objects under their cast to get to an itchy area. The patient will complain of pain, usually described as a burning type sensation. Management is removal of the offending plaster area. This may be achieved either by redoing the plaster completely or by cutting a window in the plaster over the area of pain.

The most common areas involved are the edge of plasters, bends such as the elbow and knee, and bony prominences.

Extreme positioning of the body part

Extreme positioning of a limb may result in functional compression of nerves resulting in pain and paresthesia and may be confused with a compartment syndrome. This is commonly seen in excessive palmar flexion of the wrist during the application of a plaster for distal radial fracture, flexion of the elbow in supracondylar humeral fractures, or compression of metacarpals and fingers with tight bandaging across the palm.

Removal of the plaster and reapplication with the limb in a less extreme position will relieve the pain and paresthesia should resolve soon after.

If the fracture position cannot be maintained without extreme positioning of the limb, alternative methods of holding the reduction of the fracture should be used, e.g. internal fixation.

Wound infection

If a wound problem is suspected, it must be inspected either by removal of the plaster or by cutting a window in the plaster.

Windows are also used to check sutures, skin integrity and pressure areas. Usually they are performed when there is no need to remove the cast. Generally, it is better to cut a slightly larger window than a smaller one. This allows greater access to the wound. Always replace a window; if the window is not replaced in an oedematous limb, the skin can herniate out of the cast, causing extreme pain.

CUTTING PLASTER

Plaster when dry and hard may be cut with a plaster saw. The blade of a plaster saw vibrates at high frequency with a small amplitude, so soft mobile structures such as skin will move with the blade and will not be cut. Hard structures such as plaster will not give and will be cut. If the saw is dragged it will cut both hard and soft structures: skin will be injured and a severe laceration can result.

The saw should be used with a 'dipping' technique; this is not intuitive and practical experience is important. The blade is firmly applied against the plaster until there is a loss of resistance (indicating the inner side of the plaster has been breached), the blade is pulled out, advanced along the plaster and the process repeated.

A wet plaster can be difficult to cut with a plaster saw and shears or heavy scissors will be required to divide the plaster.

The splitting of a cast is performed when the neurovascular status of the limb is compromised. It can be performed prophylactically in cases of severe trauma, where gross swelling is anticipated. When splitting a cast, it is best not to split the cast on the same side as the displacement or angulation. The cast must be split down the entire full length. The under-cast padding including all dressings must also be split. The skin must be visible from end to end.

Do not:
- Use blunt or bent blades
- Force the saw to cut
- Drag the blade
- Have wet hands
- Disregard the patient's comments.

Do:
- Reassure the patient
- Rotate the cast saw blade
- Use a firm surface to lean on
- Avoid concavities
- Avoid bloodstained areas (if possible)
- Have a firm grip on the saw.

FURTHER READING

McRae R. Orthopaedics and Fractures. Injury 1999; 31:4:278.

Solomon L, Warwick D, Nayagam S. Apley's System of Orthopaedics and Fractures. 8th ed. London: Hodder Arnold, 2001.

Wheeless Textbook of Orthopaedics; Data Trace Internet Publishing, 2008. Available from: http://www.wheelessonline.com.

CHAPTER FOURTEEN
LAPAROSCOPIC SURGERY

When you have a new hammer, suddenly everything looks like a nail.

Anon

INTRODUCTION

Soon after its introduction in 1987, laparoscopic surgery was billed as the greatest revolution in surgery since the invention of general anaesthesia. Indeed, it was predicted that over 80% of abdominal surgical procedures would be conducted laparoscopically by the turn of the century. While this became an overstatement, it is true to say that laparoscopic surgery has induced a fundamental change in the attitudes of surgeons towards operative outcomes, postoperative recovery, postoperative pain and cost effectiveness of surgical procedures.

THE CURRENT SCOPE OF LAPAROSCOPIC SURGERY

To a greater or lesser degree, laparoscopic surgery has been responsible for a resurgence in the specialty of surgery and trainees now seek it as keenly as other specialties. It has also been responsible for much harm, but the phase of using outdated operations to allow the procedure to be accomplished laparoscopically should now have passed. Critical assessment of indications, operations and results is now the norm rather than the exception.

Common procedures

Laparoscopic cholecystectomy is the laparoscopic operation most commonly performed by general surgeons. All approaching the end of their advanced general surgical training would expect to be confident with it. However, there is no doubt that the risk of bile duct injury is higher than in open surgery. The precise rate of injury varies widely. If one assumes the average (though high) rate of bile duct injury to be 0.4%, a surgeon doing one laparoscopic cholecystectomy per week may go five years without causing one.

Laparoscopic fundoplication is probably the operation of choice for gastro-oesophageal reflux but it demands greater skill than laparoscopic cholecystectomy. The operation may be accomplished by many routes, but the same tenets remain: meticulous patient selection, anatomical dissection of the hiatus, crural re-approximation and a tension-free and durable wrap are the mainstays of this operation. A wrap performed in the Nissen style previously accounted for around three-quarters of the anti-reflux surgery performed around the world, but more modern partial wraps are becoming more common.

Laparoscopic appendicectomy would seem like a natural extension of laparoscopy for right iliac fossa pain. In some institutions, over 95% of cases of appendicitis are managed this way. Critical evidence in favour of this technique is less apparent, however. Criticisms include increased cost and increased operating time. In favour of it are significantly shorter admission times, lower wound infection rates and earlier return to work. It is an ideal operation for the teaching of laparoscopic skills.

Laparoscopic inguinal hernia repair is one of the more controversial of the common procedures. It is the most susceptible to technical failures, and when difficult can be the least satisfying to complete. On the other hand, many surgeons would agree an open hernia is an enjoyable operation to perform and to teach. To supplant open inguinal hernia, laparoscopic repair will need to endure the scrutiny that the myriad of open techniques have undergone, to test both claim and counterclaim. At present, a multicentre study with surgeons experienced in laparoscopic hernia repair has shown a lower recurrence rate than traditional anterior darned repairs, and patients return to work earlier. The laparoscopic technique requires general anaesthesia and is currently regarded as most suitable for bilateral and recurrent hernias.

Within a specialised unit, advanced laparoscopic procedures can be undertaken. Unlike many equivalent open operations, these cases require investment in equipment, skills and patience. An example might be laparoscopic anterior resection of the rectum or laparoscopic total gastrectomy. This requires skills, time and staff that the equivalent open procedure does not. The optimal setting for advanced laparoscopic techniques is within a unit which is prepared to make the appropriate investment.

Research and experimental procedures

As experience with laparoscopic surgery grows, an increasing number of procedures are moving from experimental to mainstream (Table 14.1).

Table 14.1	Less commonly performed laparoscopic procedures
	Gastrointestinal bypass procedures (e.g. gastrojejunostomy)
	Gastrostomy
	Heller's cardiomyotomy
	Perforated duodenal ulcer repair
	Common bile duct exploration
	Liver cyst fenestration
	Adrenalectomy
	Pelvic lymphadenectomy
	Colectomy—right hemicolectomy, anterior resection, total colectomy
	Rectopexy
	Adhesiolysis
	Laparoscopic procedures not commonly performed but reported in the literature
	Vagotomy (truncal and highly selective)
	Pyloroplasty
	Gastropexy
	Pylorus preserving pancreatico-duodenectomy
	Hepatic resection
	Ligation of bleeding duodenal ulcer
	Cholecystojejunostomy
	Drainage of pancreatic abscesses
	Drainage of pancreatic pseudocyst
	Enterolithotomy for gallstone ileus
	Caecopexy
	Laparoscopically assisted operations
	Devascularisation of oesophageal varices
	Repair of ruptured diaphragm
	Abdominoperineal resection of rectum
	Continent catheterisable cutaneous appendico-vesicostomy
	Meckel's diverticulectomy

The literature contains numerous case reports, retrospective analyses, personal series and unusual cases. Laparoscopic retrieval of an ingested padlock from the stomach of a child was the author's personal favourite. In the culture of evidence-based medicine, such scenarios do not add to the esteem of laparoscopic surgery. Progress needs to be made through meticulous research, not thinly veiled experimental series. This should take place in centres where advances will be made the most of, rather than in places where the next five years are spent undoing the damage caused by improperly monitored procedures.

PRINCIPLES OF LAPAROSCOPIC SURGERY

Basics

In any medical field, familiarity with standard equipment is fundamental and this applies especially in laparoscopic surgery. A trainee is expected to be able to check the equipment as well as troubleshoot common problems. The ten seconds spent fixing the video image is worth more to a pupil than the six months of encouraging camera banter!

Electronics

A good quality video screen is essential. It should be mounted on an articulated arm or on a mobile trolley along with the other essential laparoscopic equipment, and should be positioned at eye level. In most cases, one screen is sufficient. A facility to lock the controls for adjusting the screen brightness, contrast and colour is useful. A recording facility is useful, and real-time digital image capture as DVD or high-definition quality represents an ideal solution.

A three-chip CCD camera is a necessity. The quality of image is vastly superior to one-chip models, especially with respect to colour representation, colour bleed and sensitivity at low light levels. The camera should connect to a camera control unit that allows automatic iris setting, white balance and gain. The use of a sterile camera sleeve obviates the need for repeated camera disinfection and improves turnaround times. Other systems available on the market and in various stages of development include three-dimensional cameras. The technology in 3D imaging is evolving but most laparoscopic surgeons would agree that two-dimensional views are adequate for most procedures.

The light source should be dedicated to laparoscopic use and regular bulb changes are important. A poorly performing light source detracts considerably from the view. Regular checks of the integrity of the light cables are also important: breaches of the outer coat may allow solution ingress, and cables with broken light fibres will not transmit light well. A light lead with an uncovered end will burn theatre drapes if left on them whilst at full power. The use of paper drapes adds to this risk. For safety, always connect the light lead to the source last, or to the eyepiece first.

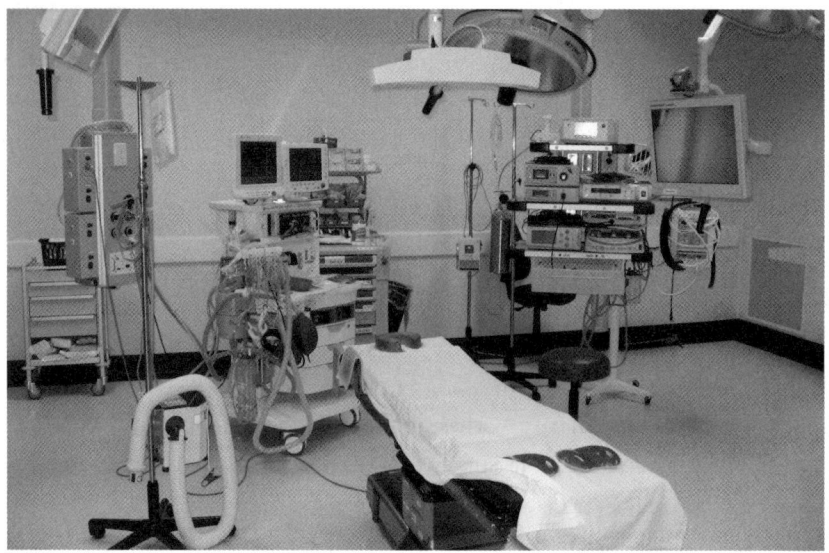

Fig 14.1 High-definition operating theatre

Setting up for laparoscopic surgery

It is important to be mindful of the setting in which any form of surgery is undertaken (e.g. Fig 14.1). A specialised unit with appropriate resources—in both skill and equipment—can undertake an array of procedures that a smaller department cannot. If safe and successful procedures are to be undertaken, the occasional laparoscopic operator needs to carefully consider his or her abilities and the backup available. Remember that the average general surgeon in the United States (doing laparoscopic surgery) performs two laparoscopic cholecystectomies per month. Opportunities to hone one's skill under these circumstances are therefore limited.

BASIC HARDWARE

Optics

Most rigid endoscopes incorporate a Hopkins rod lens, an eyepiece and optical fibres to carry light. A camera head clips onto the eyepiece. Recently, single-piece autoclavable endoscopes have become available, with a high-definition video chip at the tip of the scope, obviating the need for a rod lens.

Scopes vary in diameter, angle and field of view. The larger the diameter, the larger the light carrying elements can be. A 10 mm laparoscope gives a brighter and more detailed picture than its 5 mm partner. In addition, the 5 mm instrument is less robust, less tolerant of fogging and much more susceptible to physical bending. The instrument's angle describes the relationship between the visual axis and the light axis.

The 25° eyepiece, for example, gives an optical field centred 25° off the axis of the scope. This allows a sensation of perspective using shadowing effects, and rotation of the scope with respect to the camera allows looking around corners. However, angled scopes carry less light than 0° degree scopes. For most situations, a 25° to 30° angle is most useful and is recommended for beginners. Some special-purpose endoscopes have an enlarged field of vision, much like a wide angle lens in a camera. The greater benefit of these is their greater depth of field, reducing the need for refocusing.

Diathermy

Diathermy equipment is usually the standard monopolar diathermy available in most theatres; however, sophisticated diathermy machines with safety cut-outs to prevent capacitance coupling or arcing are available but are expensive. Where it is appropriate, bipolar diathermy is safer. See Chapter 7 for a full discussion on diathermy.

Insufflator

The basic hardware required for any laparoscopic procedure includes a machine for delivering high-flow carbon dioxide to establish and maintain pneumoperitoneum. The minimum standard equipment should be a pressure-alarmed, single-channel CO_2 insufflator. The use of volume-limited insufflators is unsafe, as they have no way of alarming when intra-abdominal pressure escalates. Modern devices measure the pressure via the insufflation tubing (single-channel) as opposed to a separate channel (dual-channel). The latter system has been shown to be unsafe as the pressure measuring tubing can inadvertently become occluded or disconnected.

The optimum intra-abdominal pressure is 12 mm Hg, which allows adequate visibility for most situations in adults. There is some evidence that this low pressure of pneumoperitoneum lowers the incidence of venous stasis and deep vein thrombosis. For pelvic laparoscopy, pressures even less than 12 mm Hg are often adequate. A pressure-alarmed insufflator will auto-regulate when the preselected pressure is reached and give an audible signal above this level. A flow rate of 6 litres per minute is a minimum; newer technologies allow rates of up to 40 l/min to be delivered under controlled circumstances. Other options include gas warming and humidification.

ENDOSCOPIC INSTRUMENTS

Basic concepts

Laparoscopic instruments that are commonly used include dissectors, scissors and various grasping devices. Many laparoscopic instruments are available as disposable after a single use, completely reusable or reusable/disposable.

Opinion varies as to the best instruments for dissection: some surgeons prefer to use an electrocautery hook while others prefer straightforward dissectors to minimise the risk of inadvertent injury. Various suction–irrigation devices are also available. Needle holders and automatic suturing devices are available for more advanced procedures, although the automatic devices are disposable and can be expensive.

Many instruments are available in a range of sizes. Early in the evolution of laparoscopic surgery, only a limited range of instruments was available in 5 mm diameter and these were particularly prone to failure. This is no longer the case and for most situations, there is now an adequate 5 mm instrument for all but a few indications. Heavy graspers and stone scoops, by their nature are invariably 10 mm in diameter. Graspers come in a bewildering array of jaw designs, and some incorporate ratchet locks (Fig 14.2). Graspers are typically straight, although angled tips exist.

All instruments should be insulated, and selections that allow the use of monopolar diathermy are an advantage. Few of these instruments are suitable for grasping bowel. This is principally because of the great mechanical advantage afforded by a long instrument, so that tearing of bowel occurs long before there is any tactile appreciation of it. For manipulating bowel, DeBakey or Hunter forceps are preferred. Other essential instruments include cholangiogram forceps.

Ports

Ports are sophisticated sleeves which traverse the abdominal wall and allow instruments to be placed and replaced without trauma or losing gas pressure. Ports begin at 5 mm diameter and go up to no less than 40 mm. They broadly divide into disposable, reusable and a combination of the two. Single-use ports can add to the cost of a procedure, and in most cases, excellent quality reusable ports exist. Concerns have been raised regarding the adequacy of sterility inside the valve and seal mechanisms of the reusable ports, and it is this mechanism that often exacts a high toll on the barrel insulation of instruments as they are passed through. Hybrid ports combining a reusable shaft/trocar assembly with a small disposable multi-adapter seal offer the best of both worlds. Ports must have a self-retaining mechanism; this may be crude as in the style of suture and stanchion, through to special alloy non-slip surfaces or threaded barrels that 'screw' into the abdominal wall.

Reusable versus disposable

Certainly in recent years, the gulf between reusable and disposable instruments has narrowed considerably. Reusable-disposable instruments have recently been introduced which can be discarded after a certain number of uses. Single-use instruments that have advantages over comparable reusables include combined sucker/irrigators and scissors. Disposable sucker/irrigators using battery-driven pumps can irrigate litres through an abdomen in minutes, allowing effective laparoscopic management of peritonitis and haemoperitoneum. Single-use scissors by their nature are sharp and cut well from the outset. They may be a luxury for short procedures, but represent a better option for operations requiring substantial dissection.

Staplers, clippers, guns and tackers

Control of ducts, bowel and vessels in laparoscopic surgery requires a range of devices. The simplest is the reusable 10 mm clip applier for control of the cystic artery and duct in cholecystectomy. Reloading requires removal from the abdomen. Common problems include the clip falling out, and the clip 'scissoring', where the clip legs cross and fail to occlude the structure; both are often caused by loose applier jaws. Disposable 10 mm clip appliers typically hold 20 clips and add to the overall cost, but in situations where close to this number of clips is necessary may represent an efficient use of resources. Several 5 mm clip appliers are available, although the jaw action differs from the 10 mm instrument.

Tackers and staplers may be necessary for hernia repairs where prosthetic mesh is inserted. Staplers apply a staple similar in appearance to a skin staple, and are available in 10 mm straight and flexible head models. A tacker is available in 5 mm and uses a corkscrew arrangement to spiral a small wire coil to hold prosthetic mesh in place. It may be preferable to staples because of its greater strength and the fact that it causes less local tissue damage. Laparoscopic staple guns are used to divide viscera and vascular pedicles. They are mostly 10–12 mm in diameter with a 30–60 mm staple line. They are typically manually operated with a single grip squeeze and are multi-load, i.e. they allow reloading after firing. Longer staple lines are achieved with multi-squeeze or gas-assisted firing. Some machines offer angled firing via a flexible head (Fig 14.2). Cartridges come with different staple lengths and spacing, reflecting their suitability for thick tissue, normal tissue and vascular purposes.

Instruments are colour-coded for this, and different cartridges of one brand are interchangeable in their own stapler. All work on the principle of an initial action to approximate the jaws, and a second action to activate the staple anvil and the blade. Note that none staple all the way to the limit of the jaws—the limit of the knife and anvil travel is marked on the jaws. Insertion of the instrument through the port requires closure of the jaws. In general, these instruments are neither cheap nor foolproof, and require a ready stock of replacement cartridges. Before opening a sterile stapling device, a supply of cartridges for that brand must be at hand.

Specimen retrieval

Once the tissue or organ has been resected, its retrieval should not be overlooked. If a gall bladder is intact, it is simple to deliver it carefully, but for a spleen, appendix or colon, delivery may present major problems. In the case of the appendix, delivery into the largest port intra-corporeally may be all that is needed. This allows it to be removed without contacting the abdominal wall. A colon specimen should be delivered through a small incision via a plastic wound protector. This device consists of a semi-rigid plastic ring and flange that is placed across the abdominal wall and its use excludes the specimen from contact with the abdominal wall. In the case of solid organs or a punctured gall bladder, a specimen retrieval bag can be inserted intra-corporeally and the specimen placed within. These are available in 10 mm or 15 mm diameters. For splenectomy, the spleen is fragmented or 'morselised' within the bag prior to delivery through the port incision.

Cost

All the necessary equipment adds substantially to the cost of an operation. If capital purchases and the cost of disposables are considered, the cost of a laparoscopic cholecystectomy compares unfavourably with the cost of an open cholecystectomy. However, length of stay is a major issue in Australasian hospitals. The cost of a stapler is equivalent to ten hours in a postoperative surgical ward. Taking length of hospital stay and time off work into account may draw the issue into sharper focus and allow the true cost comparison for a particular technique to be scrutinised more equitably.

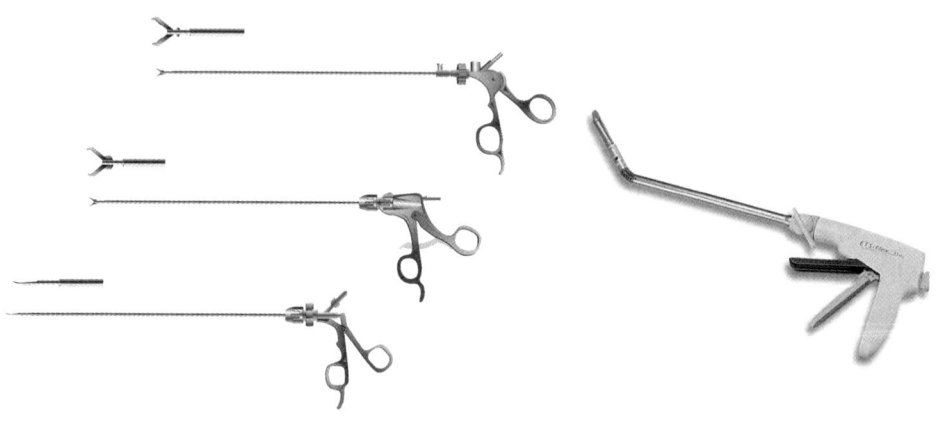

Fig 14.2 5 mm graspers in common use (left) and a flexible linear stapler (right)

THEATRE SET-UP

Lighting

The theatre lights need to be dimmed, and importantly, it should be possible to exclude all natural light. Newer theatre set ups may choose green lighting, which is supposed to increase visual acuity in dim lighting.

Scrub nurse, surgeon and screen

The surgeon should try to achieve the most familiar view of the operative field. This means standing by the right iliac fossa facing the left upper quadrant for a splenectomy, and standing by the right iliac fossa facing the left flank for left-sided colonic operations. Cholecystectomy can be performed from left or right sides. Appendicectomy is best done from the left flank looking towards the right flank. The camera should be between the surgeon's hands, and the screen should be within a field of 30° either side of the surgeon-camera-field axis. Exceptions do exist, but spatial relationships are most evident in these positions, particularly so in the lower half of the abdomen.

The positioning of the staff and cables should allow the surgeon and assistants free access towards and away from the table. This is best achieved by laying all cables, tubing and equipment across the patient's upper body, leaving the lower body free.

The scrub nurse should set up in such a position that instruments can be passed without the surgeon having to look away from the field. The scrub nurse must also have an unrestricted view of the screen which is essential for anticipation of the surgeon's requirements. The camera operator should in general be positioned on the side of the patient opposite to the surgeon. In certain circumstances, the camera operator may stand behind the surgeon, particularly for teaching purposes.

PNEUMOPERITONEUM

This is the single most dangerous step in laparoscopic surgery. More fatalities and major morbidity have arisen from the establishment of the pneumoperitoneum than any other step.

Verres needle cannulation

Closed cannulation by *Verres puncture* causes a large proportion of the complications of laparoscopy. Pneumoperitoneum established with a Verres needle is a blind procedure and may, in inexperienced hands, cause serious complications. Injury to bowel, bladder and large vessels (aorta and vena cava) have all been reported in the literature. Complications include vessel injury with haemorrhage, gas embolism and tissue infarction as well as organ injury, which are all potentially catastrophic if they go unrecognised. Verres cannulation requires blind insertion of sharp instruments twice, and insufflation without visual confirmation of satisfactory placement. Logic dictates that open cannulation should avoid all of this and it is therefore recommended that all trainee surgeons should be trained only in the open insertion technique to prevent these mostly avoidable and potentially serious complications.

Open cannulation

Open cannulation allows establishment of the pneumoperitoneum under vision using blunt insertion, and permits immediate full insufflation rates. Open cannulation is simple once learnt, and obviates blind puncture manoeuvres which cannot be accepted as safe surgical practice.

For the right-handed surgeon, open cannulation via the *Hasson technique* is best performed from the patient's right side. The umbilicus is elevated with tissue graspers and a vertical or semilunar infra-umbilical incision is made. This is deepened so the inferior limit of the umbilical cicatrix is seen. With umbilical elevation using the left hand, the cicatrix is incised vertically in the midline for a distance of around 10 mm. Note that a longer incision will cause gas leakage. Whilst maintaining the elevation, a closed pair of blunt-pointed artery forceps is inserted to the plane superficial to the peritoneum and is opened with the curve pointing downward. The largest artery forceps in the instrument set usually has the bluntest tip and lends itself best to this task. This manoeuvre occasionally needs to be repeated, but in most cases the peritoneum can now be opened and the viscera will have fallen away. The situation is checked by relaxing the left hand, and allowing the abdominal wall to descend until the viscera can easily be seen though the defect. Now the cannula is inserted using a blunt obturator, and the pneumoperitoneum can be the established at normal flow rates.

This technique allows easy establishment of the pneumoperitoneum, with a mean period of 40 seconds taken to insert the cannula and start normal gas flow. Previous surgery renders any method of cannulation difficult, but performing it under vision is the safest method. Open cannulation can also be performed easily through a small incision in either flank if a midline scar influences the surgeon not to use the umbilicus.

Port insertion and placement

Port insertion should be performed under direct vision, using the camera to check the trajectory. A small stab incision is made in the most suitable location and the port inserted. Should any resistance be encountered, the skin incision should be enlarged first as this is the most common cause of increased entry resistance. If parietal adhesions are found which prevent use of a favoured port site, then alternative port sites can be used to clear adhesions from the favoured site.

Port placement must avoid the inferior epigastric arteries, and placement in the lower abdomen must avoid bladder and iliac vessels. In thin patients, the abdominal wall should be transilluminated from the inside to demonstrate large vessels which can thus be avoided. These are general rules which govern port placement, and specific operations have a variety of well-founded port positions.

Working and visual space

Ideal port sites should allow the surgeon to work within an arc of 120°; this can be thought of as 'the visual space'. When instruments enter and leave the space via the ports, a good camera operator will keep the instrument tip constantly in view. Most of the operation takes place with the two working instruments at a 90° angle; this can be thought of as 'the working space', where movements are most precisely controlled in the visual 'fairway'. The visual or camera axis should bisect this space. This is particularly important when advanced laparoscopic skills such as suturing are needed.

LAPAROSCOPIC SKILLS

Ligating, knotting and suturing

Ligation can be by suture transfixion, loop ligation, clip application or stapling devices. *Loop ligation* can be via pre-tied suture loops or via hand-tied loops slipped in with a knot pusher. A common example is a suture loop around the appendix base. *Clips* may be applied to a structure either in continuity or following division. *Staple guns* allow the control of larger structures; for example, for dividing bowel and its vascular pedicles. The correct cartridge is essential: attempts to control the splenic pedicle with a bowel cartridge are doomed to fail.

The *endoloop ligature* is a preformed loop supplied with an introducer. This is useful for ligating pedicles where one end is free. A grasping instrument is passed through the endoloop and the pedicle is grasped; the endoloop can then tightened over the pedicle. Endoloops are most useful for ligating the appendix stump or large cystic ducts. They are rarely employed for ligating blood vessels, which would need to be divided before the endoloop could be passed over them.

Suturing can be achieved by extracorporeal or intracorporeal methods. The former allows the knot to be thrown outside the port, and by way of a knot pusher, slid down the port. Intracorporeal suturing requires the suture to be brought into the abdomen. Most laparoscopic suturing follows the general principles of open suturing. The needle with its suture material is passed into the abdomen via a port, with care taken to grasp the thread rather than the needle as it passes through the port. This is to prevent the thread being pulled off the needle if it becomes trapped in the valve mechanism of the port. A 26 mm needle will usually fit down a 10 mm port because of the curve of the needle.

Laparoscopic suturing is usually carried out with two needle holders, one in each hand, to allow safe and secure passage of the needle through the tissue. After passing the needle through the tissue with the right-hand instrument, the needle can be grasped with the left hand and then transferred back to the right hand to place the next suture. Knots can be made extracorporeally, employing a long suture, one end of which remains outside the body. The needle is passed through the port, the suture inserted and the needle is brought back through the port and a knot formed outside. The knot needs to be a lockable slip knot which is carried into the abdomen with a knot pusher and tightened to prevent it slipping. The basic extracorporeal knot is shown in Fig. 9.7. There are several variations that follow the same general principle.

Intracorporeal knots are more difficult to perform and require more practice, but are recommended for surgeons conducting laparoscopic suturing. The curved needle is passed using a needle holder and the knot tied in situ. This requires skill, but allows better knot placement; it also permits a surgeon's knot to be used, rather than having to use slip knots. There are several techniques for intracorporeal knots, but the simplest one is to form a slip knot which can be tightened to the desired tension. A reverse throw is then made to create a reef knot that locks the first knot in place.

A disposable suturing device is available that uses a small straight needle attached to a thread. The needle is passed between the right and left jaws of the instrument using a lever. It is then automatically grasped on the other side after passing through the tissue. A potential drawback of this instrument is that the tissues have to be in close approximation and one cannot 'feel' the needle passing through the tissue to ensure a substantial bite has been taken.

Retraction, dissection

Expert retraction requires the best choice of grasper, applied to the most suitable part of the viscus, with traction in the optimum direction, maintained and appropriately repositioned. It is therefore crucial to the successful completion of an operation.

Diathermy

Diathermy in laparoscopy must be employed using strict safety measures to prevent inadvertent burns that can lead to delayed perforation of hollow organs. The phenomena of capacitive coupling and arcing are well recognised and it is a surgeon's responsibility to ensure the insulation on instruments is intact before connecting them to diathermy. It is advisable that metal ports should not be used in conjunction with plastic instruments and vice versa to avoid capacitive coupling.

Laparoscopic dissection may be achieved with a monopolar hook. Bipolar diathermy does not lend itself well to dissection, but does offer certain advantages laparoscopically. In particular, it avoids current spreading outwards from the point of application. For example, it is preferred for control and coagulation of the mesoappendix, thus avoiding current conduction across the thin-walled caecum. It is also beneficial for sympathectomy, where conduction of a monopolar current along the sympathetic chain can give unpredictable results. Bipolar diathermy does not need a large indifferent electrode applied to the body surface.

Dissection

Once the pneumoperitoneum is established, the ports are in place and the diagnosis confirmed, dissection can proceed. Dissection may be performed with a diathermy hook or scissors but it cannot be emphasised too strongly that the working tip of the instrument should always be in view. Removal and reinsertion of instruments via the ports should be conducted under direct vision to prevent inadvertent injury to other organs. This is especially important if instruments are connected to diathermy.

If diathermy is used for hook dissection, the minimal amount of 'collateral damage' should be caused. This is achieved by the pulling up the hook in order to 'tent' the tissue to be diathermied away from the other tissues. Heating of adjacent tissues will thus be kept to a minimum and the 'current of injury' avoided. This is of crucial importance in dissecting ductal structures. The diathermy should be activated for the shortest possible time in these areas; short, carefully directed bursts also help to minimise local heating. In areas where structures can safely be cleared, the heel of the hook can be swept in a gentle arc across the tissues. Spot bleeding points can be dealt with using the flat side of the hook.

Cannulation

Cannulation of ducts is a necessary skill and should become routine. For example the cystic duct can readily be cannulated whenever cholangiography is important. Purpose-made cholangiogram forceps, e.g. Olsen–Reddick forceps, make this a simple step.

Maintaining vision

Laparoscopes tend to fog. There is no entirely satisfactory answer but it is preventable, and several small steps can minimise this frustrating problem. Warming the laparoscope in sterile hot water is most useful. A pre-warmed eyepiece fogs less, and the use of minimal amounts of irrigation fluid, or delaying irrigation until the last step of the procedure, also help. Coating the lens in peritoneal fluid allows a phospholipid bilayer to form and thus minimise condensation. Proprietary solution exist which achieve a similar end.

The appearance of blood in the field absorbs light and leads to picture degradation. It is best to prevent bleeding, use appropriate suction to clear blood should it appear and control it early. The picture quality can often be improved by increasing light output to maximum and opening the camera aperture to maximum. Irrigation merely disperses the blood and seldom alleviates this situation.

Organ manipulation

Appropriate traction on structures is difficult to gauge. The leverage of the long instrument can allow considerable force to be inadvertently applied to a viscus and the limited feedback may allow damage to the viscus before it is detected. Control of a structure should be through the use of a wide jawed grasper applied to the most robust part of the structure. The use of toothed graspers, while adding to the purchase on a structure, also leads to significant local trauma. Inappropriate grasping can lead to damage to the specimen so that it becomes unrecognisable histologically. Bowel can be damaged with even minimal manipulation.

ADVANCED TECHNIQUES

Resection

To carry out laparoscopic resection, it is essential to appreciate the 'dynamic viewpoint'. The camera allows the picture to be appreciated from different angles, magnified to different degrees. When combined with retraction in various directions, there are many variables in the way the field appears. For example a view of the splenic flexure can be obtained from the left paracolic gutter, from above the greater omentum and from the transverse colon. This has inherent benefits but also may cause disorientation. Anatomical landmarks, as is the case in all forms of surgery, are important, but predicting for example the direction in which the ureter will cross the operative field depends entirely on the camera angle and position. It is important at all times to recognise where the camera is situated and its direction.

Anastomoses

Anastomoses are usually achieved with a combination of stapling and suturing. A side-to-side anastomosis can be created with a linear stapler, with the remaining defect closed by sutures, typically using a continuous absorbable monofilament suture. Triangulation of instruments and an ergonomic working position are essential.

Stone retrieval

Laparoscopic exploration of the common bile duct requires skills additional to basic cholecystectomy. With appropriate equipment, the duct can be trawled via the cystic stump, allowing retrieval of common bile duct stones using a flat wire basket. Success requires visualisation of the calculus, and this can be via X-ray image intensification or flexible choledochoscopy. In the first, the stone is localised after contrast injection and delivered via the cystic stump under fluoroscopy. The choledochoscopic technique requires the introduction of the endoscope into the cystic stump, and visualisation of the calculus and 'basketing' under vision. This can be done via a 'buddy system' in which the basket is slid alongside the endoscope, or by using a very small calibre basket down the endoscope working port. This allows the stone to be basketed under direct vision.

Anaesthetic considerations

For most laparoscopic procedures an abdominal insufflation pressure of 12 mm Hg is adequate, although recently it has been shown that lower abdominal insufflation pressure causes reduced venous stasis and hence reduces the risk of deep venous thrombosis. Hypercarbia resulting from carbon dioxide absorption may require increased ventilation and anaesthetists have to be aware of this. Rarely, a patent pleuroperitoneal canal exists which causes a pneumothorax as soon as the abdomen is insufflated. Difficulties with ventilation before any dissection has begun should alert the surgeon and anaesthetist to this possibility. Procedures that require dissection of the diaphragmatic hiatus (e.g. laparoscopic fundoplication) may cause an iatrogenic breach of the pleura and lead to a pneumothorax. It is important to be aware of this potential complication. However, only very infrequently will the patient require insertion of a chest drain; most spontaneously resolve or can be aspirated with a needle.

It was previously considered that minimal-access surgery is also 'minimally invasive'. It must be remembered that the invasiveness of a procedure does not depend on the route of access because the procedure within the abdomen is exactly the same whether open or laparoscopic access is used. General anaesthesia is invariably required and a complete risk assessment must be carried out before embarking on these procedures in patients who are elderly or have significant co-morbidity.

INDEX

Page numbers followed by *f* and *t* indicate figures and tables, respectively.